Psychiatric and Behavioural Disorders in Intellectual and Developmental Disabilities

Entirely revised and updated, this new edition of a very well-received and successful book provides the essentials for all those involved in the fields of intellectual, developmental and learning disabilities, drawing both on clinical experience and on the latest research findings. An international, multidisciplinary team of experts cover the available literature in full and bring together the most relevant and useful information on mental health and behavioural problems of people with intellectual, developmental and learning disabilities and mental retardation. In addition, this book highlights the principles behind clinical practice for assessment, management and services. It offers hands-on, practical advice for psychiatrists, psychologists, nurses, therapists, social workers, managers and service providers.

Nick Bouras is Professor of Psychiatry in the Division of Psychological Medicine and Health Service Research Department at the Institute of Psychiatry King's College London and Chairman of the Mental Health Studies Programme. He is also Consultant Psychiatrist at South London and Maudsley NHS Trust and Director of the Estia Training, Research and Development Centre at Guy's Hospital, London.

Geraldine Holt is Honorary Senior Lecturer in Psychiatry at the Institute of Psychiatry, King's College London, and Consultant Psychiatrist at South London and the Maudsley NHS Trust.

From reviews of the first edition:
'A set of excellent contributors, drawn from around the world, provide generally excellent reviews and updates for this volume . . . this is an excellent and current overview that will be of interest to practitioners and investigators alike.'
Fred Volkmar, *The American Journal of Psychiatry*

'The multidisciplinary approach is central to work in this field. This book confirms that it is enjoyable and exciting . . . Each of the 25 chapters is a gem . . . I strongly recommend this as a book that should be browsed through by anyone involved in this work.'
T. P. Berney, *Journal of Child Psychology and Psychiatry and Allied Disciplines*

Psychiatric and Behavioural Disorders in Intellectual and Developmental Disabilities

Second Edition

Edited by

Nick Bouras and Geraldine Holt

King's College, London

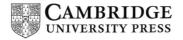

CAMBRIDGE
UNIVERSITY PRESS

CAMBRIDGE UNIVERSITY PRESS
Cambridge, New York, Melbourne, Madrid, Cape Town, Singapore, São Paulo

Cambridge University Press
The Edinburgh Building, Cambridge CB2 2RU, UK

Published in the United States of America by Cambridge University Press, New York

www.cambridge.org
Information on this title: www.cambridge.org/9780521608251

© Cambridge University Press 2007

First published 2007

Printed in the United Kingdom at the University Press, Cambridge

A catalogue record for this publication is available from the British Library

ISBN-13   978-0-521-60825-1 paperback

Contents

Part III   Treatment and therapeutic interventions

Contributors

Betsey A. Benson
Adjunct Associate Professor of Psychology
Nisonger Center, The Ohio State University
1581 Dodd Drive, Colombus, Ohio,
    43210–1296
USA

Nick Bouras
Professor of Psychiatry
King's College, London
The Institute of Psychiatry
Estia Centre
York Clinic – Guy's Hospital
47 Weston Street
London SE1 3RR
UK

Elspeth A. Bradley
Associate Professor, Department of
    Psychiatry, University of Toronto,
CANADA

Nancy N. Cain
Associate Clinical Professor of Psychiatry
300 Crittenden Blvd, Rochester, NY 14642
USA

David Clarke
Consultant Psychiatrist
North Warwickshire Primary Care Trust
Lea Castle Centre, Kidderminster
    DY10 3PP
UK

Sally-Ann Cooper
Professor of Learning Disabilities
University of Glasgow
Section of Psychological Medicine, Division
    of Community Based Sciences, Academic
    Centre
Gartnavel Royal Hospital, 1055 Great
    Western Road, Glasgow G12 ONH.
UK

Helen Costello
Senior Researcher
King's College London
The Institute of Psychiatry
Estia Centre – Guy's Hospital
66 Snowsfields, London SE1 3SS
UK

Stuart Cumella

Head of the Division of Neuroscience

Division of Neuroscience, University of
Birmingham Medical School

University of Birmingham Medical School,
Birmingham B15 2TT

UK

Dave Dagnan

Consultant Clinical Psychologist and Clinical
Director

North Cumbria Mental Health and Learning
Disability NHS Trust and Institute for
Health Research

University of Lancaster North Cumbria
Mental Health and Learning Disability
NHS Trust, Psychological Services, West
Cumberland Hospital, Hensingham,
Whitehaven, Cumbria

UK

Philip W. Davidson

Professor of Psychiatry and Paediatrics

Strong Centre for Developmental Disabilities

University of Rochester Medical Centre

601 Elmwood Avenue, Rochester NY 14642

USA

Robert Davis

Associate Professor

The Centre for Developmental Disability
Health Victoria, Department of General
Practice Monash University, Suite 202, 3
Chester Street, Oakleigh, Vic. 3166

AUSTRALIA

Shoumitro Deb

Clinical Professor of Neuropsychiatry &
Intellectual Disability

Division of Neuroscience, University of
Birmingham

University of Birmingham, Division of
Neuroscience, Department of Psychiatry

Queen Elizabeth Psychiatric Hospital,
Mindelsohn Way

Birmingham B15 2QZ

UK

Philip Dodd

Consultant Psychiatrist in the Psychiatry of
Learning Disability, St. Michael's House,
Dublin

St. Michael's House, Adare Green, Coolock,
Dublin 17

IRELAND

Elisabeth M. Dykens

Associate Director, Kennedy Center for
Research on Human Development and
Professor of Psychology and Human
Development

Peabody College Vanderbilt University

230 Appleton Place, Box 40, Nashville, TN
37203

USA

Niki Edwards

Clinical Coordinator and Lecturer

Queensland Centre for Intellectual &
Developmental Disability School of
Population Health The University of
Queensland, Mater Hospital, South
Brisbane 4101

AUSTRALIA

Chris Hatton
Professor of Psychology, Health and Social
    Care
Institute for Health Research, Lancaster
    University, Lancaster LA1 4YT
UK

Susan M. Havercamp
Assistant Professor of Psychiatry
Center for Development & Learning,
    University of North Carolina, CB#7255,
    Chapel Hill, NC, 27599–7255
USA

Jessica Hellings
Associate Professor of Psychiatry
University of Kansas Medical Center
3901 Rainbow Blvd, Kansas City, Kansas,
    66160
USA

Colin Hemmings
Consultant Psychiatrist
South London and the Maudsley NHS Trust
Department of Mental Health in Learning
    Disabilities and Estia Centre
York Clinic, Guy's Hospital, London SE1 3RR
UK

John Hillery
Consultant Psychiatrist, Stewarts Hospital,
    Palmerstown, Dublin 20
IRELAND

Robert M. Hodapp
Professor of Special Education
Kennedy Center for Research on Human
    Development
Peabody College, Vanderbilt University
230 Appleton Place, Box 328, Nashville, TN
    37203
USA

Anthony J. Holland
Professor of Learning Disabilities
The Health Foundation
University of Cambridge
Developmental Psychiatry, Learning
    Disabilities Unit, Douglas House, 18B
    Trumpington Road, Cambridge CB2 2AH
UK

Sheila Hollins
Head of Division of Mental Health
Professor of Learning Disability
St. George's, University of London
Cranmer Terrace
London SW17 0RE
UK

Geraldine Holt
Consultant Psychiatrist, South London &
    Maudsley NHS Trust, The Institute of
    Psychiatry
Estia Centre
York Clinic – Guy's Hospital
47 Weston Street
London SE1 3RR
UK

Bryan King
Professor and Vice Chair of Psychiatry and
    Behavioural Sciences
University of Washington
Washington
USA

Nick Lennox
Associate Professor
Queensland Centre for Intellectual &
    Developmental Disability School of
    Population Health The University of
    Queensland
Mater Hospital, South Brisbane 4101
AUSTRALIA

William R. Lindsay
Consultant Forensic Clinical Psychologist
The State Hospital
Clinical Psychology Department,
  Wedderburn House, 1 Edward Street,
  Dundee DD1 5NS
UK

Fiona Lobban
Senior Lecturer in Clinical Psychology
Division of Clinical Psychology, Liverpool
  University, Liverpool
UK

Yona Lunsky
Assistant Professor, Department of
  Psychiatry, University of Toronto
Dual Diagnosis Program, Centre for
  Addiction and Mental Health
1001 Queen Street West, Toronto, Ont. M6J
  1H4
CANADA

Jonathan Mason
Clinical Psychologist
Cedar House, Dover Rd, Barham,
  Canterbury, Kent CT4 6PW
UK

Caroline Mohr
Consultant Clinical Psychologist
Centre for Developmental Psychiatry and
  Psychology, Monash University,
  Melbourne, Victoria, Australia
Haumietiketike, P.O. Box 50–233, Porirua,
  Wellington, NEW ZEALAND.

Glynis Murphy
Professor of Clinical Psychology
Institute for Health Research
University of Lancaster
Lancaster LA1 4YT
UK

Jean O'Hara
Consultant Psychiatrist
South London and the Maudsley NHS Trust
Department of Mental Health in Learning
  Disabilities and the Estia Centre
York Clinic, Guy's Hospital, London SE1
  3RR
UK

Georgina Parkes
Specialist Registrar
South West London and St George's Mental
  Health NHS Trust
Division of Mental Health
St George's, University of London, Cranmer
  Terrace, London SW17 ORE
UK

Max Pickard
Consultant Psychiatrist in Mental Health of
  Learning Disabilities
South London and the Maudsley NHS Trust
  and the Estia Centre
York Clinic, Guy's Hospital, London SE1 3RR
UK

R. Matthew Reese
Clinical Associate Professor of Paediatrics
Developmental Disabilities Center
University of Kansas Medical Center
3901 Rainbow Blvd, Kansas City, Kansas
  66160
USA

Dene Robertson
Consultant Psychiatrist
King's College London, The Institute of
  Psychiatry, Section of Brain Maturation
De Crespigny Park, London SE5 8AF
UK

Celine Saulnier
Associate Research Scientist in Clinical
    Psychology
Child Study Center, Yale University School of
    Medicine
P.O. Box 207900, New Haven, CT
    06520–7900
USA

Stephen Schroeder
Emeritus Director and Professor
    Schiefelbush Institute for Life Span Studies
University of Kansas
3901 Rainbow Blvd, Kansas City, Kansas
    66160
USA

Chrissoula Stavrakaki
Professor of Psychiatry
737 Manor Avenue
Ottawa-Ontario K1M 0E4
CANADA

Peter Sturmey
Professor of Psychology
Department of Psychology, Queens College
    and The Graduate Centre, City University
    of New York
USA

Bruce Tonge
Professor of Psychiatry, Monash University
Centre for Developmental Psychology &
    Psychiatry, Monash Medical Centre
Clayton VIC. 3168
AUSTRALIA

Jennifer Torr
Senior Lecturer in Mental Health
The Centre for Developmental Disability
    Health Victoria, Department of General
    Practice, Monash University, Suite 202,
    3 Chester Street, Oakleigh, Vic. 3166
AUSTRALIA

Fred Volkmar
Irving B. Harris Professor of Child
    Psychiatry, Pediatrics, and Psychology
Child Study Center, Yale University School of
    Medicine, P.O. Box 207900, New Haven,
    CT 06520–7900
USA

Germain Weber
Professor of Psychology, Department of
    Clinical, Biological and Differential
    Psychology, Faculty of Psychology,
University of Vienna, Universitaetsstrasse 7,
    A-1010 Vienna
AUSTRIA

Preface

People with intellectual disabilities and mental health problems have the same right to high standards of assessment, treatment, and as good a quality of life as other people. Historically, the mental health problems of people with intellectual disabilities have had a low priority in health care systems around the world. Consequently the treatment facilities have been insufficient, the training of staff underdeveloped and the care offered far from the best to meet their mental health needs. This is further compounded by the fact that the mental health problems of people with intellectual disabilities are often very complex, difficult to diagnose and require specialist multiprofessional involvement.

The potential for comprehensive and effective care of people with intellectual disabilities and mental health problems has improved greatly in recent years with developments in the way that people with disabilities are viewed within society, increased understanding of psychological processes and with advances in neuroscience, genetics and neuro imaging. There are now more effective treatment methods including behaviour therapy, psychopharmacology, psychosocial interventions and psychotherapy.

This second edition of the book *Psychiatric and Behavioural Disorders in Developmental Disabilities and Mental Retardation* is fully revised and offers an up-to-date account in the field. In this edition we have replaced the term 'mental retardation' with 'intellectual disabilities' as the latter has gained widespread international recognition and acceptance.

Several new chapters have been added on mental health assessment and monitoring tools for people with intellectual disabilities, interdisciplinary multimodal assessment for mental health problems, the interface between medical and psychiatric disorders, personality disorders, mental health problems in people with autism and related disorders, mental health and epilepsy among adults with intellectual disabilities, psychosocial interventions and psychodynamic approaches.

New contributors drawn from the broad international multiprofessional context of intellectual disabilities and mental health have re-written several of the latter chapters in this edition. Some topics are approached from different points of view, offering a variety of perspectives and dimensions.

On reflection, looking back at the very first book, *Mental Health in Mental Retardation* published in 1994, we can see the significant progress that has occurred in the fields of intellectual disabilities and mental health. Though research continues constantly to appear in our areas of professional interests including psychiatry, psychology, genetics, paediatrics, occupational therapy, speech and language therapy and social work, more research including randomized controlled trials is necessary to assess clinical effectiveness. Also, vigorous evaluation of service models and international comparative research will facilitate further advances and practices.

For this book, thanks are owed to all contributors, to Mary Spiller for her invaluable assistance in helping us with the editing, and to Pauline Graham of Cambridge University Press for her advice and support.

Part I

Assessment and diagnosis

Diagnosis of mental disorders in people with intellectual disabilities

Peter Sturmey

Introduction

Classification of mental disorders in people with intellectual disabilities (ID) continues to be a very active field since the last edition of this book (Sturmey, 1999). This chapter reviews the importance and functions of classification as well as psychometric properties that any adequate classification system must have. It then goes on to review classification in relation to intellectual disabilities, mental health and classification of mental health issues in people with ID. The final section highlights the changes that have occurred and areas for future development.

The importance and functions of classification

Classification is often seen as a hallmark of science: atomic theory and the Linnaean system advanced their respective folk technologies into sciences. Yet, nineteenth-century Alienists were reluctant to classify madness beyond insanity and mental deficiency. As psychiatry strived towards scientific respectability, classification progressed vigorously, especially in the twentieth century. Kraepelin (Kihlstrom, 2002) developed taxonomy of insanity into 15 aetiological classes. In the end he had to admit that the effort was in vain, and that classification by course and prognosis was more promising. The precursors of the *Diagnostic and Statistical Manual* (DSM) implied aetiology, but were based on presenting symptoms, as putative causes could not be observed. Presenting symptoms continue to be cardinal features of DSM and the *International Classification of Disease* (ICD). Critics of the early DSM-I and II noted that they were both explicitly psychoanalytical in orientation and did not guide the diagnostician as to the specific symptoms and were hence unreliable. Later editions of DSM made three important changes. First, it was not explicitly theoretical (although implicitly it adopted a medical model of mental disorders).

Psychiatric and Behavioural Disorders in Intellectual and Developmental Disabilities, ed. Nick Bouras and Geraldine Holt. Published by Cambridge University Press. © Cambridge University Press 2007.

Second, it addressed the issue of reliability by operationalizing symptoms, and the number and combinations of symptoms necessary for diagnosis. Third, instead of adopting a model of diseases where all similar diseases shared common features, it adopted a stochastic model wherein a certain number of symptoms were required, but no one symptom was required. Hence, in DSM-II all psychoses were characterized by problems in reality testing, whereas in DSM-IV there is no such commonality among psychotic disorders (Kihlstrom, 2002).

Classification of mental disorders and ID has become longer and progressively more detailed, whereas this trend is not observed in classification of physical illnesses. Houts (2002) noted that from DSM-I to DSM-IV the number of diagnoses increased from 106 to 365 and the number of pages increased from 128 to 886. (From these unhappy data we can observe that DSM grows at the rate of approximately six new diagnoses and 16 pages per year. If the growth is mercifully linear then we might predict a DSM-V in say 2010 containing 461 diagnoses, including 96 new ones, with 1142 pages!)

Classification serves several, diverse purposes (see Table 1.1). Problems arise in a single classification system that accommodates multiple functions. For example, a system of classification of ID based on aetiology might be highly useful for prevention, but might have no use for guiding habilitation.

Necessary properties of classification systems

Any adequate classification scheme must have certain properties. These include being publicly verifiable and open to inspection by more than one person, measuring what it purports to measure, practicality, completeness, acceptability, and usefulness. Reliability refers to a number of related but distinguished properties, including stability across observers, stability over time and internal consistency. Validity refers to the extent to which a measure accurately and coherently measures what it purports to measure. Table 1.2 gives definitions, examples and associated statistics of these properties. Reliability and validity criteria can be applied to a variety of aspects of measurement including diagnostic decisions, such as whether or not someone has a mental disorder, or what type of disorder it is. They can also be applied to psychometric instruments (e.g. Aman, 1990; Deb, *et al.*, 2001, Finlay, 2005; Sturmey, *et al.*, 1991), structured diagnostic interviews (Moss, *et al.*, 1993; Patel *et al.*, 2001) as well as to clinical decision-making, such as a decision to place someone on a psychotropic medication.

Most research emphasizes reliability and validity, but there are also other important properties of a classification system. Classification systems must be both complete and efficient to use. Practitioners face the paradoxical needs of a classification system that efficiently addresses the relatively small number of common

Table 1.1 Some of the functions of psychiatric classification.

Purpose	Example
Service record keeping	Diagnoses or levels of disability are entered into a record to indicate reasons for treatment or change in disability in response to intervention.
Statistical	A school district surveys the numbers of students with ID and self-injury in order to determine staff training and other policy needs.
Communicating with third parties	A label such as 'Mood Disorder NOS' is used to summarize a cluster of presenting symptoms and to explain aggressive behaviour.
Reimbursement for services	Coverage for in-patient services is denied because the client's symptoms do not meet covered diagnosis.
Research	A research protocol specifies that all participants will meet DSM-IV criteria for mild or moderate ID and post-traumatic stress disorder.
Basis for screening instrument	Structured interview such as the PASADD (Moss *et al.*, 1993; Patel *et al.*, 2001) and psychometric instruments are based on standardized diagnostic criteria in order to screen for those people who truly meet diagnostic criteria.
Summarizing symptoms	Instead of listing a large number of specific observable behaviours, a client is said to be manic.
Aetiology	The cause of ID is classified as 'Non-Organic/cultural familial' or 'Organic'. If 'Organic' is coded then one of several classes is checked such as infections, acquired brain damage, or genetic; if 'genetic' is coded, one of 800 or so specific causes is coded.
Prognosis	Down syndrome has an increased risk of Alzheimer's disease after age 40; Lesch–Nyhan syndrome does not.
Legal purposes	A client is found incompetent to stand trial because of mild ID and personality disorder.
Service planning, monitoring and evaluation	Statistical returns to the US Department of Education indicate that the number of students with ID has dropped by nearly 50% in ten years, but the number of children with autism spectrum disorders has greatly increased. Additional resources are provided for a variety of services related to autism spectrum disorders.
Determining blameworthiness	A child with ID is removed from school because it is determined that his aggressive behaviour was not caused by ID or any mental health diagnosis.

Table 1.2 The various types of reliability and validity of classification systems.

Property	Definition	Examples	Associated statistics
Inter-rater reliability	Independent observers agree on the presence or absence of a symptom or diagnosis.	Two interviewers agree that the client has depressed mood. Two researchers scoring a videotaped standardized interview agree that a client meets research diagnostic criteria for a psychotic disorder. Two team members, both present in an interview, agree that a client no longer meets diagnostic criteria after treatment was successful.	Cohen's kappa between two diagnosticians recording the presence or absence of a diagnosis exceeds 0.7. Pearson correlations between ratings of number of depressive symptoms is 0.9 or greater.
Test–retest reliability	When a condition truly does not change over time the observer gives the same result.	A client who has Antisocial Personality Disorder or Alzheimer's disease continues to meet diagnostic criteria at each monthly review. A client who has a mood disorder is correctly diagnosed by a general physician and the diagnosis is confirmed one week later by a consultant psychiatrist.	Cohen's kappa between diagnoses at first and second evaluations by one diagnostician exceed 0.7. Pearson correlations between scores generated by a psychometrician ratings of mood one week apart correlate 0.9 or greater.
Internal consistency	Individual criteria that go to make a diagnosis are all closely related to the presence or absence of a diagnosis.	All people who present with an individual symptom of depression, score higher on a scale to measure depression and vice versa.	All item-total (minus item) point biserial correlations exceed 0.3 and Cronbach's alpha exceeds 0.6 for a newly developed scale to measure depression. Behavioural items that do not correlate with presence of depression are dropped from a new scale.

Face validity	Content appears to measure what the test purports to measure.	Members of a committee all agree that t[he] proposed items on a test appear to measure psychosis.
Content validity	The instrument samples all the relevant domains of the construct it purports to measure. (Usually relates to tests of achievement.)	A measure of depression samples cognit[ive] affective, and vegetative symptoms of depression.
Criterion validity	Scores on test predict some other relevant aspect of behaviour.	Scores on a measure of depression are correlated with a measure of social sk[ill]
Construct validity	The degree to which a test score measures the construct it purports to measure.	People with an anxiety disorder diagnosis respond better to anxiolytic than an antidepressant medication. People with a mood disorder diagnosis respond better to an antidepressant than an anxiolytic medication.

inferred from a wide range of information about a measure.

disorders and the need for a comprehensive assessment. A classification system must be acceptable to a wide range of audiences with different needs and interests and must be quick, efficient and useful. For example, a classification system should rapidly guide clinical decision-making and lead to better client outcome than would have occurred without the classification system.

Criteria for ID

ID is defined in a variety of legal, professional and research contexts. Most criteria for ID usually refer to (a) significantly below average intelligence, (b) deficits in adaptive behaviours that (c) occur during the developmental period. These criteria have been operationalized in a number of ways. The intelligence quotient (IQ) cut-off was previously operationalized as 85, and more recently as up to 75, 70 and 69. Further, the application of these cut-offs varies dramatically depending upon the test used, the validity of the sample used to standardize the test, the years since the test was standardized (Flynn, 1984, 1985, 1987; Lynn *et al.*, 1987) and attention to cultural and linguistic variables in the assessment. The developmental period has been defined as 18, 21 and 22 years. Measures of adaptive behaviour may also suffer from psychometric and conceptual inadequacies similar to measures of intelligence.

There is also evidence accumulating that practitioners and services are highly susceptible to social trends in diagnosis. In the United States the number of children classified as having ID has reduced dramatically and the use of other diagnoses such as specific learning disabilities, developmental disabilities, autism and speech and language delays have greatly increased (US Department of Education, 2002). Children who do in fact meet the psychometric criteria for having ID are knowingly and erroneously classified as have specific learning disabilities unless they have maladaptive behaviour or fail to learn to read or write (Keogh *et al.*, 1998; MacMillan *et al.*, 1996, 1998). MacMillan has argued that special education practitioners are not concerned with the accuracy of labels. Rather, as the client fails to obtain the needed services with the current diagnosis, a new diagnosis is obtained to gain access to additional resources. Thus, practitioners, unconcerned about the niceties of diagnostic criteria, but very concerned about providing services to clients, use diagnostic labels as heuristic devices to access progressively more services for clients in need. In contrast to the changes in the USA, in England the numbers of full-time children in segregated special education fell from 90 000 to only 86 777 and the number of segregated schools fell from 1171 to 1088 from 1997 to 2003 (Department of Education and Skills, 2003: Table 15). We might ask how did the USA lose so many children with ID and the United Kingdom lose so few?

These findings suggest that diagnosis of ID is continually changing. This reflects developing social practices and service ideologies, changing test characteristics, population changes and changes in incidence and case finding.

Criteria for mental disorders

The ICD-10 defines mental disorders as

... clinically significant conditions characterised by alterations in thinking, mood (emotions) or behaviour associated with personal distress and/or impaired functioning. Mental and behavioural disorders are not just variations within the range of "normal", but are clearly abnormal or patho-logical phenomena. One incidence of abnormal behaviour or a short period of abnormal mood does not, of itself, signify the presence of a mental or behavioural disorder ... such abnormali-ties must be sustained or recurring and they must result in some personal distress or impaired functioning. ... [and] are also characterized by specific symptoms and signs, and usually follow a more or less predictable natural course, unless interventions are made.

The DSM-IV contains a broadly similar definition. Both definitions invoke a num-ber of similar concepts, such as changes from pre-morbid functioning, personal distress, patterns of symptoms and recognizable courses of illnesses and exclusion of culturally acceptable deviations in behaviour.

The application of the concept of a mental disorder to people with ID presents several challenges. First, the diagnosis must be made in a person whose behaviour is already restricted and unusual compared to the general population because they have ID. Hence, a decision must be made that a further change in behaviour has occurred beyond that which was already present prior to the onset of the alleged mental disorder. The difficulty of this decision is reflected in a number of potential problems such as intellectual distortion, psychosocial masking, cognitive disinte-gration, baseline exaggeration (Sovner, 1986), diagnostic overshadowing, and other confusions regarding the difficulty in accurately recognising psychoses (Hurley, 1996), (see Table 1.3).

A second problem is that making a diagnosis of a mental disorder involves many subjective judgments including judgments concerning the clinical significance of the change in behaviour, the certainty that other causes for the change, such as provocative practices by carers or undetected physical illnesses, have accurately been ruled out, the accuracy of third-party reports, the tolerance of third parties for deviant behaviour, and judgments over the cultural appropriateness of behaviour.

A third problem is that mental health referrals typically are initiated by the client themselves. However, in the case of referrals from people with ID, most referrals are initiated by distressed carers, rather than distressed clients, usually in response to externalizing maladaptive behaviours, such as aggression, self-injury and tantrums.

Table 1.3 Some common problems in making psychiatric diagnoses in people with intellectual disabilities.

Phenomenon	Definition	Example
Intellectual distortion (Sovner, 1986)	Concrete thinking and impaired communication result in poor communication about their own experience.	Client describes self as 'scared' instead of 'mad' because of poor verbal skills.
Psychosocial masking (Sovner, 1986)	Impoverished social skills and life experiences result in unsophisticated presentation of a disorder or misdiagnosis of unusual behaviour as a psychiatric disorder.	Giggling and silliness is misdiagnosed as psychosis.
Cognitive disintegration (Sovner, 1986)	Bizarre behaviour is presented in response to minor stressors that could be misdiagnosed as a psychiatric disorder.	A client is highly disruptive and complains a lot after a preferred staff member leaves, but is diagnosed with schizophrenia.
Baseline exaggeration (Sovner, 1986)	Prior to the onset of a disorder there are high levels of unusual behaviours, making it difficult to recognize the onset of a new disorder.	A person who already had poor social skills and was withdrawn becomes more so and begins to experience other signs and symptoms of depression. This is missed because staff reports are inaccurate and staff turn-over means that no-one is aware of the overall change in the person's functioning.
Misdiagnosis of developmentally appropriate phenomenon (Hurley, 1996)	Developmentally appropriate behaviours that are unusual for the client's chronological age are misdiagnosed as a psychiatric disorder.	Solitary play, talking to oneself and imaginary friends are taken as evidence of psychosis.
Passing (Edgerton, 1967)	People with ID learn to cover up disability and pass for normal.	Unusual personal experiences are not reported or are ascribed to physical problems.
Diagnostic overshadowing	Unusual behaviour is erroneously ascribed to ID, rather than a true mental disorder.	Poor social skills and withdrawal are ascribed to ID rather than a psychosis.

Indeed, these challenging behaviours, rather than typical mental disorders, are often the reason for the prescription of psychotropic medication in this population (Holden & Gitelson, 2004; Singh *et al.*, 1997). Hence, internalizing disorders, such as anxiety and depression, may be missed as they do not cause distress for carers, and clinicians may receive pressure to make an inappropriate diagnosis in order to justify the use of psychotropic medication to treat a challenging behaviour.

A fourth problem relates to the presentation of clients with chronic and severe challenging behaviours who take multiple psychotropic medications and who continue to present significant problems. Often such clients do not meet standardized diagnostic criteria, take multiple psychotropic medications, have long but incomplete and contradictory records, and perhaps do not receive adequate behavioural services. Management of such cases is further complicated by the distress and frustration of carers. Disentangling such diagnostic problems is extremely difficult.

Critiques of classification

If classification of mental disorders has become a major academic industry, then critiques of psychiatric classification have become an important subsidiary effort. Criticism includes disparagements that revisions to psychiatric classification are more rhetoric than science (Kirk & Kutchins, 1992) or bad science (Beutler & Malik, 2002a, 2002b; Kihlstrom, 2002; Kirk & Kutchins, 1992; Malik & Beutler, 2002) influenced by political pressure (Bayer, 1987). Less subtle voices have referred to diagnosis as 'the quackery of labels' and a 'psychiatric cash cow'.

Intellectual disabilities

The World Health Organization (1992) and DSM-IV admonish us to note that diagnoses classify behaviour not people. Many diagnostic and administrative labels that refer to ID often have negative connotations, and formerly neutral or technical terms rapidly become perverted into terms of disparagement which may negatively affect how carers interact with clients and what kinds of service clients receive. The trend to declassify children with ID and to use alternate more acceptable labels in the US may reflect this concern. Such observations challenge diagnosticians to recognize the harm done by labelling people and to ensure that there are benefits that flow from the label that outweigh its costs. Merely to label someone correctly with a negative label is to do them harm; there is an ethical obligation to negate that harm by providing positive consequences for the person so labelled.

Other concerns over the use of labelling reflect concerns over social justice issues, such as inappropriately labelling ethnic minorities or perhaps also boys with negative labels. Intellectual disabilities are predominantly mild ID of no known organic aetiology (Yeargin-Allsopp *et al.*, 1997), which are mostly identified during the school years (Murphy *et al.*, 1995). Studies conducted in the US in the 1960s indicated that African-American and Hispanic children were disproportionately labelled as having ID (Maheady *et al.*, 1983). Data indicating large differences in the prevalence of ID from state to state (Center for Disease Control, 1996) could indicate either true difference in the prevalence of ID or differences in local practices in labelling children with ID. Yeargin-Allsopp *et al.* (1995) conducted a case-controlled study comparing the prevalence of ID in black and white American children aged ten in the metropolitan Atlanta region. They found an unadjusted Black–White Odds Ration (OR) of 2.6, which when adjusted for five socio economic variables fell to 1.8. Further, the Black–White adjusted OR was 1.2 for children aged below six years, indicating no difference between the two groups, but rose to 2.5 for children aged eight to ten years. Thus, more black than white children aged over six years were labelled with mild ID, even when some socioeconomic factors were controlled for. The residual difference may merely reflect variables that were not measured in the study that future research might identify. However, the possibility that the cumulative effects of biased practices in preschool and school services and other accumulated social disadvantage lead to underachievement in American black children must also be recognized as possible causes.

Current British statistics indicate similar potential problems. The label 'special educational needs' (SEN) is applied at differing rates to children from different ethnic backgrounds and further, receiving a statement of SEN is also related to ethnicity. For example, the proportion of children with a statement of SEN ranged from 1.2% to 2.6% and 3.0% for children of Indian origin, travellers of Irish heritage and Gypsy/Roma backgrounds respectively. Thus, the proportion of children with SEN varied by a factor of 2.5 across different ethnic groups. Furthermore, whereas only 13.7% of children with an Indian background had no written statement, approximately half the children of travelling Irish and Gypsy/Roma heritages with SEN had no written statement (Department of Education and Skills, 2003). Thus, large disparities in access to special education were associated with ethnicity. Thus, if a negative 'SEN' label accrues stigma to the child but does not bring services that might ameliorate the child's developmental problems, the process of labelling without service delivery raises serious ethical issues.

Many communities have become more mobile, and ethnically, culturally and linguistically diverse. The question of how to conceptualize and accurately label ID, especially mild ID, will continue to be a challenge.

Mental disorders

The application of standardized diagnostic criteria for mental disorders in people with ID raises numerous problems. People with ID have almost always been excluded from field trials of standardized diagnostic criteria, raising the question of whether their results apply to this population. Many diagnostic criteria require self-reports of thoughts, feelings, physiological states, past events and reactions to these events. These require adequate language discrimination and memory skills. People with ID often have poor skills in these areas, making it difficult or, in the case of people with limited or no verbal skills, impossible to meet unmodified diagnostic criteria. This is reflected in the widespread use of modified diagnostic criteria in the literature (Sturmey, 1993). People with ID may have sufficient verbal skills to report adequately, but still may have response styles such as response acquiescence that limit the accuracy of the information provided. Hence, clinical interviewers may have to modify their interviewing behaviours to use simplified language, check for response acquiescence, using clear anchoring events, check for understanding, giving breaks and so on (Finlay, 2005). These problems have been widely recognized, but not been well documented. Opinions have been variously expressed that some (or most) people with mild, (or perhaps) moderate and perhaps not (or perhaps) some people with severe ID could be adequate informants! Future research should focus on developing objective and reliable criteria for adequately participating in a psychiatric interview and then apply them systematically to people with ID.

As a significant proportion of people with ID are not adequate informants, diagnosticians rely on third parties to act as informants. Third parties can sometimes act as accurate informants for other people's private events and histories, but such information should be treated with caution. Any of us would have a hard time reporting a typically developing person's personal experiences, as we can only do so from inferring them from the things that other people do and say: interpreting the behaviour of people with atypical development is even more challenging. Third-party informants may only know the client for a short period of time or be able to observe them in one setting. Third-party informants may have their own strong opinions as to the cause or actual diagnosis responsible for the distressing behaviour or may not have the language and discrimination skills to report the relevant information to professionals accurately. Many clinicians see psychiatric history as an essential element of a diagnostic work up (Deb & Iyer, 2005). However, some clients have long and complex histories that may be poorly or incompletely documented or may not be available.

Comment

The diagnosis of ID, especially mild ID, remains controversial. The dominant biomedical models of disability are challenged by a heterogeneous condition with no single clear aetiology or indeed, in most cases, no known aetiology at all. Hence, trends in labelling people with ID, and especially mild ID, are likely to be driven by a variety of social trends, ideology and policy rather than biomedical discoveries.

The application of standardized classification schemes of mental disorders to people with ID has numerous problems, especially with people with moderate through to profound ID. In response to these problems a variety of alternative approaches have been developed over the last ten years.

Alternative approaches to classification

Modified criteria

Standardized psychiatric classification schemes appear inflexible in their use of explicit symptom counts and rule outs, but do also contain considerable flexibility. For example, DSM-IV's use of 'not otherwise specified' categories for each of the major groups of disorders, the 'unspecified Mental Disorder (non psychotic)' and the plethora of 'Other Conditions' that may be the focus of clinical attention all give the diagnostician considerable leeway in making a diagnosis of some kind. Szymanski and King (1999) boldly state that '. . . every behavioural presentation that is serious enough to cause significant discomfort or dysfunction, can be characterized by a DSM-IV designation, even if a relatively non-specific one or a V code is used' (p. 12S). So there it is: according to Szymanski and King (1999) a standardized psychiatric diagnosis is always possible for aggression, self-injury and non-compliance that causes 'significant discomfort or dysfunction'. Not all of us agree!

Despite all this flexibility in standardized classification systems several alternative approaches have been developed. Pragmatically, a clinician may limit the problems of third-party informants and instead focus on more objective signs, such as weight change and changes in other vegetative functions that are closely related to the core signs and symptoms of a disorder. Others have modified standardized diagnostic criteria for people with ID, developed behavioural equivalents or used functional assessment and analysis to better understand the presenting problems.

Individual recommendations

Some researchers and practitioners have proposed modifications to standardized diagnostic criteria for mental disorders in people with ID and there are many examples of such recommendations (Cain *et al.*, 2003; Davis *et al.*, 1997; Marston *et al.*, 1997; Clarke & Gomez, 1999; Moss *et al.*, 1997; Ross & Oliver, 2003; Szymanski & King, 1999). These recommendations for modifications are useful sources of hypotheses, but are difficult to evaluate. They may reflect a useful and valid insight or idiosyncratic and erroneous personal experience. Only through reliability and validity trials can the value of such proposals be evaluated. It is worth noting that almost all these recommendations have not been empirically evaluated. Tsiouris *et al.* (2003) demonstrated that such recommendations may not be confirmed by empirical research.

The British Royal College of Psychiatrists, voicing dissatisfaction with the application of ICD-10 criteria to people with ID, set up a working group of experts to review ICD-10 criteria and conduct a comprehensive literature search. Subsequently a series of reviews were published in the areas of non-affective psychoses (Melville, 2003), delirium (Simpson, 2003), attention deficit hyperactivity disorder (Seager & O'Brien, 2003), anxiety disorders (Bailey & Andrews, 2003), depressive disorders (Smiley & Cooper, 2003) and eating disorders (Gravestock, 2003), as well as a classification of problem behaviours (O'Brien, 2003) and discussion of the application of DC-LD (see below for definition) to behavioural phenotypes (Clarke, 2003). The working group then made recommendations for modified diagnostic criteria (Cooper et al., 2003) resulting in the publication of the *Diagnostic Criteria for Psychiatric Disorders for Use with Adults with Learning Disabilities* (DC-LD: Royal College of Psychiatrists, 2001). The developers of DC-LD also conducted a field trial in which 52 field investigators applied the DC-LD criteria to 709 people with ID. They found 96.3% agreement between DC-LD criteria and clinical opinion (Cooper et al., 2003).

The development of DC-LD was relatively explicit, research based, systematic and did include a field trial that indicated some preliminary validity data. Although widely discussed in Britain, its empirical basis, including basic questions of reliability and validity, remains to be demonstrated. Although Cooper et al. (2003) reported 96.3% agreement between DC-LD criteria and clinical opinion, the meaning of this observation is unclear. For example, details on agreement between DC-LD and clinical opinion on individual diagnoses were not reported. Further, the very high agreement between DC-LD criteria and clinical opinion seems odd: new diagnostic criteria that are more valid than old diagnostic criteria should have moderate, rather than near-perfect concurrent validity. Future research on DC-LD should address basic issues such as reliability and validity.

Behavioural equivalents

Charlot (2005) reviewed the meanings and logic of behavioural equivalents within the context of mood disorders and these observations apply generally to this problem. She noted that 'behavioural equivalents' were used in at least two ways: to connote an atypical presentation of a symptom or disorder and as an alternative diagnostic criterion that is not closely related to standardized diagnostic criteria. Charlot (2005) noted that the notion of behavioural equivalents already has an extensive use in a variety of other contexts such as childhood 'masked depression' where it is assumed that observable behaviours, such as school refusal and somatic complaints, were evidence of depression in the absence of meeting full diagnostic criteria. Despite the extensive interest in behavioural equivalents of depression in children and adolescents, it is notable that behavioural equivalents were *not* adopted in DSM-IV. Rather DSM-IV criteria for mood disorders are applied with only minor modifications to children and adolescents.

Treatment of symptoms

Some psychiatrists and researchers have moved away from treating mental disorders and in their place have begun to treat psychiatric symptoms. In this way they apparently sidestep the issue of diagnosis, although the issues of reliably identifying the symptom and the validity of treatments indicated by a symptom still remain.

Comment

There are now several proposed modifications to standardized diagnostic criteria and a burgeoning literature on the use of behavioural equivalents. However, the rationale and empirical criteria for reliability and validity for these modifications have not been made explicit or systematically applied. A surprising and continuing absence from the literature are data-based studies clearly documenting the extent and nature of problems in applying ICD and DSM criteria to people with ID. There are at least two kinds of problems: (a) the criteria are not reliable with this population, and (b) the criteria cannot be applied because the clients lack the necessary skills to meet the diagnostic criteria. It is widely assumed that people with mild ID and some people with moderate ID can report symptoms, and some people with moderate and most, if not all, people with severe and profound ID cannot. Systematic data on this impression would be useful; for example, it might be the case that some people with mild ID may not be good reporters. Likewise, the absence of reliability data on both applying standardized and modified diagnostic criteria with verbal and non-verbal clients is a significant lacuna that inhibits evaluation of both standardized and modified diagnostic criteria.

Functional assessment and analysis

Diagnostic models of understanding and treating psychiatric and behavioural disorders use an essentialist model of explanation in which the cause of the unusual behaviour is located inside the person and is usually some relatively enduring structural property of the person. Prototypical examples of this structuralist approach include medical models of acute illnesses, neurotransmitter dysfunction models of mental disorders, brain abnormality explanations of unusual behaviours and personality traits including intelligence as explanations of observable behaviour (Sturmey, 1996).

Skinner (1953) criticized such approaches on a number of grounds. These included logical grounds, such as the circularity of the arguments evoked by structuralists. For example, a client who presents with angry aggressive behaviour is inferred to have an 'impulse control disorder', as evidenced by their angry aggressive behaviour. When asked what caused them to hit someone, the unobservable impulse control disorder is invoked as the cause of that behaviour. Other versions of this logical error include invoking unobserved neurotransmitter dysregulation, brain damage, kindling and so on to explain observable behaviour. Skinner termed this logical error as evoking an 'explanatory fiction'. A second important logical error related to evoking explanatory fictions to explain behaviour is that the experimenter never manipulates these variables, since they cannot be observed by anyone other than the person themselves. In place of these explanatory fictions, Skinner placed functional relationships at the core of understanding and changing behaviour. If an experimenter can manipulate some observable variable systematically and observe a reliable relationship between it and observable behaviour then the possibility of changing the behaviour and understanding the reasons for change are possible. Independent variables that can be manipulated include antecedent events that occur immediately before the behaviour, consequences that occur immediately after the behaviour and establishing operations, such as deprivation and satiation that change the value of a stimulus as a reinforcer. In this approach emphasis is placed on the function, not the form, of the presenting problem. Functional approaches ignore the topography of the presenting problem as a source of information for how to understand and intervene; rather, they look at the function to guide intervention.

This model has been successful in providing explanations of and treatment for challenging behaviours in people with ID including self-injury (Kahng et al., 2002), aggression (Gardner, 2002), many problems associated with autism spectrum disorders (Sturmey & Fitzer, in press) and a wide range of other maladaptive behaviours (Smith et al., in press.). There is an extremely large evidence base supporting its use, reflected in meta-analyses of hundreds of peer-reviewed papers (Carr et al., 1999; Didden et al., 1999; Scotti et al., 1991; Shogren et al., 2004) and recommendations for treatments based on its used from several consensus panels (New York State Department of Health, 1999a, b, c; Surgeon General, 1999; Rush & Frances, 2000). Functional analysis has been used as the basis for interventions for a wide range of clinical problems (Sturmey, 1996, 2005). A variety of mental disorders in people with ID have been successfully analyzed and treated using functional analysis including mood (Sturmey, 2005), psychotic speech (Mace et al., 1988), substance-abuse disorders (Sturmey et al., 2003) and anxiety disorders (Matson, 1981a, b).

Conclusion

Many of the issues identified in recent years continue to be actively researched questions (Sturmey, 1999). We still do not know enough about the reliability and validity of psychiatric diagnosis in people with ID. This is a basic question that largely remains unanswered. Large numbers of people with ID take psychotropic medications ostensibly for psychiatric diagnoses, but the basis for much of this practice remains uncertain. Large numbers of people with ID who present with challenging behaviours still fail to receive effective behavioural services and receive psychiatric diagnosis and psychotropic medication by default.

The last few years have seen considerable interest in the areas of modified psychiatric classification systems specifically tailored for use with people with ID and a similar increase in research into the use of behavioural equivalents.

Despite advancement, a number of basic questions remain unanswered. One principal question is the reliability of psychiatric diagnosis in people with ID. The reliability of individual psychometric instruments has been extensively addressed, yet this fundamental issue remains an elephant in the middle of the room that we dare not speak of. Do psychiatrists and psychologists independently agree whether a person has a mental disorder? Do they reliably agree on whether the presenting problem is a mental disorder or a challenging behaviour that is primarily learned? Do diagnosticians agree what kind of mental disorder is present in someone with ID? We do not know and without this information the field is hamstrung! Psychiatry and psychology cannot defend themselves against the accusation that the entire endeavour of psychiatric diagnosis in people with ID is a house built on sand and that prescription of psychotropic medication is not diagnosis driven. There is no gold standard against which to validate psychometric instruments and interviews. Professional training is weak as trainees merely learn the idiosyncrasies of their mentor, rather than a true and public psychiatric classification system. Future research must address this issue.

Summary points

- Classification of mental disorders must be reliable and valid.
- Classification serves multiple purposes.
- Labels associated with classification usually have a negative connotation; thus there is an ethical obligation that classification should bring with it compensatory benefits to the person classified.
- Alternative approaches to standardized classification schemes include modified diagnostic criteria, individual recommendations, DC-LD, behavioural equivalents and treatment of symptoms, rather than syndromes.
- Functional approaches to treatment of unusual behaviour rejects structuralist approaches, such as classification of mental disorders, and focuses on the environmental determinants of observable behaviour that can be manipulated.

- Functional approaches have an extensive evidence base and support from several consensus panels and have been widely successful in treating a large range of maladaptive behaviours in people with ID.

REFERENCES

Aman, M. G. (1990). *Assessing psychopathology and behavior problems in persons with mental retardation: A review of available instruments.* Rockville, MD: US Department of Health and Human Services.

Bailey, N. M. & Andrews, T. M. (2003). Diagnostic Criteria for Psychiatric Disorders for use with Adults with Learning Disabilities/Mental Retardation (DC-LD) and the diagnosis of anxiety disorders: A review. *Journal of Intellectual Disabilities Research,* **47**, 50–61.

Bayer, R. (1987). *Homosexuality and American Psychiatry. The Politics of Diagnosis. With a New Afterword on AIDS and Homosexuality.* Princeton, NJ: Princeton University Press.

Beutler, L. E. & Malik, M. L. (2002a, eds.). *Rethinking the DSM. A Psychological Perspective.* Washington, DC: American Psychiatric Association.

Beutler, L. E. & Malik, M. L. (2002b.) Diagnosis and treatment guidelines: The example of depression. In: L. E. Beutler & M. L. Malik (eds.), *Rethinking the DSM. A Psychological Perspective,* (pp. 251–78). Washington, DC: American Psychiatric Association.

Cain, N. N., Davidson, P. W., Burhan, A. M. *et al.* (2003). Identifying bipolar disorder in individuals with intellectual disability. *Journal of Intellectual Disability Research,* **47**, 31–8.

Carr, E. G., Horner, R. & Turnbull, A. P. (1999). *Positive Behavior Support in People With Developmental Disabilities: A Research Synthesis (Monograph (American Association on Mental Retardation)).* Washington, DC: American Association on Mental Retardation.

Center for Disease Control (1996). State-specific rates of mental retardation – United States 1993. *Mortality and Morbidity Weekly Review,* **45**(03), 61–5.

Charlot, L. (2005). Use of behavioral equivalents for symptoms of mood disorders. In P. Sturmey (ed.), *Mood Disorders and People with Mental Retardation.* Kingston, NY: National Association for the Dually Diagnosed Press.

Clarke, D. (2003). Diagnostic Criteria for Psychiatric Disorders for use with Adults with Learning Disabilities/Mental Retardation (DC-LD) and psychiatric phenotypes. *Journal of Intellectual Disabilities Research,* **47**, 43–9.

Clarke, D. J. & Gomez, G. A. (1999). Utility of modified DCR-10 criteria in the diagnosis of depression associated with intellectual disabilities. *Journal of Intellectual Disabilities Research,* **43**, 413–20.

Cooper, S. A., Melville, C. A. & Einfeld, S. L. (2003). Psychiatric diagnosis, intellectual disabilities and Diagnostic Criteria for Psychiatric Disorders for use with Adults with Learning Disabilities/Mental Retardation (DC-LD). *Journal of Intellectual Disabilities Research,* **47**, 3–15.

Davis, J. P., Judd, F. K. & Herrman, H. (1997). Depression in adults with intellectual disability. Part 2. A pilot study. *Australian and New Zealand Journal of Psychiatry,* **31**, 243–51.

Deb, S. & Iyer, A. (2005). Clinical Interviews. In P. Sturmey (ed.), *Mood Disorders in People with Mental Retardation.* Kingston, NY: National Association for the Dually Diagnosed Press.

Deb, S., Matthews, T., Holt, D. & Bouras, N. (2001). *Practice Guidelines for the Assessment and Diagnosis of Mental Health Problems in Adults with Intellectual Disability.* Brighton: Pavilion Press.

Department of Education and Skills (2003). *Statistics of Education: Special Needs in England, January 2003. Issue no. 09/03, November 2003.* London: The Stationary Office.

Didden, R., Duker, P. C. Z. & Korzilius, H. (1999). Meta-analytic study on treatment effectiveness for problem behaviors with individuals who have mental retardation. *American Journal on Mental Retardation,* **101**, 387–99.

Edgerton, R. B. (1967). *The Cloak of Competence.* Los Angeles, CA: University of California Press.

Finlay, W. M. L. (2005). Psychometric assessment of mood disorders in people with intellectual disabilities. In P. Sturmey (ed.). *Mood Disorders in People with Mental Retardation.* Kingston, NY: National Association for the Dually Diagnosed Press.

Flynn, J. R. (1984). The mean IQ of Americans: Massive gains 1932 to 1978. *Psychological Bulletin,* **95**, 29–51.

Flynn, J. R. (1985). Wechsler intelligence tests: do we really have a criterion of mental retardation? *American Journal on Mental Deficiency,* **90**, 236–44.

Flynn, J. R. (1987). Massive IQ gains in 14 nations: What IQ tests really measure. *Psychological Bulletin,* **101**, 171–91.

Gardner, W. I (2002). *Aggression and Other Disruptive Behavioral Challenges: Biomedical and Psychosocial Assessment and Treatment.* Kingston, NY: National Association for the Dually Diagnosed Press.

Gravestock, S. (2003). Diagnosis and classification of eating disorders in adults with intellectual disabilities: the Diagnostic Criteria for Psychiatric Disorders for use with Adults with Learning Disabilities/Mental Retardation (DC-LD). *Journal of Intellectual Disabilities Research,* **47**, 72–83.

Holden, B. & Gitlesen, J. P. (2004). Psychotropic medication in adults with mental retardation: prevalence and prescription practices. *Research in Developmental Disabilities,* **25**, 509–21.

Houts, A. C. (2002). Discovery invention and the expansion of the modern *Diagnostic and Statistical Manuals of Mental Disorders.* In: L. E. Beutler & M. L. Malik (eds.), *Rethinking the DSM. A Psychological Perspective,* (pp. 17–68). Washington, DC: American Psychiatric Association.

Hurley, A. D. (1996). The misdiagnosis of hallucinations and delusions in persons with mental retardation: A neurodevelopmental perspective. *Seminars in Neuropsychiatry,* **1**, 122–33.

Kahng, S., Iwata, B. A. & Lewin, A. B. (2002). Behavioral treatments of self-injury, 1964–2000. *American Journal on Mental Retardation,* **107**, 212–21.

Keogh, B. K., Forness, S. R. & MacMillan, D. L. (1998). The real world of special education. *American Psychologist,* **53**, 1161–2.

Kihlstrom, J. F. (2002). To honor Kraeplin: From symptoms to pathology in the diagnosis of mental illness. In: L. E. Beutler & M. L. Malik (eds.), *Rethinking the DSM. A Psychological Perspective,* (pp. 279–304). Washington, DC: American Psychiatric Association.

Kirk, S. A. & Kutchins, H. (1992). *The Selling of DSM: The Rhetoric of Science in Psychiatry.* New York, NY: Lindine de Gruyter.

Lynn, R., Hampson, S. L. & Mullineux, J. C. (1987). A long-term increase in the fluid intelligence of English children. *Nature*, **328**, 797.

Mace, F. C., Webb, M. E., Sharkey, R. W., Mattson, D. M. & Rosen, H. S. (1988). Functional analysis and treatment of bizarre speech. *Journal of Behavior Therapy and Experimental Psychiatry*, **19**, 289–96.

MacMillan, D. L., Gresham, F. M. & Bocian, K. M. (1998). Discrepancy between definitions of learning disabilities and school practices: An empirical investigation. *Journal of Learning Disabilities*, **31**, 314–26.

MacMillan, D. L., Gresham, F. M., Siperstein, G. N. & Bocian, K. M. (1996). The labyrinth of IDEA: School decisions on referred students with subaverage intelligence. *American Journal on Mental Retardation*, **101**, 161–74.

Maheady, L., Towne, R., Algozzine, B., Mercer, J., & Ysseldyke, J. (1983). Minority overrepresentation: A case for alternative practices prior to referral. *Learning Disability Quarterly*, **6**, 448–56.

Malik, M. L. & Beutler, L. E. (2002). The emergence of dissatisfaction with the DSM. In: L. E. Beutler & M. L. Malik (eds.), *Rethinking the DSM. A Psychological Perspective*, pp. 3–16. Washington, DC: American Psychiatric Association.

Marston, G. M., Perry, D. W. & Roy, A. (1997). Manifestations of depression in people with intellectual disabilities. *Journal of Intellectual Disability Research*, **41**, 476–80.

Matson, J. L. (1981a). Assessment and treatment of clinical fears in mentally retarded children. *Journal of Applied Behavior Analysis*, **14**, 287–94.

Matson, J. L. (1981b). A controlled outcome study of phobias in mentally retarded adults. *Behavior Research and Therapy*, **19**, 101–7.

Melville, C. A. (2003). A critique of the use of Diagnostic Criteria for Psychiatric Disorders for use with Adults with Learning Disabilities/Mental Retardation (DC-LD) chapter on non-affective disorders. *Journal on Intellectual Disabilities Research*, **47**, 16–25.

Moss, S., Ibbotson, B., Prosser, H. *et al.* (1997). Validity of the PAS-ADD for detecting psychiatric symptoms in adults with learning disabilities (mental retardation). *Social Psychiatry and Psychiatric Epidemiology*, **32**, 344–54.

Moss, S., Patel, P., Prosser, H. *et al.* (1993). Psychiatric morbidity in older people with moderate and severe learning disability. I: Development and reliability of the patient interview (PAS-ADD). *British Journal of Psychiatry*, **163**, 471–80.

Murphy, C. C., Yeargin-Allsopp, M., Decoufle, P. & Drews, C. D. (1995). The administrative prevalence of mental retardation in 10-year-old children in metropolitan Atlanta, 1985 through 1987. *American Journal of Public Health*, **85**, 319–23.

New York State Department of Health (1999a). *Clinical Practice Guidelines: Report of the Recommendations. Autism/Pervasive Developmental Disorders. Assessment and Intervention for Young Children (Age 0–3 Years)* (Publication No. 4215). Albany, NY: New York State Department of Health.

New York State Department of Health (1999b). *Clinical Practice Guidelines: Quick Reference Guide. Autism/Pervasive Developmental Disorders. Assessment and Intervention for Young Children (Age 0–3 Years)* (Publication No. 4216). Albany, NY: New York State Department of Health.

New York State Department of Health (1999c). *Clinical Practice Guidelines: The Guideline Technical Report. Autism/Pervasive Developmental Disorders. Assessment and Intervention for Young Children (Age 0–3 Years)* (Publication No. 4217). Albany, NY: New York State Department of Health.

O'Brien, G. (2003). The classification of problem behaviors in Diagnostic Criteria for Psychiatric Disorders for use with Adults with Learning Disabilities/Mental Retardation (DC-LD). *Journal of Intellectual Disabilities Research*, **47**, 32–7.

Patel, P., Goldberg, D. & Moss, S. (2001). Psychiatric morbidity in older people with moderate and severe learning disability. II: The prevalence study. *British Journal of Psychiatry*, **163**, 481–91.

Ross, E. & Oliver, C. (2003). The assessment of mood in adults who have severe or profound mental retardation. *Clinical Psychology Review*, **23**, 225–45.

Royal College of Psychiatrists (2001). *OP48. DC-LD: Diagnostic Criteria for Psychiatric Disorders for use with Adults with Learning Disabilities/Mental Retardation.* London: Gaskell.

Rush, A. J. & Frances, A. (2000). The Expert Consensus Guideline Series: Treatment of Psychiatric and Behavioral Problems in Mental Retardation. *American Journal on Mental Retardation*, **105**, 159–228.

Scotti, J. R., Evans, I. M., Meyer, L. H. Z. & Walker, P. (1991). A meta-analysis of intervention research with problem behavior: Treatment validity and standards of practice. *American Journal on Mental Retardation*, **96**, 233–56.

Seager, M. C. & O'Brien, G. (2003). Attention deficit hyperactivity disorder: Review of ADHD in learning disability – the Diagnostic Criteria for Psychiatric Disorders for use with Adults with Learning Disabilities/Mental Retardation (DC-LD) criteria for diagnosis. *Journal of Intellectual Disabilities Research*, **47**, 26–31.

Shogren, K. A., Faggella-Luby, M. N., Bae, S. J. & Wehmeyer, M. L. (2004). The effects of choice making as an intervention for problem behavior: A meta-analysis. *Journal of Positive Behavioral Interventions*, **6**, 228–37.

Simpson, N. (2003). Delirium in adults with intellectual disabilities. *Journal of Intellectual Disabilities Research*, **47**, 38–42.

Singh, N. N., Ellis, C. R. & Wechsler, H. (1997). Psychopharmaco-epidemiology of mental retardation: 1966 to 1995. *Journal of Child and Adolescent Psychopharmacology*, **7**, 255–66.

Skinner, B. F. (1953). *Science and Human Behavior.* New York NY: Free Press.

Smiley, E. & Cooper, S. A. (2003). Intellectual disabilities, depressive episodes, diagnostic criteria and Diagnostic Criteria for Psychiatric Disorders for use with Adults with Learning Disabilities/Mental Retardation (DC-LD). *Journal of Intellectual Disabilities Research*, **47**, 62–71.

Smith, R. G., Vollmer, T. R. & St. Peter, C. (in press). Functional approaches to assessment and treatment of problem behavior in persons with autism and related disabilities. In P. Sturmey & A. Fitzer (eds.). *Autism Spectrum Disorders: Applied Behavior Analysis Evidence and Practice.* Austin, TX: PROED Inc.

Sovner, R. (1986). Limiting factors in the use of DSM-II with mentally ill/mentally retarded persons. *Psychopharmacology Bulletin*, **22**, 1055–9.

Sturmey, P. (1993). The use of ICD and DSM criteria in people with mental retardation: A review. *The Journal of Nervous and Mental Disease*, **181**, 39–42.

Sturmey, P. (1996). *Functional Analysis in Clinical Psychology.* London: Wiley.

Sturmey, P. (1999). Classification: Concepts, progress and future. In N. Bouras, (ed.), *Psychiatric and Behavioral Disorders in Developmental Disabilities and Mental Retardation,* pp. 3–17. Cambridge: Cambridge University Press.

Sturmey, P. (2005). Behavioral conceptualization and treatment of depression in people with mental retardation. In P. Sturmey (ed.), *Mood Disorders in People with Mental Retardation.* Kingston: National Association for the Dually Diagnosed Press.

Sturmey, P. & Fitzer, A. (in press). *Autism Spectrum Disorders: Applied Behavior Analysis Evidence and Practice.* Austin, TX: PROED Inc.

Sturmey, P., Reed, J. & Corbett, J. A. (1991). Psychometric assessment of psychiatric disorders in people with learning disabilities (mental handicap): A review of measures. *Psychological Medicine,* **21**, 143–155.

Sturmey, P., Reyer, H., Lee, R. & Robek, A. (2003). *Substance-Related Disorders in Persons with Mental Retardation.* Kingston, NY: National Association for the Dually Diagnosed Press.

Surgeon General (1999). *Mental Health: A Report of the Surgeon General.* Washington, DC: Department of Health and Human Services.

Szymanski, L. & King, B. H. (1999). Practice parameters for the assessment and treatment of children, adolescents and adults with mental retardation and comorbid mental disorders. *Journal of the American Academy of Child and Adolescent Psychiatry,* **38**, (Suppl.) 5–31S.

Tsiouris, J. A., Mann, R., Patti, P. J. & Sturmey, P. (2003). Challenging behaviours should not be considered as depressive equivalents in individuals with intellectual disability. *Journal of Intellectual Disability Research,* **47**, 14–21.

US Department of Education. (2002). *Twenty-Second Annual Report to Congress on the Implementation of the Individuals with Disabilities Education Act.* Washington, DC: US Government Printing Office.

World Health Organization (1992.). *The International Classification of Diseases (10th edn).* Geneva: WHO.

Yeargin-Allsopp, M., Drews, C. D., Decoufle, P. & Murphy, C. C. (1995). Mild mental retardation in black and white children in metropolitan Atlanta: a case-control study. *American Journal of Public Health,* **85**, 324–8.

Yeargin-Allsopp, M., Murphy, C. C., Cordero, J. F., Decoufle, P. & Hollowell, J. G. (1997). Reported biomedical causes and associated medical conditions for mental retardation among 10-year-old children in metropolitan Atlanta, 1985 to 1987. *Developmental Medicine and Childhood Neurology,* **39**, 142–9.

2

Mental health assessment and monitoring tools for people with intellectual disabilities

Caroline Mohr and Helen Costello

Introduction

Assessing the presence of mental health problems in individuals with intellectual disabilities (ID) is a complex process. Increased clinical and research attention in recent years has resulted in the development of a range of assessment instruments aimed at improving the identification and diagnosis of psychiatric and behavioural disorders in this population. The routine use of valid and reliable assessment and monitoring tools may make a significant contribution to improving the quality of care. Yet, currently there is no consensus about which assessment instruments should be used.

The aim of this chapter is to provide an overview of the characteristics and psychometric properties of what the authors consider to be the best available assessment and monitoring tools. The chapter describes the approaches employed for the development of assessment instruments, describes the key features of six checklists and rating scales and summarizes evidence about their validity and reliability. In doing so, the strengths and limitations of available assessment instruments are highlighted, and recommendations for using assessment and monitoring tools are made.

Developing assessment and monitoring tools

While the precise function of instruments may vary, the central aim of assessment and monitoring tools is to increase the validity and reliability with which the presence and severity of the signs, or symptoms, of mental health problems are measured over a given period. Standardized instruments help to ensure that individuals referred to mental health services receive a comprehensive and objective assessment, less subject to factors such as 'diagnostic overshadowing' (Reiss *et al.*,

Psychiatric and Behavioural Disorders in Intellectual and Developmental Disabilities, ed. Nick Bouras and Geraldine Holt. Published by Cambridge University Press. © Cambridge University Press 2007.

1982) and variations in the opinions of individual carers and clinicians (Einfeld & Tonge, 1992).

Given the high levels of undetected, and therefore untreated, mental health problems in individuals with ID (Deb *et al.*, 2001a; Moss, 1999), improving the accuracy and sensitivity of the identification and referral process are also a priority. The routine use of monitoring tools by carers, such as brief mental health screens, may help to increase access to mental health services and to ensure that all individuals with potential mental health problems are identified, evaluated and treated.

Assessment and monitoring tools imply greater uniformity in the measurement of mental health problems in people with ID and adherence to explicit conceptual frameworks. As such, their use provides a common discourse among researchers and clinicians, enhances the comparison and interpretability of research findings and thus helps in addressing current conflicts in the evidence base.

Assessment instruments may focus on specific disorders, or they may be used to assess the presence of a range of mental health problems. Available instruments include adaptations of tools used with the general population and with children, such as the Zung Self-rating Anxiety Scale (SAS) (Zung, 1971) and those that have been specifically developed for individuals with ID such as the Reiss Screen for Maladaptive Behaviour (RSMB) (Reiss, 1988). They may be completed by clinicians, carers or by individuals with ID themselves. However, owing to the communicative limitations of many people with ID, the majority of instruments focus on the collection of information from carers, such as family members and staff, either through clinician completion or carer self-report.

Holland and Koot (1998) highlight an important distinction between those instruments seeking to 'identify the nature and extent of problem behaviours, and which are essentially descriptive in nature' and those that 'investigate, at least partially, aetiology (e.g. a particular pattern of behaviours, or evidence of loss of function)'. This distinction between instruments assumes practical importance when the question of how to devise rating scales and checklists is addressed.

Instruments that delineate and quantify disturbed behaviour while remaining free of attachment to a theoretical framework or assumptions about causality are most likely to be developed using 'bottom up' methodology (Achenbach, 1998; Einfeld & Tonge, 1992). Rating scales and checklists developed using this descriptive–empirical approach are more likely to contain elements of the Dimensional model (Streiner & Norman, 1995) and 'allow one to commence with fewer assumptions regarding the relation between ID, behaviour problems and psychiatric disorders, or their classification' (Einfeld and Tonge, 1992).

'Bottom up' approaches to developing checklists entail collating a large pool of items describing emotional and behavioural problems followed by a series of studies to refine wording and to establish reliability, validity and factor structure. Examples include the Aberrant Behaviour Checklist (ABC) (Aman & Singh, 1985) and the Developmental Behaviour Checklist-Primary Care Version (DBC-P) (Einfeld & Tonge, 1992). By making no assumptions about why particular problems occur, or occur together, such rating scales or checklists contribute to the accumulation of clinical expertise and research data in a way that allows discoveries to be made about the ways a population or an individual may be influenced by the greatest and most diverse range of factors (Einfeld & Tonge, 1992).

The second type of instrument referred to by Holland and Koot (1998), those exploring aetiology, includes psychiatric assessments and is most often developed using 'top down' methods (Tonge & Einfeld, 1992), using existing diagnostic frameworks, typically DSM-IV (American Psychiatric Association, 1994) or ICD-10 (World Health Organization, 1992), as a starting point from which to select items that are 'reworded' in behavioural terms. Instruments developed in this way include the Psychiatric Assessment Schedule for Adults with Developmental Disabilities (PAS-ADD) (Moss *et al.*, 1993) and the Psychopathology Inventory for Mentally Retarded Adults (PIMRA) (Matson, 1988).

At present there is no research evidence to suggest whether the 'bottom up' or 'top down' approach will prove to be most useful. Both methods of developing rating scales and checklists have validity and, although differently sourced, have a contribution to make to the accumulation of knowledge. Ultimately, a lack of a suitable 'gold standard' against which checklists can be measured hinders the development of validated measures.

If modified or unmodified tools are used, it appears that this is an option mainly applicable to people with mild ID. Researchers have reported making extensive changes to the content, the format and the presentation of items in standardized instruments when using them with people with an ID. Yet, most studies have not had sufficient resources to be able to conduct revalidation and reliability studies using the modified instruments (Deb *et al.*, 2001b). Assessing the impact of changing presentation formats, such as reading checklists out loud, on the results obtained is vital. Further validation and normative studies are also required in order to measure the impact of cultural differences on instruments used in different countries and translated into other languages. Such studies need to be undertaken before modified rating scales and checklists can be used with confidence.

At the same time, there has been a great deal of debate in the literature concerning the application of DSM-IV (APA, 1994) or ICD-10 (WHO, 1992) with individuals across the entire spectrum of ID. For example, Einfeld and Tonge (1992) claimed that there was 'substantial lack of agreement that the standard diagnostic and classification systems provide the most useful account of the behavioural and emotional problems of children with an IQ below the mild range of intellectual disabilities'.

This lack of agreement about diagnostic systems in children also applies to work with adults with ID and remains largely unresolved 14 years later.

The application of standard psychiatric diagnostic criteria to adults with severe and profound levels of ID is not supported at this time by experienced researchers (Aman, 1991; Tonge *et al.*, 1996). For people with a moderate or greater degree of ID, specially developed carer- or clinician-completed instruments are probably required. An alternative solution may be to devise a separate diagnostic framework specifically for adults with an ID, or to modify existing categories of disorder to take account of the differences caused by ID. The DC-LD (Diagnostic Criteria for Use with Adults with Learning Disabilities/Mental Retardation) (Royal College of Psychiatrists, 2001) is one example of a new set of diagnostic categories specifically designed for individuals with moderate to profound ID (see Chapter 1). These criteria are based on the ICD framework and were developed on the basis of expert clinical consensus. Assessment and monitoring tools based on these criteria are awaited.

Key characteristics of assessment and monitoring tools

The following review includes those assessment instruments that were regarded as 'promising' in Aman's (1991) review of psychopathology checklists for individuals with ID and that have since been widely used. Two scales developed since 1991 have also been included: the PAS-ADD Checklist (Moss *et al.*, 1998) that has been used in many recent publications and the DBC-A (for adults) (Mohr *et al.*, 2004) as it was derived from the frequently used DBC-P for children and adolescents with ID. All of these instruments assess the presence of a range of mental health problems and are based on information collected from informants such as family members and direct care staff. They include checklists and rating scales completed by clinicians during interviews with carers and those completed independently by carers.

The Psychopathology Instrument for Mentally Retarded Adults (PIMRA)

The PIMRA (Matson *et al.* 1984) is a structured interview designed for completion by a mental health professional. Two versions are available, an informant version for completion by carers (PIMRA-I) and a self-report version, to be completed with the individual with ID where possible. It has a rating scale format comprising 58 items drawn from the major categories of DSM-III, and is organized into eight subscales: Schizophrenia, Affective Disorder, Psychosexual Disorder, Adjustment Disorder, Anxiety Disorder, Somatoform Disorder, Personality Disorder and Inappropriate Adjustment. Each item is scored either 'yes' or 'no', and 75% of the scale must be completed for a valid result to be obtained. For diagnosis, at least four items on each subscale should be scored positively, although Matson (1988) advocates a degree of flexibility in accordance with the rules of DSM-III and experience of the mental health professional. A time frame over which to assess the presence of behaviours is not provided.

Aberrant Behaviour Checklist (ABC)

The ABC (Aman & Singh, 1985) was designed to be brief and suitable for repeated use. Item descriptions are provided in a glossary (Aman *et al.*, 1986) which raters are asked to study prior to completion. The 58 items on the checklist were drawn from case notes and other popular rating scales used with people with ID and were factorially derived. Each item is rated on a 4-point scale indicating severity (Aman *et al.*, 1986). A manual provides normative data for different age groups and levels of intellectual disability (Aman *et al.*, 1986). A version with modified language has been devised for individuals residing in community settings (Marshburn & Aman, 1992).

Reiss Screen for Maladaptive Behaviour (RSMB)

The RSMB (Reiss, 1988) is a rating scale designed for completion by two or more carers and does not require training. It consists of 38 psychiatric symptoms with brief accompanying definitions and examples. Each item is rated on a 3-point scale (0 = no problem, 1 = problem, and 2 = major problem). Perhaps confusingly, the manual asks carers to rate symptoms, such as hallucinations, as problems even when they are controlled by treatment. A total of 26 items contribute to the eight subscales: Aggressive Behaviour, Autism, Psychosis, Paranoia, Depression (B) (behavioural signs), Depression (P) (physical signs), Dependent Personality Disorder, Avoidant Disorder.

The Diagnostic Assessment for the Severely Handicapped Scale (DASH)

Based upon a mixture of DSM-III-R criteria, other instruments and previous studies, the DASH Scale (Matson *et al.* 1991a) was designed for individuals with severe and profound levels of ID. It comprises 84 items grouped into 13 clinical scales (anxiety; mood disorder – depression; mood disorder – mania; autism; schizophrenia; stereotypes; self-injurious behaviours; elimination disorders; eating disorders; sleep disorders, sexual disorders, organic syndromes; impulse control and miscellaneous problems). Administered by clinicians, DASH is multidimensional and requires carers to report on the severity, frequency and duration of individual items during the past two weeks. For subscales 1–5, endorsement of more than half of the subscales items is used as a diagnostic index. For subscales 6–13, endorsement of at least one subscale item with a severity of 1 or 2 is used as a diagnostic index. A later version of the scale (DASH-II) with modifications to the wording of 9 items became available after 1991.

Psychiatric Assessment Schedule for Adults with Developmental Disabilities (PAS-ADD) Checklist

The PAS-ADD Checklist (Moss *et al.* 1998) is a more recently developed instrument and is one of a family of three assessment instruments developed from the Schedules for Clinical Assessment in Neuropsychiatry (SCAN) (WHO, 1994). The PAS-ADD Checklist focuses exclusively on Axis I disorders and was designed for completion by carers with no knowledge of psychopathology. Its aim is to help carers to recognize mental health problems and to make informed referral decisions. It comprises a 'life events' section and a 'problems' section comprising 29 items worded in everyday language, describing behaviours associated with mental health problems along with examples. Each item is rated on a 4-point scale according to frequency and whether or not it has been a problem for the person in the previous 4-week period. Items are grouped into 5 subscales that combine to produce scores for 'affective/neurotic disorder', 'possible organic condition' and 'psychotic disorder'. Scores in excess of the threshold scores provided indicate that an individual is at risk of having a mental health problem and that referral for further psychiatric assessment is required.

The Developmental Behaviour Checklist for Adults (DBC-A)

The Developmental Behaviour Checklist for Adults (DBC-A) (Mohr *et al.* 2004) is a carer-completed checklist of emotional and behavioural disturbance in adults with ID adapted from the DBC-P for children and adolescents with ID (Einfeld & Tonge, 1992) allowing for the continuity of assessment for people with ID across the whole life span. Replicating the development of the DBC-P, the DBC-A was modified using 'bottom up' processes. It comprises 106 items with a reading level suitable for carers with a primary level of education. It takes a carer, who knows the person with ID well, approximately 15 minutes to complete. Items are rated on a three point scale: 0 = not true, 1 = somewhat or sometimes true, 2 = very true or often true. It has six factorially derived subscales and a cut-off score for psychiatric caseness.

Psychometric properties of assessment and monitoring tools

Tables 2.1 and 2.2 summarize available data about the reliability and validity of the selected assessment and monitoring tools. The studies from which data were drawn are listed in the reference list at the end of the chapter. Inevitably, the divergent methodologies employed, such as variations in sample size (ranging from 15 to 648), and the differing populations on which studies were based, limit to some extent, the comparison of psychometric properties of alternative instruments. Also, while extensive data are available for some instruments such as the PIMRA, it is sparser for more recently developed instruments such as the PAS-ADD Checklist and the DBC-A. These summaries are therefore intended to guide mental health professionals in selecting rating scales and checklists for clinical and research purposes, by providing an overview of the strengths and limitations of each instrument and highlighting current gaps in knowledge about their performance.

Internal consistency and reliability

Internal consistency

Table 2.1 shows that the internal consistencies of the instruments is largely adequate, with Cronbach's alpha values ranging from 0.6 to 0.95 for total scales. Greater variation is reported for individual subscales, alpha values are generally lower (ranging from −0.1 to 0.77) and poor internal consistency is reported for some individual items. For example, a few items on the PIMRA failed to correlate with whole scale or subscale scores (Aman *et al.*, 1986; Senatore *et al.*, 1985; Sturmey & Ley, 1990; Watson *et al.*, 1988), and Moss *et al.* (1998) report an alpha value of 0.51 for the psychosis scale on the PAS-ADD checklist. However, where the purpose of a scale is to identify at-risk individuals and to assess the presence of a possible disorder rather than to indicate its precise nature, low inter-correlations do not imply that instruments are unsuitable for use as screening instruments.

Test–retest and inter-rater reliability

Studies have used a range of techniques to measure test–retest and inter-rater reliability (including the level of percentage agreement, correlations and Cohen's Kappa). In some cases, substantial variation is reported across different studies of the same instrument. For example, subsequent studies of the PIMRA (Watson *et al.*, 1988) and of the ABC (Aman, 1991) both discount the higher findings of previous studies. At the same time, the test–retest reliability of some instruments, such as the PAS-ADD checklist, has not been investigated.

Aman (1991) reports that the inter-rater reliability of the RSMB is 'generally very acceptable' and that 'acceptable, but not high levels' of inter-rater reliability ($r = 0.50$ to low 0.60) have come from several studies of the ABC (Aman & Singh, 1985; Ono, 1996; Rojahn & Helsel, 1991). A study of test–retest reliability, inter-rater reliability and internal consistency conducted by Sturmey *et al.* (1995) concluded that the RSMB 'appeared to have moderate to good psychometric robustness'. A

Table 2.1 Internal consistency and reliability of assessment and monitoring tools.

Psychometric properties	Internal consistency		Reliability		
			Test–retest		Inter-rater t = total score, ss
Checklists (*n* of studies)	Total scale	Subscales	Total scale	Subscales	= subscales
PIMRA (13)	0.64 to 0.9	−0.1 to 0.77	0.65 to 0.91	−0.15 to 1.0	0.4 to 0.77 ss
ABC (9)	0.94	0.78 to 0.94	–	0.84 to 0.99	0.58 to 0.78 t
RSMB (8)	0.8 to 0.92	0.46 to 0.87	0.75	0.5 to 0.7	0.6 to 0.81 t 0.5 to 0.8 ss
DASH (9)	0.86	0.2 to 0.84	% 0.84 to 0.91	–	% 0.95 to 0.85 t
PAS-ADD Checklist (2)	0.87	0.51 to 0.84			0.79 t 0.55 to 0.60 (r) ss
DBC-A (3)	0.95	0.61 to 0.89	0.75 to 0.85	–	0.72 t

later study of the RSMB based on 134 individuals 'representative of the administratively defined Swedish group of people with ID' (Gustafsson & Sonnander, 2002) found that inter-rater agreement (r) on total scores between two raters was 0.60.

Data were collected using the DASH for 506 people with severe (32%) and profound (62%) ID (Aman, 1991). Inter-rater reliability was assessed from two ratings of 29 residents made within three hours. The percentage level of agreement was reported to be generally high, with the exception of a few items related to irritability and frustration. Using a later version of the DASH (DASH-II), Matson and Smiroldo (1997) found an alpha value of 0.79 for the Mania subscale and item total correlations ranged from 0.42 to 0.76. Using Kappa, perhaps a stronger test of reliability because it takes chance agreement into account, Linaker (1991) reported that the level of agreement in terms of caseness was 0.64 for the PIMRA and Moss et al. (1998) reported 0.54 (95% CI 0.34–0.75) for the PAS-ADD Checklist. For the DBC-A, higher test–retest reliability was found between pairs of family carers (0.85, 95% CI 0.75–0.91) than between pairs of paid carers (0.75, 95% CI 0.55–0.86) in a large institutional setting (Mohr et al., 2004).

Criterion group and concurrent validity

Criterion group validity

Validity studies of the PIMRA have yielded mixed and conflicting results (Table 2.2). Early work on the factor structure (Aman et al., 1986; Matson et al., 1984; Watson *et al.*, 1988) suggested between two and four factors, but a later study (Linaker, 1991) described nine factors, some of which resembled earlier factors. There is evidence to suggest that both forms of the PIMRA are able to distinguish between individuals with and without diagnosed psychopathology (Senatore *et al.*, 1985; van Minnen *et al.*, 1994).

However, using subject response to medication as a measure of criterion group validity, Swiezy *et al.* (1995) found no significant correlations between the PIMRA subscales and drug responsiveness. Linaker and Helle (1994) report that although the PIMRA correctly identified schizophrenia in 71% of psychiatric patients without ID, its accuracy varied greatly depending on what form the illness took (disorganized, paranoid or schizoaffective). Swiezy *et al.* (1995) compared PIMRA results for 65 adults with mild to moderate ID with an assessment interview by a psychologist using 'a set of items derived from the schizophrenia and depression sections of the DSM-III-R'. They concluded that the PIMRA-I schizophrenia and depression subscales were valid, although this seems hardly surprising with both assessments 'derived' from DSM criteria.

The psychometric properties of the ABC have been widely studied and its validity is well established. The factor structure of the ABC has been confirmed in several countries (Newton & Sturmey, 1988; Ono, 1996), in different residential settings (Aman *et al.*, 1995) and with children (Rojahn & Helsel, 1991). Criterion group validity has been addressed in specific groups. For example, individuals previously found to have lower levels of behavioural disturbance, such as those with Down syndrome (Aman *et al.*, 1987) and those taking most psychoactive medications (Aman *et al.*, 1995; 1987) received significantly lower scores on the ABC. In contrast, individuals with a diagnosis of schizophrenia (Aman *et al.*, 1987) received higher scores. Yet, the ABC contains items describing observable and behavioural phenomena (exceptions are: Mood changes rapidly; Depressed mood; Irritable) and there are many emotional and experiential aspects of psychopathology not covered in the 58 items.

Validity studies of the RSMB have established that 'validity is good insofar as the instrument is used for the identification of any psychopathology' (Aman, 1991). As the principle role of the RSMB is to establish the need for further mental health evaluation, the lack of validity data on subscales may be less important (Aman, 1991). Aman (1991) expressed concern about the small standardization sample, the seemingly arbitrary choice of cut-off scores, and the presence of diagnostic subscales, which he argued could be used for diagnostic purposes even though the tool was not designed for this purpose. Although the RSMB is the only checklist to have been studied using confirmatory factor analysis, disagreement about its factor structure is evident. For example, Reiss (1988) and Havercamp and Reiss (1997) described eight clinical subscales although Sturmey *et al.* (1996) suggested a one-or three-factor solution. Yet, several limitations in the latter study were identified by Reiss (1997) (e.g. small and homogeneous samples) who recommended that future studies should employ confirmatory factor analytic techniques on large samples of 300 or more people from a diverse population. A comparison of RSMB results and psychiatric opinion for 21 individuals with ID in Sweden found agreement in 81% of cases, with significant chance-corrected agreement (Gustafsson & Sonnander, 2002).

A factor analysis of the DASH conducted by Matson et al. (1991b) yielded six factors accounting for 39% of the variance ($n = 506$). Matson et al. (1991b) concluded 'coherent taxonomies or psychiatric problems among individuals with profound and severe ID might be derived from a combination of factor analytic and clinically derived scales' (Matson et al., 1991b). Substantial variation is reported in studies addressing criterion group validity of the DASH. Matson and Smiroldo (1997) report that the DASH-II mania subscale correctly identified 90.9% of individuals with independently diagnosed mania and 100% of the control subjects ($n = 22$).

Matson et al., (1998) found that the autism/PDD subscale successfully identified autism ($n = 51$). Bamburg et al. (2001) report that the schizophrenia subscale correctly identified schizophrenia in verbal, but not in non-verbal, individuals ($n = 60$). Matson et al. (1997c) found that only 7 of the 33 individuals identified by the anxiety subscale received an anxiety disorder diagnosis from a clinician. Matson et al., (1997b) report that overall 83% of individuals with a DSM-IV diagnosis of Stereotypy and Self-injury were correctly identified and that there were no false negatives ($n = 123$). Individuals with high scores on the stereoptypies subscale had lower scores on the Vineland Adaptive Behaviour Scales (Nihira et al., 1975). A total of 73% of individuals with a clinical diagnosis of depression were identified by the depression subscale in a study conducted by Matson et al. (1999).

Factor analysis, performed on 201 PAS-ADD Checklists, generated eight factors, which were '. . . readily interpretable in psychiatric terms' (Moss et al., 1998) and accounted for 65% of the variance. In a sample of 59 individuals, selected to cover a broad range of conditions and degrees of severity of disorder, the likelihood of identification rose with the severity rating received from the psychiatrist, and depended on the disorder being one of those covered by the PAS-ADD Checklist. This included 26% of subjects with no disorder, 56% with a mild disorder, and 92% with a severe disorder.

Using the PAS-ADD Interview (Moss et al., 1993) as a 'gold standard' ($n = 93$), the best agreement was obtained when any symptom reported was allocated a '1', and summed to form an overall score, disregarding the scoring algorithm and threshold sores on the three subscales (Simpson et al., 1998). A study by Taylor et al. (2004) of 1155 adults with ID living in community, residential and hospital settings in a county in northern England provides normative data for the PAS-ADD Checklist in relation to gender, age and type of residence. As the rates of mental disorders found were consistent with previous studies of general populations of individuals with ID using over-inclusive screening instruments, the authors conclude that the PAS-ADD Checklist is an easy to use and sensitive tool for identifying mental health cases in this population. However, further investigation of the instrument's specificity is recommended. A recent independent replication study by Sturmey *et al.* (2005) of a community sample of 226 adults with ID reported that the PAS-ADD Checklist was sensitive to differences between diagnostic groups and had an overall sensitivity of 66% and specificity of 70%.

The factor structure of the DBC-A was investigated in a study of 508 people with ID, and a six-factor solution adopted. When compared with the DBC-P factor structure, this finding indicates that both checklists have a stable and factorially valid structure when employed in studies of people with ID of all ages (Mohr *et al.*, 2004). Criterion group validity of the DBC-A is reported from a study of 70 people referred to a specialist health clinic for adults with ID. Clinician ratings of the presence and severity of psychopathology were highly correlated, and DBC-A total scores were significantly different between groups with high versus low levels of psychopathology ($t(69) = 4.48, p < 0.000$) (Mohr *et al.*, 2004). In the same study the optimal DBC-A total cut-off score for psychiatric caseness was established with acceptable sensitivity and specificity for screening purposes. The collection of normative data is proceeding at the time of publication.

Concurrent validity

Working with an earlier version of the RSMB (The Checklist of Emotional Problems with Mentally Retarded Adults, CHEMRA) Davidson (1988) found a high correspondence with PIMRA total scores. Likewise, van Minnen *et al.* (1994) reported a significant correlation between RSMB and PIMRA-I (Informant version) total scores, and mainly significant correlations between subscales on both instruments. Comparing the RSMB, the PIMRA and the ABC, Sturmey and Bertman (1994) reported 'modest to good concurrent validity', although some apparently homologous scales such as the schizophrenia subscale on the RSMB and PIMRA did not correlate significantly. Sturmey and Bertman (1994) found a significant correlation between RSMB and ABC total scores and some subscale scores, although this finding was not supported by a study by Walsh and Shenouda (1999), possibly owing to sample differences (Walsh & Shenouda, 1999).

McDaniel *et al.* (1999) studied a small institutional sample of people with mild to moderate ID, for whom the PIMRA-I and the RSMB were administered twelve months apart to assess the robustness of, and the relationship between, the two scales in the area of personality disturbance. Although lower than the Sturmey and Bertman (1994) finding, a significant correlation was found between total scores

Table 2.2 Criterion group validity and concurrent validity of assessment and monitoring tools.

Checklists	Criterion group validity	Concurrent validity
PIMRA (13)	+ file psychiatric disorder + for schizophrenia Schizophrenia subscale with DSM 0.43 Affective subscale with DSM 0.58	RSMB/PIMRA total scores 0.83 PIMRA/ABC total score 0.73
ABC (9)	-----	+ ABS and presence of behaviour disorder ABC/PIMRA total scores 0.73 ABC/DASH total scores 0.75 ABC/RSMB from 0.16 to 0.67
RSMB (8)	+ any 'psychopathology' on files + psychiatrist diagnosis + behaviour program in place + 'diagnosed' psychopathology	RSMB/PIMRA total scores 0.6 RSMB/ABC total scores 0.5 Low RSMB depression subscales with two measures of depression

DASH (9)	+ Mania subscale with clinician diagnosis
	+ Higher DASH = lower adaptive
	  behaviour
	Mixed results with depression subscale
	  + schizophrenia subscale only with verbal
	  patients
		DASH/ABC total scores 0.75
		CARS/DASH autism subscale 0.69

PAS-ADD Checklist (2)	Identifies 26% no disorder (false positive) Identifies 56% with mild problems Identifies 92% with severe problems PAS-ADD and clinician ratings of severity 0.54 Specificity = 66%, sensitivity = 70%	–
DBC-A (3)	DBC-A with clinicians ratings of severity 0.52 Total score = 4.48, Receiver Operating Characteristics (ROC) 0.77 (specificity = 69%, sensitivity = 79%)	DBC-A/ABC total scores 0.63 DBC-A/PAS-ADD total scores 0.61

on both checklists and some support was evident for the concurrent validity of subscales and persistence across time of personality difficulties.

Concurrent validity of the ABC 'has been determined by moderate relationships in the expected direction with adaptive behaviour, maladaptive scales and direct observations' (Aman, 1991). For example, Sturmey and Ley (1990) demonstrated moderate to strong correlations between total scores and many of the subscales in a small study of the PIMRA and ABC. A study comparing ABC and DASH-II scores conducted by Pacalawskyji *et al.* (1997), found 'a relatively high degree of overall concurrent validity' and many significant subscale correlations between the two scales. This finding raises many interesting points of comparison between these essentially differently derived checklists, and they conclude that 'when used together for clinical purposes [the two scales] should complement each other nicely' (Pacalawskyji *et al.*, 1997). Matson *et al.* (1998) report a significant correlation between DASH-II Autism/PDD subscale scores and the Childhood Autism Rating Scale ($r = 0.69$, $p < 0.0001$) and DSM-IV diagnosis ($r = 0.87$, $p < 0.0001$).

The DBC-A has been used in two studies with the ABC ($n = 77$) and PAS-ADD Checklist ($n = 70$). A moderate positive correlation was found between the DBC-A and ABC ($r = 0.63$, $p < 0.001$) and the PAS-ADD Checklist ($r = 0.61$, $p < 0.01$) (Mohr *et al.*, 2004).

Using checklists and rating scales constructively

When a carer completes a checklist they are providing information that may be a biased or incomplete picture of what may be a complex situation. Some checklist developers recommend completion by two carers separately, and that the results be compared (e.g. Reiss, 1988). Another way to collect information from multiple carers might be to ask them to complete the rating scale as a 'consensus document', after discussion amongst themselves. Sometimes the different information given by different carers is important clinically, and reflects real differences in the way a person behaves in different settings or when cared for by different people. If possible these differences need to be identified and understood (Achenbach *et al.*, 1987).

Carer-completed checklists and rating scales cannot be used to make a diagnosis of a specific psychiatric disorder. Aman (1991) cautioned against this use of rating scales, particularly those with subscales containing items derived from diagnostic criteria. Even when a carer selects a cluster of items that appears to point to a diagnosis such as depression it does not indicate that the person actually has this disorder. The individual may be physically unwell, or have a related disorder, or no disorder at all. At best a checklist result might indicate the need for a clinical assessment and raise the possibility of the presence of a disorder.

A checklist completed at a certain time is a snapshot of the current or recent situation. A person's mental health can change even in the absence of known interventions or changes in circumstance. Therefore repeated use of a checklist might provide a useful method to track change. In addition the suggested rating period of any checklist (such as six months or two weeks) may not give a clear picture of the presentation of a person with ID.

A checklist used to screen for emotional and behavioural disorders should be followed, where indicated, by assessment with a specialist in the area. When used in clinical practice, checklists and rating scales should only form part of a comprehensive assessment of the mental health of a person with an ID, and should never be relied upon solely to provide a diagnosis (Einfeld & Tonge, 2002). A comprehensive mental health assessment of a person with ID should include, wherever possible: an interview of the patient, opportunities to observe the person in a home or work setting, interviews with carers, an appropriate medical review, tests and investigations and the selective use of a range of assessment instruments. This process may take longer to complete than mental health assessments of people without disabilities. (See also Chapter 3 by O'Hara and Chapter 17 by Reese *et al.*)

Conclusion

Clinicians and researchers looking for a checklist or rating scale with sound psychometric properties to assist in the process of assessing psychopathology in adults with ID will find that all of the instruments reviewed here have something to offer. However, they also have practical, psychometric and theoretical limitations. For example, although described as carer-completed checklists, manuals for the PIMRA and DASH-II also suggest that a 'trained' interviewer administer them (Matson, 1988; Matson *et al.*, 1991b). This increases the costs of completion in terms of time and money.

Nevertheless, when used within the context of a comprehensive assessment of mental health, there are a number of distinct advantages derived from using rating scales and checklists for people with ID. In an era of evidence-based practice, assessment and monitoring tools may make a significant contribution to measuring the prevalence of mental health problems and outcomes of psychiatric and behavioural interventions at an individual, local and national level. In turn, this helps to ensure that mental health services accurately reflect the needs of the population, that they conform to national standards and that they provide value for money.

Summary points

- Two types of assessment instruments: those that identify and describe the nature and extent of problem behaviours, and those that investigate aetiology.
- Two approaches to development: 'bottom-up' and 'top-down' methods
- Assessment and monitoring tools may help to increase the validity and reliability of measuring mental health problems in people with ID, although they also have practical, psychometric and theoretical limitations.

- To ensure the comprehensive assessment of mental health, rating scales and checklists need to be used in tandem with interviews with the individual with ID and their carers, observations and appropriate medical reviews, tests and investigations.

REFERENCES

Achenbach, T. M. (1998). Diagnosis, assessment, taxonomy, and case formulations. In *Handbook of child psychopathology*, ed. T. H. Ollendick and M. Hersen. New York, Plenum Press: pp. 63–87.

Achenbach, T. M., Mc Conaughy, S. H., & Howell, C. T. (1987). Child/adolescent behavioural and emotional problems: Implications of cross-informant correlations for situational specificity. *Psychological Bulletin*, **101**, 213–32.

Aman, M. G. (1991). Assessing psychopathology and behaviour problems in persons with mental retardation. Rockville, MD: U.S. Department of Health and Human Services.

Aman, M. G., Burrow, W. H. & Wolford, P. L. (1995). The Aberrant Behavior Checklist – Community: Factor validity and effect of subject variables for adults in group homes. *American Journal on Mental Retardation*, **100**(3), 283–92.

Aman, M. G., Richmond, G., Bell, J. C. & Kissel, R. C. (1987). The Aberrant Behavior Checklist: Factor structure and the effect of subject variables in American and New Zealand facilities. *American Journal of Mental Deficiency*, **91**(6), 570–8.

Aman, M. G. & Singh, N. N. (1985). Psychometric characteristics of the Aberrant Behavior Checklist. *American Journal of Mental Deficiency*, **89**(5): 492–502.

Aman, M. G., Watson, J. E., Singh, N. N., Turbott, S. H. & Wilsher, C. P. (1986). Psychometric and demographic characteristics of the Psychopathology Instrument for Mentally Retarded Adults. *Psychopharmacology Bulletin*, **22**(4), 1072–6.

American Psychiatric Association (1994). *Diagnostic and Statistical Manual of Mental Disorders.* Washington, DC: American Psychiatric Association.

Bamburg, J. W., Cherry, K. E., Matson, J. L. & Penn, D. (2001). Assessment of schizophrenia in persons with severe and profound mental retardation using the Diagnostic Assessment for the Severely Handicapped-II (DASH-II). *Journal of Developmental and Physical Disabilities*, **13**(4), 319–31.

Davidson, M. (1988). Psychometric Characteristics of the Checklist of Emotional Problems with Mentally Retarded Adults (CHEMRA). Unpublished doctoral dissertation, University of Illinois, Chicago.

Deb, S., Matthews, T., Holt, G. & Bouras, N. (2001b). *Practice Guidelines for Assessment and Diagnosis of Mental Health Problems in Adults with Intellectual Disability.* Brighton: Pavilion.

Deb, S., Thomas, M. & Bright, C. (2001a). Mental disorder in adults with intellectual disability. 1: Prevalence of functional psychiatric illness among a community-based population aged between 16 and 64 years. *Journal of Intellectual Disability Research*, **45**, 495–505.

Einfeld, S. L. & Tonge, B. J. (1992). *Manual for the Developmental Behaviour Checklist (DBC)(Primary Carer version)*. Melbourne: School of Psychiatry, University of New South Wales, and Centre for Developmental Psychiatry, Monash University, Clayton, Victoria.

Gustafsson, C. & Sonnander, K. (2002). Psychometric evaluation of a Swedish version of the Reiss Screen for Maladaptive Behavior. *Journal of Intellectual Disability Research*, **46**(3), 218–29.

Havercamp, S. M. & Reiss, S. (1997). The Reiss Screen for Maladaptive Behavior: Confirmatory factor analysis. *Behavior Research and Therapy*, **35**(10), 967–71.

Holland, A. J. & Koot, H. M. (1998). Mental health and intellectual disability: An international perspective. *Journal of Intellectual Disability Research* **42**(6): 505–12.

Linaker, O. M. (1991). DSM-III diagnoses compared with factor structure of the Psychopathology Instrument for Mentally Retarded Adults (PIMRA), in an institutionalized, mostly severely retarded population. *Research in Developmental Disabilities*, **12**, 143–53.

Linaker, O. M. & Helle, J. (1994). Validity of the schizophrenia diagnosis of the Psychopathology Instrument for Mentally Retarded Adults (PIMRA): A comparison of schizophrenic patients with and without mental retardation. *Research in Developmental Disabilities*, **15**(6), 473–86.

Marshburn, E. C. & Aman, M. G. (1992). Factor validity and norms for the Aberrant Behavior Checklist in a community sample of children with mental retardation. *Journal of Autism and Developmental Disorders*, **22**(3), 357–73.

Matson, J. L. (1988). *The PIMRA Manual*. Orland Park, IL: International Diagnostic Systems, Inc.

Matson, J. L., Coe, D. A., Gardner, W. I. & Sovner, R. (1991b). A factor analytic study of the Diagnostic Assessment for the Severely Handicapped Scale. *The Journal of Nervous and Mental Disease*, **179**(9), 553–7.

Matson, J. L., Gardner, W. I., Coe, D. A. & Sovner, R. (1991a). A scale for evaluating emotional disorders in severely and profoundly mentally retarded persons. Development of the Diagnostic Assessment for the Severely Handicapped (DASH) Scale. *British Journal of Psychiatry*, **159**, 404–9.

Matson, J. L., Kazdin, A. E. & Senatore, V. (1984). Psychometric properties of the Psychopathology Instrument for Mentally Retarded Adults. *Applied Research in Mental Retardation*, **5**, 81–9.

Matson, J. L., Kiely, S. L. & Bamburg, J. W. (1997b). The effect of stereotypies on adaptive skills with the DASH-II and Vineland Behavior Scales. *Research in Developmental Disabilities*, **18**(6), 471–6.

Matson, J. L., Rush, K. S., Hamilton, M. *et al.* (1999). Characteristics of depression as assessed by the Diagnostic Assessment for Severely Handicapped-II (DASH-II). *Research in Developmental Disabilities* **20**(4), 305–13.

Matson, J. L. & Smiroldo, B. B. (1997). Validity of the Mania Subscale of the Diagnostic Assessment for the Severely Handicapped-II (DASH-II). *Research in Developmental Disabilities*, **18**(3), 221–5.

Matson, J. L., Smiroldo, B. B., Hamilton, M. & Baglio, C. S. (1997c). Do anxiety disorders exist in persons with severe and profound mental retardation? *Research in Developmental Disabilities*, **18**(1), 39–44.

Matson, J. L., Smiroldo, B. B. & Hastings, T. L. (1998). Validity of the Autism/Pervasive Developmental Disorder Subscale of the Diagnostic Assessment for the Severely Handicapped-II. *Journal of Autism and Developmental Disorders*, **28**(1), 77–81.

McDaniel, W. F., Turner, M. D. & Johns, M. R. (1999). Long-term associations among personality disorder scales of the Reiss Screen for Maladaptive Behaviour and the Psychopathology Inventory for Mentally Retarded Adults. *Developmental Disabilities Bulletin*, **27**(2), 32–41.

Mohr, C., Tonge, B. J. & Einfeld, S. L. (2004). *Manual for the Developmental Behaviour Checklist – Adult Version*. Melbourne: Monash University, Centre for Developmental Psychiatry & Psychology.

Moss, S. (1999). Assessment: conceptual issues. In *Psychiatric and Behavioural Disorders in Mental Retardation*, ed. N. Bouras. Cambridge: Cambridge University Press, pp. 18–37.

Moss, S. C., Patel, P., Goldberg, D., Simpson, N. & Lucchino, R. (1993). Psychiatric morbidity in older people with moderate and severe learning disability. I: Development and reliability of the patient interview (PAS-ADD). *British Journal of Psychiatry*, **163**, 471–80.

Moss, S. C., Prosser, H., Costello, H. *et al.* (1998). Reliability and validity of the PAS-ADD Checklist for detecting psychiatric disorders in adults with intellectual disabilities. *Journal of Intellectual Disability Research*, **42**(2), 173–83.

Newton, J. T. & Sturmey, P. (1988). The Aberrant Behavior Checklist: A British replication and extension of its psychometric properties. *Journal of Mental Deficiency Research*, **32**, 87–92.

Nihira, K., Foster, R., Shellhaas, M. & Leland, J. (1975). *AAMD Adaptive Behavior Scale Manual (Rev.)*. Washington, DC: American Association on Mental Deficiency.

Ono, Y. (1996). Factor validity and reliability for the Aberrant Behavior Checklist-Community in a Japanese population with mental retardation. *Research in Developmental Disabilities*, **17**(4), 303–9.

Pacalawskyji, T. R., Matson, J. L., Bamburg, J. W. & Baglio, C. S. (1997). A comparison of the Diagnostic Assessment for the Severely Handicapped-II (DASH-II) and the Aberrant Behavior Checklist. *Research in Developmental Disabilities*, **18**(4), 289–98.

Reiss, S. (1982). Psychopathology and mental retardation: Survey of a developmental disabilities mental health program. *Mental Retardation* **20**: 128–32.

Reiss, S. (1988). *The Reiss Screen for Maladaptive Behavior Test Manual*. Worthington, OH: IDS Publishing Corporation.

Reiss, S. (1997). Comments on the Reiss Screen for Maladaptive Behavior and its factor structure. *Journal of Intellectual Disability Research*, **41**(4), 346–54.

Rojahn, J. & Helsel, W. J. (1991). The Aberrant Behavior Checklist with children and adolescents with dual diagnosis. *Journal of Autism and Developmental Disorders*, **21**(1), 17–28.

Royal College of Psychiatrists. (2001). *DC-LD. Diagnostic Criteria for Psychiatric Disorders for Use with Adults with Learning Disabilities/Mental Retardation*. Occasional Paper 48. London: Gaskell.

Senatore, V., Matson, J. L. & Kazdin, A. E. (1985). An inventory to assess psychopathology of mentally retarded adults. *American Journal of Psychiatry*, **89**, 459–66.

Simpson, N. (1998). *Prevalence of Psychiatric Disorders in Adults with Learning Disabilities*. Paper presented at the Second International Medical Aspect of Mental Health Meeting, Manchester, England.

Streiner, D. L. and G. R. Norman (1995). *Health Measurement Scales. A Practical Guide to Their Development and Use*. Oxford: Oxford University Press.

Sturmey, P. & Bertman, L. J. (1994). Validity of the Reiss screen for maladaptive behavior. *American Journal on Mental Retardation*, **99**(2), 201–6.

Sturmey, P., Burcham, K. J. & Perkins, T. S. (1995). The Reiss Screen for Maladaptive Behavior: Its reliability and internal consistencies. *Journal of Intellectual Disability Research*, **39**(3), 191–5.

Sturmey, P., Jamieson, J., Burcham, J., Shaw, B. & Bertman, L. (1996). The factor structure of the Reiss Screen for Maladaptive Behavior in institutional and community populations. *Research in Developmental Disabilities*, **17**(4), 285–91.

Sturmey, P. & Ley, T. (1990). The Psychopathology Instrument for Mentally Retarded Adults. *British Journal of Psychiatry*, **156**, 428–30.

Sturmey, P., Newton, J. T., Cowley, A., Bouras, N. & Holt, G. (2005). The PAS-ADD Checklist: An independent replication of its psychometric properties in a community sample. *British Journal of Psychiatry*, **186**, 319–23.

Swiezy, N. B., Matson, J. L., Kirkpatrick-Sanchez, S. & Williams, D. E. (1995). A criterion validity study of the schizophrenia subscale of the Psychopathology Instrument for Mentally Retarded Adults (PIMRA). *Research in Developmental Disabilities*, **16**(1), 75–80.

Taylor, J. L., Hatton, C., Dixon, C. & Douglas, C. (2004). Screening for psychiatric symptoms: PAS-ADD checklist norms for adults with intellectual disabilities. *Journal of Intellectual Disability Research*, **48**, 37–41.

Tonge, B. J., Einfeld, S. L., Krupinski, J. *et al.* (1996). The use of factor analysis for ascertaining patterns of psychopathology in children with intellectual disabilities. *Journal of Intellectual Disability Research*, **40**(3), 198–207.

van Minnen, A., Savelsberg, P. M. & Hoogduin, K. A. L. (1994). A Dutch version of the Psychopathology Inventory for Mentally Retarded Adults (PIMRA). *Research in Developmental Disabilities*, **15**(4), 269–78.

Walsh, K. K. & Shenouda, N. (1999). Correlations among the Reiss screen, the Adaptive Behavior Scale Part II, and the Aberrant Behavior Checklist. *American Journal on Mental Retardation*, **104**(3), 236–48.

Watson, J. E., Aman, M. G. & Singh, N. N. (1988). The Psychopathology Instrument for Mentally Retarded Adults: Psychometric characteristics, factor structure, and relationship to subject characteristics. *Research in Developmental Disabilities*, **9**, 277–90.

World Health Organization (1992). ICD-10 International statistical classification of disease and related health problems (10th edn). Geneva: World Health Organization.

World Health Organization (1994). *Schedules for Clinical Assessment in Neuropsychiatry Version 2*. Geneva: World Health Organization.

Zung, W. K. (1971). A rating instrument for anxiety disorders. *Psychosomatics*, **12**, 371–9.

3

Inter-disciplinary multi-modal assessment for mental health problems in people with intellectual disabilities

Jean O'Hara

Introduction

The advantages of a co-ordinated, inter-disciplinary approach to the assessment, diagnosis, treatment and management of mental health problems in individuals with intellectual disabilities (ID) are generally accepted. However, the degree of co-ordination, and the timeliness of assessments and interventions can make it difficult to pull the various strands of information together. Without this co-ordination and overview, the histories of individuals with ID tend to remain fragmented, lost and forgotten. This may then be perpetuated by poorly documented clinical notes, incomplete personal, social and treatment histories, inadequate mental state and physical state examinations or investigations, and minimal attempts to document an understanding of why a person is presenting with a particular set of problems or needs, at a particular time in their lives.

The theory and research evidence behind assessment of mental health, self-injurious behaviours, challenging needs and the importance of excluding underlying physical health problems are covered elsewhere in this volume (see Chapters 5 by Lennox, 7 by Stavrakaki and Lunsky, 8 by Clarke, 9 by Lindsay, 13 by Saulnier and Volkmar, 14 by Hillery and Dodd, 10 by Cooper and Holland and 11 by Murphy and Mason). Diagnostic criteria, rating scales and interview schedules are also covered elsewhere (see Chapter 2 by Mohr and Costello). A comprehensive review of rating instruments can also be found in Lecavalier & Aman (2005). This chapter focuses on the practical approach to inter-disciplinary, multi-modal mental health assessments of individuals with ID.

The referral

It is important to clarify the reason for the referral if the information is not obvious. This is helpful for two reasons:

Psychiatric and Behavioural Disorders in Intellectual and Developmental Disabilities, ed. Nick Bouras and Geraldine Holt. Published by Cambridge University Press. © Cambridge University Press 2007.

(a) Unlike the general population, individuals with ID tend to access health services, and particularly mental health services, because someone else thinks it is appropriate for them to do so. The judgment about whether someone with a particular set of symptoms or behaviours becomes a 'case for referral' may be socially defined and influenced by interpersonal factors as well as the social environment (Goldberg & Huxley, 1980). The referral then may not be for the individual identified, but for the system around the individual, e.g. the community home, day centre, carers.

(b) Resources for specialist mental health assessments are often limited, and need to be targeted for those most in need. Referrers may need support to negotiate the variety of health and social services available for individuals with ID, and clarification of the referral question might help in facilitating access to a more appropriate service.

Screening phase

The screening phase allows questions to be asked, and information to be gathered, about risk and eligibility. Agreed eligibility criteria and priorities, based on level of risk identified at the time of referral, will help teams establish consistency and levels of response. Table 3.1 is an example of priority levels agreed by an inter-disciplinary health team for adults with ID, developed by the author. The prioritization criteria have been in use for the past six years, and are consistently applied, whether the referral is for mental health or physical health need. (The service was not designed to provide for emergencies, and any such referrals were signposted to the most appropriate service.)

The assessment process

Venue

Consideration needs to be given to the most appropriate setting in which to see the individual referred. Clearly, if the person is housebound, or has significant transport difficulties, it would be important to arrange a visit to the home. If the referral information suggests that particular behaviours are more likely to occur in a given setting, then it would be important to assess those behaviours in that setting as well as elsewhere. If the individual is coming to you, should it be in a clinic environment, at a familiar community base perhaps, or at school, college or day centre? Finding a suitably accessible venue that is both safe and containing is an important initial step.

Table 3.1 Prioritization criteria agreed by an inter-disciplinary health team in East London.

Priority level	Need identified at referral	Response time
Level one	• Unassessed risk suggesting serious or potentially serious risk of harm to self or others, and no other service is able to respond. • Unassessed risk suggesting serious or potentially serious deterioration in complex health need and no other service is able to respond. • Relapse or deterioration in health owing to immediate or unplanned change in health or social care arrangements in the community. • Immediate issues relating to planned admissions and discharges from acute hospitals and mental health wards.	Within ten working days (often the service responded within 48 hours).
Level two	• Assessed/known risk of harm to self or others where other services are responding. • Deterioration or noticeable change in complex health needs but no immediate risk • Deterioration or noticeable change owing to planned change in social or health care arrangements in the community. • Issues relating to planned admissions and access to health services.	Within six weeks.
Level three	• Health promotion and prevention to maintain health and to minimize risk to self or others. • Skill maintenance and development of new skills to enhance quality of life. • Issues relating to clients placed out of area who are no longer the responsibility of this health team.	Within 3 months.
	• No referred health needs but reason to establish whether a person has ID. • No referred health need but reason to establish presence of a syndrome or disorder relating to intellectual disability.	Within 3 months.

Other factors taken into consideration may include: presence/extent/robustness of support networks; number of dependants/caring responsibilities.

Who should be there?

The presence of a trusted carer, advocate or friend can often facilitate not only attendance, but also the interview process itself and the care plan that follows. There may be a need for a person fluent in sign language, or for an interpreter to be present, as well as family members and other care staff. In many services, good clinical practice dictates that two clinicians from different disciplines are involved in the initial assessment stage. This might include the referrer, when appropriate, particularly if they are members of another health or mental health care team. It is important, however, to keep numbers to a minimum, and to assign a lead assessor who ensures that key issues are covered, especially if the assessment is curtailed for any reason.

The first contact

It may be that the individual with ID is not even aware that a referral has been made. Receiving a letter to come for an assessment with strangers is hardly going to facilitate engagement with the process. Likewise, paid carers or family members may bring an individual for an appointment without knowing what it is all about, or having the background information. Expectations may differ between the individual with ID, the person accompanying them, those performing the assessment, and the interpreter or signer, as well as the referrer! An introductory phone call to the home, an explanatory sentence in the appointment letter or an accessible version of the appointment letter, may all help to facilitate this process.

It goes without saying that issues about confidentiality need to be borne in mind (e.g. the individual may not wish a carer or family member to be present at the interview), and that information should be shared on a strictly need-to-know basis, particularly if the individual lacks capacity to consent to information being shared with others.

Brief assessment screen

This may involve direct or indirect contact with the referrer and/or the individual referred. The aim is to form an initial impression of the risks involved in a given situation, and which services would be most appropriate to respond to the needs identified (Figure 3.1). It might be obvious that the individual is confused and irritable because of a physical disorder; it might be the case that the person's placement in the community is breaking down because of their carer's poor health or it might be the case that someone is actively suicidal or responding to command hallucinations and requires psychiatric inpatient admission.

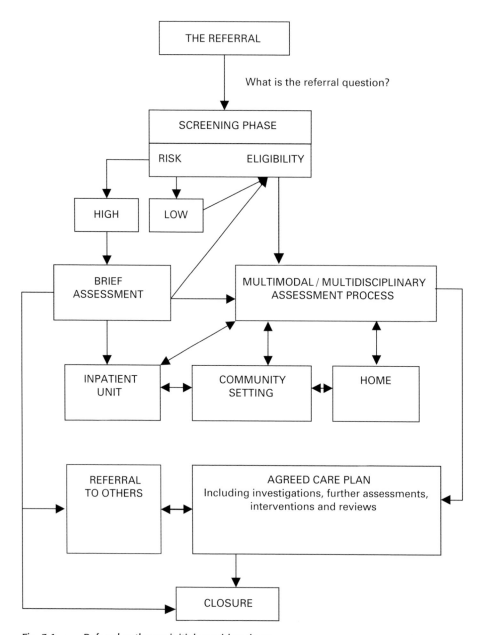

Fig. 3.1   Referral pathway: initial considerations.

Inter-disciplinary assessment

Inter-disciplinary assessments have traditionally been the bread and butter of community ID teams in the United Kingdom, but it often involved multiple individual consultations or simultaneous assessments that rarely linked with one another. This resulted not only in the individual with ID and his or her family

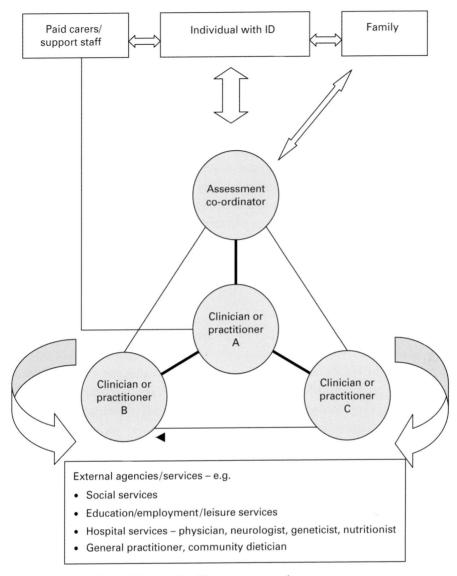

Fig. 3.2   A multi-modal mental health assessment pathway.

often being asked the same questions time and again, but also a feeling of being overwhelmed and confused with assessments. The purpose of team working is to enrich the overall understanding of the person's situation. The process needs to be co-ordinated in such a way that it continues to engage the individual and the network of support surrounding them. (An example of this is provided in Figure 3.2.)

For example, if we are considering the possibility of a drug-induced psychosis, it would be important not only to have a psychiatric assessment, but also a physical assessment and a urine screen for illicit drugs. These three components need to occur concurrently. It would be pointless from a diagnostic perspective to have the urine drug screen request sitting on a waiting list for a year.

One way of co-ordinating inter-disciplinary assessments is through local agreements for clinical pathways. Originally developed as a structured inter-disciplinary plan for the care of patients with a specific clinical problem such as cancer, it describes a time line, categories of care or intervention, outcome criteria and a record of variance to allow deviations to be documented and analysed (Campbell *et al.*, 1998). Central to clinical pathways is a named practitioner who is assigned to co-ordinate the assessment process and to help the individual referred understand where they are along the assessment route, and what to expect next. Care pathways in the assessment of dementia and in the assessment of epilepsy are recent developments within the field of ID.

The clinical interview

History taking: the narrative

There are various psychiatric assessments available (e.g. Rush & Frances, 2000; Deb *et al.*, 2001). They are all similar in their guidance, outlining useful areas to focus on in the history taking, and the need for an inter-disciplinary, multi-modal assessment process in order to explain the possible inter-relationship between biological, psychological, social and environmental factors (Gardner & Sovner, 1994). All stress the importance of a reliable, longitudinal history including the use of previous records and interviews with family members and carers. However, all too often in clinical practice, the individual's life history that may be accessible is patchy and incomplete.

A good psychiatric history should include:

- **Family history**: of ID, psychiatric illness, epilepsy, physical illnesses, as well as the quality of relationships between family members.
- **Personal and developmental history**: obstetric and birth/perinatal history, developmental history and milestones, aetiology of ID (if known) and how this news was shared with the family; how the family managed a child with ID, education and employment history, friendships, psychosexual development.
- **Communication**: preferred communication style, use of objects of reference, signs or symbols-based systems, facilitated communication.
- **Medical history**: past and present, recurrent problems, sensory impairments, epilepsy. It has been well documented that there is a disparity in health care for individuals with ID and that many medical problems are under-diagnosed (U.S. Public Health Services, 2001; NHS Scotland, 2004; Ouellette-Kuntz *et al.*, 2004). (Please also refer to Chapters 5 and 15.)

- **Psychiatric history**: previous contact with mental health services, diagnoses, inpatient admissions, treatments and interventions used and their outcome, assessments of risks to self, others and the environment and any forensic issues/problems.
- **Treatment history**: it is well recognized that individuals with ID may have unexpected reactions, side effects, or interaction effects to psychotropic medications (Reiss & Aman, 1998), and that many medications can impair cognitive functioning, lower seizure threshold or cause psychiatric symptoms such as depressed mood, agitation and hallucinations. It is also important to establish who reviews the prescription, who administers medication, and what usually happens if a dose is missed. Recent changes in medication and known allergies should also be sought.
- **Social history**: current and previous social circumstances, living circumstances, social supports, leisure and vocational opportunities, benefits and who helps to manage finances if appropriate.
- **Drug and alcohol history**: use of tobacco, alcohol and illicit drugs, and whether there are issues of exploitation, vulnerability and substance misuse or excessive caffeine intake, in the form of coffee and tea or carbonated drinks.
- **Premorbid personality**: include previous level of functioning in different areas of adaptive behaviours. It is important to remember that when the individual presents to you they may not be at their usual level of functioning.
- **Life events**: the impact of stressors and negative life events have been significantly correlated with increased aggression, destructive behaviours, affective and neurotic disorders. Psychosocial stressors identified include transitions and major life changes, interpersonal loss or rejection, illness or disability, social strain, lack of support, victimization and frustration as well as exploitation and abuse (Rush & Frances, 2000; Hastings *et al.*, 2004; Hollins & Esterhuyzen, 1997; Sequeira & Hollins, 2003).
- **History of the presenting symptom or behaviour**: including a description of the symptom in the person's own words if possible, or the behaviour as witnessed by others; any change in behaviours, when and where they occur; any aspects that might result in improvement or worsening; how long it has been going on for; what strategies have been used to help and their effectiveness, level of distress or risk involved; the individual's and his/her carers' understanding of the problems and expectations from the assessment.

The outline above suggests key components to be covered within an initial interdisciplinary assessment. It may be that eliciting such information requires a number of visits, or involvement from other team members for a more detailed assessment. For example, there may be a need for a fuller understanding of the person's social situation and support network or his/her communicative abilities, or investigation into aspects of the environment and how the individual with ID might anticipate changes in the daily routine. There might be a need to have a better idea of how the person manages everyday life, or how a particular behaviour might be used to communicate distress, or the significance of a sensory impairment. Clinicians with skills in such assessments need to be involved in a planned way, to add to the assessment and understanding of the individual's presentation.

Asking about symptoms

Presenting symptoms are the cardinal features of diagnostic classifications used in mental health (see Chapter 1 by Sturmey). How these symptoms are elicited from an individual with ID may present considerable difficulties because of the person's cognitive and linguistic abilities. It is well recognized that individuals with ID form a very heterogeneous population. Some will have verbal and language skills which lend themselves to the standard clinical interview situation, albeit with some minor adaptation. Others may find abstract concepts difficult, or be unable to label an emotion or feeling, while some may not be able to understand the questions asked, or be non-verbal or preverbal. Some individuals may be unable to identify that something is wrong, e.g. that it is not the usual state for someone to have dysuria, epileptic auras or command hallucinations. Until they are aware of this, they are unlikely to try to communicate their symptoms to others.

In clinical psychiatric practice, much of the diagnostic process depends on the interaction of factors, such as:

- What people say they are experiencing.
- What others say about them.
- How they are seen to behave.
- The history of their complaint or symptoms.

Kendell (1973) has shown that traditionally psychiatrists rely mostly on what the patient says, and not on observational skills. The actual words that the patient has chosen to use in response to a question may have considerable significance or importance in the answer (Moss, 1999). If one does not have the vocabulary or language necessary to express them, this level of complexity in human interaction is not available to aid the diagnostic process.

Interviewing an individual with ID is not fundamentally different from interviewing anyone else. However, interviews are different from everyday conversation, and as such there is a risk that the clinician dominates the interaction, and the individual with ID withdraws (Ambalu, 1997). This may be further exacerbated by previous experiences of intrusive questioning, the perceived power imbalance between the interviewer and interviewee, not understanding the questions asked, not feeling heard or understood or just wanting the interaction to end.

Effective interviewing of the person with an ID necessitates several considerations (Hurley *et al.*, in press; Perry, 2004; Tassé *et al.*, 2005, Bradley & Lofchy, 2005). These include:

- Try to involve the individual as much as possible or appropriate – talking to him or her directly rather than to care providers.
- Introduce yourself. Explain the process and what is going to happen.
- Try to establish a positive relationship – be sensitive to and encourage the use of 'comforters' such as a preference to stand instead of sit; respect avoidance of eye contact; show warmth and positive regard; ask permission before intruding into someone's personal space; provide reassurance during the process.
- Find ways of communicating effectively – through words, pictures, signs, symbols or other media. Consider the words used. Questions should be short, simple, unambiguous phrases. When talking about time events, locate these within the person's experience. Abstract concepts should be avoided. The development of the PAS-ADD (Moss *et al.*, 1993) has shown that individuals with ID can tackle quite complex propositions, provided the questions are appropriately structured. Sometimes questions are used to re-establish rapport rather than for information gathering.
- Acquiescence and suggestibility – both are more commonly found in individuals with ID. Each may be influenced by the attitude of the person being interviewed and his/her own expectations. Many individuals with ID have negative expectations of clinical interviews, so try to maximize their confidence and sense of security (Moss, 1999).
- Validity of responses – should be evaluated within the context of potential response biases such as responsiveness, acquiescence, and consistency.
- Recall and detail – even the more linguistically able person, who coped well with simple short questions, might experience difficulty in connecting sentences into a longer narrative. There may be omissions, inappropriate segments joined together and difficulty narrating events in their correct temporal sequence. This may be heightened when discussing uncomfortable or threatening topics.
- Attention and concentration – poor attention and concentration spans, hyperactivity, ritualistic behaviours, distractibility, anxiety, cognitive impairments may all influence how long the individual is able to engage with the assessment process. It may be necessary to plan for a series of short interviews over a period of time as well as prepare for such eventualities.
- Linguistic and phonological problems – individuals with ID may have sufficient verbal skills, but the way they respond might limit their accuracy owing to poor grammar, pronoun reversal or abnormal intonations which can lead to misunderstanding. They may have articulation or pronunciation problems, e.g. because of

malformation of the oral cavity, cerebral palsy or hearing loss. Some individuals may have little or no expressive language.

- Check comprehension – it is important to recap frequently. This allows re-engagement with the assessment process and focuses attention back to the interview. It also provides an opportunity for checking and understanding, and for adding detail.
- Understandably, many individuals with ID may attempt to hide or minimize their disability, negotiating the world wearing a *cloak of competence* (Edgerton, 1967) which may not be obvious.
- Sensory impairments – may not be obvious either. Their presence may not only affect the assessment process and the clinical discourse, but symptoms and behaviours may be as a direct result of these impairments.

Sovner (1986) used the terms *baseline exaggeration, intellectual distortion, psychosocial masking* and *cognitive disintegration* to describe the main difficulties in interpreting symptoms during the mental health interview. Another challenge is the tendency of clinicians to interpret signs of co-existing psychiatric problems as an inherent feature of the ID, otherwise known as *diagnostic overshadowing* (Reiss *et al.*, 1982). (See also Chapter 1 by Sturmey.) It is crucial that symptoms be interpreted within the context of the developmental delay and the individual's life experiences. Grandiose ideas are more likely to be attempts to compensate for poor self-esteem, and being seen to talk to oneself may be caused by the person remembering or fantasizing about a conversation rather than being manifestations of an underlying psychiatric disorder (Einfeld, 2001).

The adaptations to the standard clinical interview outlined will necessitate extra time, not only for the interview itself but for the preparation and thought that needs to go into making this a worthwhile experience for both parties concerned. Flexibility in the process is the key.

Aspects of a multi-modal mental health assessment

Clinicians within teams have individual strengths and clinical skills, some of which are specific, and some of which overlap with clinicians from other disciplines. The role of the assessment co-ordinator is to prioritize and co-ordinate such involvement and to ensure that they all come together to provide a holistic understanding of why the individual is presenting with a particular set of problems at this particular time (Figure 3.2). It is beyond the scope of this chapter to look at all the different functions of team members, or the various models of team working. Instead, we will address key components of a mental health assessment, and omit assessments of ID and functioning. (See also Chapter 2 by Mohr and Costello.)

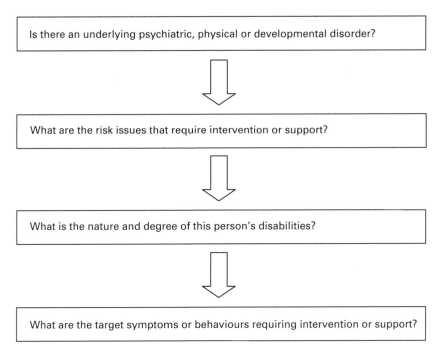

Fig. 3.3   Key assessment questions.

The mental state examination

Let us address the first key assessment question suggested in Figure 3.3. In Chapter 1 by Sturmey we are reminded that a mental disorder is a clinically significant condition characterized by:

- Alteration in thinking
- Alteration in mood (emotion)
- Alteration in behaviour
- And that these alterations are associated with personal distress and/or impairment of usual functioning. Symptoms are not just a variation within a normal range, but clearly abnormal or pathological.

Implicit in this is the need to establish *changes in premorbid functioning, personal distress, and a pattern of symptoms that is outside the cultural norm for a particular community.* A psychiatric diagnosis may therefore be susceptible to social trends (e.g. the definition of ID, attention deficit hyperactivity disorder, autism). The reader is also reminded that just because one may not be able to diagnose a psychiatric disorder (because symptoms elicited do not reach diagnostic standards as defined by operational criteria) it may not follow that the disorder does not exist. This issue is particularly important when agreeing a clinical management plan.

Alterations in thinking

Impaired cognitive and linguistic skills may present major obstacles in trying to elicit alterations in thinking through a standard mental state examination. Trying to elicit passivity phenomenon for example, by asking if someone else makes them do things is often met with a positive response, as individuals with ID have little autonomy in their daily lives and experience minimal choice.

Scenario:

A young man with mild ID, absence seizures and a history of poor trusting relationships becomes paranoid as he believes someone has come into his flat and tampered with his milk. It happens whilst he is at home, with doors and windows locked. There is no sign of a forced entry and nothing is missing. It took a while for his psychiatric team to establish that this was because of absence seizures. It had started when the patient was about to make himself a cup of tea. He had an absence seizure, and had forgotten that he had already taken the top off the milk bottle. His concrete thinking made it difficult for him to understand and accept what had happened.

Scenario:

A man of Black African origin presents with mild ID and a poorly documented history of psychotic illness (characterized by auditory hallucinations, religious beliefs and fears about being dirty and doing things 'the right way'). He was on psychotropic medication. Re-assessment of his history and mental state, interviews with family members and carers, confirmed that his beliefs were in keeping with those of his family and his community, and that his auditory hallucinations were in fact his way of reminding himself what staff had told him to do about his personal hygiene care. His medication was gradually withdrawn.

Scenario:

A woman with mild ID presents with increasing irritability and threatens to phone her solicitor if anyone tries to intervene. She lives in a highly supported community placement, and is unable to recognize numbers or use the telephone independently. Her threats are grandiose and out of keeping with her life experience. She presented with a hypomanic disorder which was missed by generic mental health services.

An inability to describe emotions in words (alexithymia) and concrete thinking may give rise to experiences being described in unusual ways and this can be mistaken for psychotic disorders. This is particularly important as co-morbid autism contributes to even more atypical presentations than ID alone (Bradley & Lofchy, 2005). Obsessional thoughts are hard for individuals with ID to describe, and although compulsions are more readily observed, it can be difficult to distinguish them from stereotypies, tics and autism (Smiley, 2005). Despite these diagnostic problems, Cooper (1997) found a prevalence rate of 2.5% for obsessive-compulsive disorder in ID, with ordering being the most common feature. We are also reminded that hallucinations are not always indicative of psychiatric disorder (Ohayon, 2000). For individuals with ID there may be an additional organic component. Distinguishing such phenomenology from pseudo-hallucinations may present even more challenges than in the general population.

Alterations in mood

Alterations in mood are more observable. However, inability to sustain eye contact or limited facial expression may be owing to an underlying cerebral palsy rather than an abnormality of mood. It is always important to ask the individual with ID how they are feeling in themselves, and to use the words they have chosen when checking back with them that you have understood what has been conveyed. Idiosyncratic use of language and gestures, difficulties distinguishing more complex emotional concepts such as irritability and anxiety, may result in false assumptions and misunderstanding. Recognizing a persistent change in mood requires information about the individual's 'usual self'. Biological symptoms, such as sleep disturbance, or changes in appetite, which often accompany affective disorders, will also need to be considered, as will increases in maladaptive or self-injurious behaviours.

Scenario:
A 40-year-old woman with severe ID and a history of depressive disorder was referred by her GP because there were concerns about her physical and mental health. She was reported to be low in mood, with periods of tearfulness and distress. She had recently withdrawn from her usual social activities, started picking at her skin and needed a great deal of encouragement to eat at mealtimes, having lost her ability to use a knife and fork. There was also a history of recurrent urinary tract infections and unwitnessed falls. Extended inter-disciplinary assessment by clinicians, who had known her in the past, revealed that this was not a relapse into a depressive illness, but rather the result of neglect and sexually abusive experiences within the care home.

Alterations in behaviour

The above scenarios also involved alterations in behaviour, and this of course is one feature that can be recorded. A comment on behaviour in standard mental state examinations is usually not sufficient, and it is here that mental health assessment in individuals with ID departs from standard psychiatric practice. Observational skills are paramount, not just in terms of recording unusual or abnormal behaviours, but also in terms of noting dynamics between individuals, conflicts and tensions, attitudes to disability, the language used, expressed emotions, and the transference and counter-transference issues which may be present. Note too, behaviours which might be concordant with the individual's developmental disability; behaviours such as echolalia (a normal stage in language development), lack of eye contact (in autism); self-stimulatory behaviours, particularly in those individuals with additional sensory impairments.

Scenario:

A young woman with mild ID and language delay has been receiving therapy for some time to increase her self-esteem and communication skills. Her support staff were delighted when she went on her first group holiday with her day centre. She became more extrovert, joining in with activities and talking in an animated way. This improvement lasted a few weeks until she became overactive, over talkative and disinhibited. She eventually required psychiatric admission for a severe manic episode.

Scenario:

A young woman with profound ID was living in a traditional long-stay hospital. She was non-verbal, doubly incontinent and suffered with epilepsy. She relied on familiar members of staff and visiting family to care for all her needs. A psychiatrist was called because she had been pulling out clumps of hair from her head. Staff were unable to identify any obvious precipitants or pattern to this behaviour, and her physical health was reported to be good. Physical examination however, revealed she was five months pregnant, and her behaviours occurred in response to the fetus kicking (O'Hara, 1989).

The role of observation

Behaviour problems are often the reason for referrals for mental health assessments. Posture, movement, gesture, facial expression, eye contact, touch and personal space are all important non-verbal communicators, affected not only by cultural and ethnic considerations, but by underlying disabilities and mental disorders. The relationship between behaviour and mental health problems is a complex one (see Chapters 4 by Hemmings, 14 by Hillery & Dodd and 19 by King).

Observation is not only about accurate noticing, watching and noting. From a psychodynamic perspective it is also about being aware of unconscious processes which can be brought to the clinical intercourse by the individual with ID, their carers and the clinician. Although beyond the scope of this chapter, it is mentioned to remind the reader that this approach may provide another mode of understanding and assessing the individual's situation. (See also Chapter 21 by Parkes and Hollins.)

A behavioural approach is concerned with identifying current internal and external conditions that influence the occurrence and persistence of problem behaviours (Gardner *et al.*, 2001). A functional assessment (FA) is the process by which variables that impact on the occurrence of behaviours are identified. It uses direct observation through the antecedent-behaviour-consequence technique, assessments of data obtained by third-party reports, and analogue assessments where contingencies are identified through direct environmental manipulation. In individuals with severe and profound ID, it has been suggested that behaviours such as aggression, self-injury and disruptive episodes, may serve the same functions as socially acceptable forms of verbal and non-verbal communication. Other psychological approaches are discussed elsewhere and include positive behaviour supports (see Chapter 18 by Benson and Havercamp) and psychosocial interventions (see also Chapter 20 by Dagnan).

It would be important to share behavioural hypotheses with other members of the team, so that, for example, the impact of pharmacological therapy or the introduction of a facilitated communication strategy can also be taken into account. Unrecognized physical health morbidity (see Chapter 5 by Lennox) or the treatment of an underlying medical condition may also have considerable impact on the person's presentation (Charlot & Silka, 2001). Such an integrative multi-modal approach allows the formulation of a bio-psycho-social view of human behaviour and mental health.

Conclusion

There are significant barriers to appropriate and effective mental health evaluations for individuals with ID. A mental health assessment is not the domain of one discipline alone. Providing professionals with specific specialized training increases the likelihood that they will make a more accurate diagnosis (Day, 1992; King et al., 1995).

Individuals with ID present with complex symptoms, behaviours and needs that are often difficult to elicit and understand. Diagnostic reliability of psychiatric disorders reduces with increased levels of cognitive and language impairment (Moss et al., 2000). Maintaining an open and sceptical attitude with constant re-evaluation of the working diagnosis is a must (Ruedrich & Hurley, 2001). However, whether or not symptoms and behaviours reach diagnostic significance does not detract from the fact that intervention may be required. Understanding how the presentation might be a synthesis of vulnerability factors (biological, psychological, social and environmental), precipitating factors (again biological, psychological, social and environmental), and maintaining factors, is a complex task and requires a co-ordinated multi-modal and inter-disciplinary approach to assessment (Figure 3.4). This can then be developed into an inter-disciplinary diagnostic formulation and a co-ordinated multi-modal care plan, which allows for review of efficacy and effectiveness of treatment and risk management.

Summary points

- The assessment of mental health problems in individuals with ID necessitates a co-ordinated multi-modal and inter-disciplinary approach.

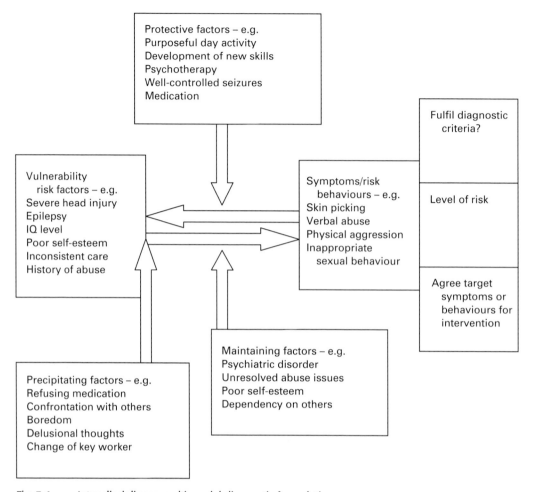

Fig. 3.4   Inter-disciplinary, multi-modal diagnostic formulation.

- Individuals with more severe cognitive and language limitations often cannot self-report the presence of symptoms. Without this self-reporting, it becomes more difficult to reliably diagnose many mental health problems.
- Behavioural symptoms associated with mental health problems may be observed – such as motor agitation, sleeplessness, irritability. However, research is needed to establish the relationship between specific signs, symptoms and behaviours with the presence of physical or mental health problems across the intellectual spectrum.
- Biological, psychological and psychosocial factors may mimic or cause mental health problems and these factors need to be addressed as part of an effective assessment and intervention programme.

REFERENCES

Ambalu, S. (1997). Communication. In *Adults with Learning Disabilities: A Practical Approach for Health Professionals*, ed. J. O'Hara & A. Sperlinger, Chapter 4, pp. 45–60. Chichester: John Wiley & Sons.

Bradley, E. & Lofchy, J. (2005). Learning disability in the accident and emergency department. *Advances in Psychiatric Treatment*, **11**, 45–57.

Campbell, H., Hotchkiss, R., Bradshaw, N. & Porteus, M. (1998). Integrated Care Pathways. *British Medical Journal*, **316** (7125), 133–7.

Charlot, L. and Silka, V. R. (2001). Creating a continuum of intensive psychiatric services for individuals with dual diagnosis: a perspective on the Massachusetts Experience. III. Inpatient psychiatric care. *The National Association for the Dually Diagnosed Bulletin*, Jan/Feb Vol. 4 No. 1, 7–9.

Cooper, S. A. (1997). Epidemiology of psychiatric disorders in elderly compared to younger adults with learning disabilities. *British Journal of Psychiatry*, **170**, 375–80.

Day, K. (1992). Mental health care for the mentally handicapped in four European countries: The argument for specialized services. *Italian Journal of Intellectual Impairment*, **5**, 3–11.

Deb, S., Matthews, T., Holt, G. & Bouras, N. (2001). Practice Guidelines for the Assessment and Diagnosis of Mental Health Problems in Adults with Intellectual Disability. Brighton: Pavilion.

Edgerton, R. B. (1967). Cloak of competence: stigma in the lives of the mentally retarded. Berkeley, CA: University of California.

Einfeld, S. L. (2001). Systematic management approach to pharmacotherapy for people with learning disabilities. *Advances in Psychiatric Treatment*, **7**, 43–9.

Gardner, W. I., Graeber-Whalen, J. L. & Ford, D. R. (2001). Behavioral therapies: individualizing interventions through treatment formulations. In *Treating Mental Illness and Behavior Disorders in Children and Adults with Mental Retardation*, ed. A. Dosen and K. Day. Washington, DC: American Psychiatric Press Inc.

Gardner, W. I. & Sovner, R. (1994). Self-injurious behaviours, diagnosis, and treatment: a multimodal approach. Willow Street, PA: VIDA Publishing.

Goldberg, D. & Huxley, P. (1980). *Mental Illness in the Community*. London: Tavistock Publications.

Hastings, R. P., Hatton, C., Taylor, J. L. *et al.* (2004). Life events and psychiatric symptoms in adults with ID. *Journal of Intellectual Disability Research*, **48**, 42–6.

Hollins, S. & Esterhuyzen, A. (1997). Bereavement and grief in adults with learning disabilities. *British Journal of Psychiatry*, **170**, 497–501.

Hurley, A. D., Levitas, A., Lecavalier, L., Pary, R. J. & King, B. H. (in press). Assessment and diagnostic procedures. In R. J. Fletcher, E. Loschen & P. Sturmey (eds.), *Diagnostic Manual for the Dually Diagnosed*. Kingston, NY: National Association for the Dually Diagnosed Press.

Kendell, R. E. (1973). Psychiatric diagnoses: a study of how they are made. *British Journal of Psychiatry*, **122**, 437–45.

King, B. H., Szymanski, L. S. & Weisblatt, S. (1995). *Psychiatry and Mental Retardation: A Curriculum.* Washington, DC: American Psychiatric Association.

Lecavalier, L. & Aman, M. G. (2005). Rating instruments. In J. L. Matson R. B. Laud & M. L. Matson (eds.), *Behaviour Modification for Persons with Developmental Disabilities: Empirically Supported Treatments.* Vol. 1, pp. 160–89. Kingston, NH: National Association for the Dually Diagnosed Press.

Moss, S. (1999). Assessment: conceptual issues. In *Psychiatric and Behavioural Disorders in Developmental Disabilities and Mental Retardation*, ed. N. Bouras. Chapter 2, pp. 18–37. Cambridge: Cambridge University Press.

Moss, S., Bouras, N. & Holt, G. (2000). Mental health services for people with intellectual disability: a conceptual framework. *Journal of Intellectual Disability Research*, **44**, 97–107.

Moss, S. C., Patel, P. & Prosser, H. *et al.* (1993). Psychiatric morbidity in older people with moderate and severe learning disability (mental retardation). Part I: Development and reliability of the patient interview (the PAS-ADD). *British Journal of Psychiatry*, **163**, 471–80.

NHS Scotland (2004). *People with Learning Disabilities in Scotland: Health Needs Assessment Report.* Glasgow: NHS Health Scotland.

O'Hara, J. (1989). Pregnancy in a severely mentally handicapped adult. *Journal of Medical Ethics*, **15**, 197–99.

Ohayon, M. M. (2000). Prevalence of hallucinations and their pathological associations in the general population. *Psychiatry Research*, **97** (2–3), 153–64.

Ouellette-Kuntz, H., Garcia, N., Lewis, S. *et al.* (2004). *Addressing health disparities through promoting equity for individuals with intellectual disability.* Canadian Institute of Health Research. Kingston, Canada: Queen's University.

Perry, J. (2004). Interviewing people with intellectual disabilities. In E. Emerson, C. Hatton, T. Thompson and T. R. Parmenter (eds.), *The International Handbook of Applied Research in Intellectual Disabilities*, pp. 116–31. New York, NY: John Wiley & Sons Inc.

Reiss, S. & Aman, M. G. (1998). *Psychotropic Medication and Developmental Disabilities: The International Consensus Handbook.* Worthington, OH: IDS Publishing.

Reiss, S., Levitan, G. W. & Szysko, J. (1982) Emotional disturbance and mental retardation: Diagnostic overshadowing. *American Journal of Mental Deficiency*, **86**, 567–74.

Ruedrich, R. L. & Hurley, A. D. (2001), Expert consensus guideline series: Treatment of psychiatric and behavioural problems in mental retardation. *American Journal of Mental Retardation*, **105**, 159–228.

Rush, A. J. & Frances, A. (eds.) (2000). Editors: Expert consensus guideline series: treatment of psychiatric and behavioural problems in mental retardation. *American Journal of Mental Retardation (special issue)*, **105**, 159–228.

Sequeira, H. & Hollins, S. (2003). Clinical effects of sexual abuse on people with learning disability: critical literature review. *British Journal of Psychiatry*, **183**, 13–19.

Smiley, E. (2005). Epidemiology of mental health problems in adults with learning disability: an update. *Advances in Psychiatric Treatment*, **11**, 214–222.

Sovner, R. (1986). Limiting factors in the use of DSM-III criteria with mentally ill/mentally retarded persons. *Psychopharmacology Bulletin*, **22**, 1055–9.

Tassé, M. J., Schalock, R., Thompson, J. R. & Wehmeyer, M. (2005). Guidelines for interviewing people with disabilities: Supports Intensity Scale. Washington, DC: American Association on Mental Retardation.

U.S. Public Health Service (2001). Closing the Gap: A National Blueprint for Improving the Health of Individual with Mental Retardation. Report of the Surgeon General's Conference on Health Disparities and Mental Retardation. Washington, DC.

4

The relationships between challenging behaviours and psychiatric disorders in people with severe intellectual disabilities

Colin Hemmings

Introduction

Knowledge continues to increase about psychiatric disorders in people with intellectual disabilities (ID). The overwhelming bulk of the research activity has concentrated on those individuals with mild ID. Yet even though people with severe (and profound) ID make up less than 10% of the total ID population (Fryers and Russell, 2004), they provide a disproportionate amount of referrals to specialist ID services (Day, 1985). The major reason for referral of those with more severe ID is for problem (or 'challenging') behaviours, such as aggressive, self-injurious and destructive behaviours. They tend to have more frequent and more severe challenging behaviours compared with those with milder ID (Emerson and Bromley, 1995; Jacobsen, 1982). It has long been established that there are multiple factors associated with these behaviours (McClintock *et al.*, 2003). These include physical health problems, epilepsy, behavioural phenotypes, and communication and sensory difficulties. Some challenging behaviours may also be developmentally appropriate behaviours in a person with more severe ID.

In some people with more severe ID, challenging behaviours can be associated with psychiatric symptoms and disorders. Many clinicians have suggested that some of these behaviours may be either caused or exacerbated by the coexisting psychiatric disorders. If this hypothesis is supported then improved detection (and treatment) of the associated psychiatric disorders may potentially reduce both the human suffering and the economic burden that challenging behaviours cause. However, the inter-relationships between challenging behaviours and psychiatric symptoms have until recently remained a relatively neglected area of research. This has been, at least in part, because of the conceptual difficulties researchers face. Ultimately, a fully comprehensive summary of these inter-relationships cannot be given without wider consideration of how cognitive, emotional and behavioural problems in

Psychiatric and Behavioural Disorders in Intellectual and Developmental Disabilities, ed. Nick Bouras and Geraldine Holt. Published by Cambridge University Press. © Cambridge University Press 2007.

people with ID should be conceptualized and classified, and how these problems should be assessed in those people with more severe ID. Although this chapter will briefly consider such wider issues, it will mainly concentrate on the ways these inter-relationships have been explored so far, with particular emphasis on some more recent studies. This chapter will also consider how further research in this area could proceed.

Definitions

The terms 'severe ID' and 'profound ID' used in this chapter refer to the ICD-10 definitions; that is, together referring to adults with an IQ less than 35. However few studies investigating the inter-relationships have concentrated just upon those with severe and profound ID. The term 'challenging behaviours' (rather than 'problem behaviours') is used in this chapter because of its widespread usage in the field of ID. There is no universal definition, but for one often cited, see Emerson (1995).

Why should such associations be expected?

It is now widely accepted that there is an increased prevalence of psychiatric disorders in people with ID. Furthermore, the majority of the factors that predispose to, precipitate and perpetuate psychiatric disorders in people with ID (in particular structural brain damage) become more prevalent as the severity of ID increases (Cooper and Bailey, 2001). It is reasonable therefore to expect an increased prevalence rate of psychiatric symptoms in people with more severe ID compared with those with milder ID. The evidence though from existing studies has been conflicting (Cooper and Bailey, 2001). For example, Lund (1985) and Gostason (1985) reported higher rates of psychiatric symptoms in more severe ID, but other studies have found higher rates in individuals with mild ID (e.g. Iverson and Fox, 1989; Jacobson, 1990). Findings that people with severe ID have fewer psychiatric symptoms may only reflect the low sensitivity of rating instruments for this group. Such evidence supports the possibility that psychiatric symptoms may manifest in atypical ways in more severe ID, and thus be frequently missed using language-based assessments following standard diagnostic criteria. If schizophrenia is considered as an example, higher rates have been found in people with mild ID compared with the general population. Lowest rates of all have been found in the group with severe ID (Lund, 1985). Reid (1972) influentially stated that schizophrenia could not be reliably diagnosed much below an IQ of 45. However, just because a disorder cannot be diagnosed reliably and easily may not mean that it does not exist. For example, it may be being missed because of altered presentation. Anxiety disorders too have tended to be diagnosed less frequently in people with more severe ID.

In this patient group only behavioural symptoms can be assessed reliably and this makes it difficult for all the criteria of an anxiety disorder to be met (Matson *et al.*, 1997).

How might any such associations be caused?

Moss, Kiernan and Emerson (1999) have argued that the relationships between psychiatric symptoms and challenging behaviours can work in three different ways. First, some challenging behaviours might actually be atypical symptoms of a mental illness. For example, Bodfish *et al.* (1995) argued that self-injurious behaviours (SIB) might be manifestations of obsessive-compulsive disorder in people with severe ID. Second, some challenging behaviours may occur as a secondary feature of a psychiatric disorder alongside the core features. For example, someone unable to express feelings may manifest them as behaviours (Meins, 1995). Third, psychiatric disorders may produce the conditions for the expression of challenging behaviours that are maintained by operant behavioural processes (Emerson, 1995). For example, depression may be associated with a resistance to socialize, thus turning social activities into negative reinforcers. Lowry (1993) had previously argued similarly that events in the environment might become aversive when an individual experiences a particular psychiatric symptom. Cooper *et al.* (2003) have also argued that, although more typically any existing challenging behaviours are exacerbated by superimposed psychopathology, some symptoms of psychiatric disorders can be a reduction of behaviours. For example, in a person with long-standing aggression, a disorder such as depression could cause this to reduce as well as increase. It is also possible that challenging behaviours may contribute to psychiatric symptoms such as low mood, rather than being indicative of them (Ross and Oliver, 2002).

What problems have researchers faced?

(i) Difficulties in assessment

There is a consensus that psychiatric disorders can generally be reliably assessed in people with mild ID and, furthermore, that standard diagnostic criteria such as ICD-10 and DSM-IV may be used (Meins, 1995). It remains difficult however to make a definitive diagnosis of psychiatric disorder in people with severe ID (King *et al.*, 1994). First, as ID becomes more severe there are increasing problems in the use of predominantly language-based standard diagnostic criteria because the person's capacity for verbal communication typically becomes limited or absent. Some symptoms such as excessive guilt or lowered self-esteem then become at best only partially assessable, if at all. Second, the actual manifestations of psychiatric disorders are widely considered to change as the severity of ID increases. This may be a result of the person's developmental level as well as other factors such as the increased co-morbidity with physical and sensory problems. 'Atypical' psychiatric symptoms in this population group may thus also include features such as irritable mood, social withdrawal and psychomotor agitation, as well as 'increase or onset of maladaptive behaviours' and/or 'decrease of adaptive behaviours' (Sovner and Lowry, 1990). These atypical features have been collectively termed 'behavioural equivalents' (Clarke and Gomez, 1999). Attempts to investigate these have been hampered by circular reasoning. There has been much criticism of the practice of describing behaviours as 'symptoms' then using these 'symptoms' to show that as behaviours are increased, associated psychiatric disorders also increase (McBrien, 2003). However, to some extent such circular reasoning is not easily avoidable in the absence of reliable biological markers of psychiatric disorders.

(ii) Inconsistent terminology and classification

As in the entire field of research into psychiatric disorders in people with ID, there has been a lack of consensus regarding important definitions. There have also been inconsistencies between the types of diagnostic criteria and assessment instruments used. A particular problem is the lack of universal definition for the commonly used term 'challenging behaviours'. Decreased adaptive behaviours, such as loss of skills or reduced communication, are usually not thought of as 'challenging behaviours' although they have often been included (along with other atypical features such as irritable mood) in research into 'behavioural equivalents'. There also do not exist clear definitions of individual problem behaviours either. Although widely used without clarification, an umbrella term such as 'self-injurious behaviours' encompasses behaviours with sometimes little in common (Rojahn, 1994).

There are ongoing further differences of opinion between what should be regarded as 'psychiatric' and as 'behavioural'. For example, 'psychiatric' disorders as defined by DSM-IV and ICD-10 encompasses 'behavioural disorders' as well as 'developmental' disorders such as autism. The core question is: how exactly should clusters of problem behaviours in individuals be described and classified? Whether or not behaviours cluster meaningfully as 'behaviour disorders' and then whether they should be considered 'psychiatric' remain unsettled debates, although a major problem is that many erroneously equate 'psychiatric' with 'biological'. There is thus no wider consensus that problem behaviours are best considered as mental health issues (Einfield and Aman, 1995) although many, such as Einfield and Tonge (1999), maintain that there is no sustainable (or useful) practical distinction between challenging behaviours and psychiatric disorders.

(iii) Lack of integrated approaches

Problem behaviours can be viewed through many perspectives, including developmental, sociological and behavioural (Reid, 1980). These perspectives are not mutually exclusive for no single perspective is able to provide a complete explanation of behaviour. Many clinicians have tended to view challenging behaviours in two main ways. They see them either as biologically 'driven' and 'psychiatric' or as simply (and tautologically) 'behavioural' and therefore as having little or no psychiatric significance (Reid, 1994). Sovner and Hurley (1999) have described the 'fiction' of the false dichotomy between the 'biological' and the 'behavioural'. In this dichotomy, if behaviour is thought to be 'behavioural' then it is often considered to have a function, but if considered 'psychiatric' any possible functional component is disregarded. But as Gardner and Cole (1990) have highlighted, just because some behaviours are biologically 'driven' the environment can still reinforce them or they can provide some function for the individual that may make them amenable to behavioural interventions in multimodal assessment and management. Conversely, Lowry (1997) has proposed the term 'behavioural overshadowing' to emphasize the identification of psychopathology only as 'learned behaviour' rather than also as a possible symptom or sign of mental illness.

What approaches have been used?

In order to try to substantiate expert clinical opinion approaches have been drawn from various methodologies, including case reports as well as cross-sectional, intervention and factor/cluster analytic studies. Some important examples of each are described here.

(i) Case reports

Lowry and Sovner (1992) published case reports of two adults with profound ID showing how the symptoms of their rapid cycling bipolar disorders fluctuated with self-injurious and aggressive behaviours over time. In the first case, SIB only occurred during episodes of depression. The SIB appeared to be communicative and demand avoidant, but only occurred when typical symptoms of lowered mood, appetite and activity levels were present. In the second case, aggression in a woman with ID was associated with manic phases, while she became mute in the depressive phases. The aggression appeared to be related to irritability. In a similar study using behavioural monitoring, Sovner et al. (1993) showed associations between SIB and chronic depression in a man with severe ID and a man with profound ID. In both cases, treatment with fluoxetine improved both depressive symptoms and SIB. The authors therefore argued that severe problem behaviours might sometimes be a 'state-dependent' secondary feature of affective disorder.

(ii) Cross-sectional studies

The most common approach has been 'checklist' type cross-sectional studies using either standard or modified diagnostic criteria. Depression has often been the psychiatric disorder most commonly suggested to be associated with challenging behaviour using this approach (McBrien, 2003). Meins (1995) found that 'behavioural equivalents' such as SIB, aggression, tantrums, and screaming were more common in people with severe ID and depression compared with those with more mild ID. Marston *et al.* (1997) compared adults with varying levels of ID who had had an ICD-10 depressive syndrome and those who had not. The core symptoms of depressed affect and sleep disturbance were found in the depressed group across all levels of ID. However, they also found that, with increasing ID, there was a move towards 'behavioural equivalents' such as aggression, screaming and SIB. But there has been a recent backlash against the idea of using 'behavioural equivalents' as core diagnostic criteria (Tsiouris *et al.*, 2003; McBrien, 2003).

There have been four recent cross-sectional surveys with relatively large sample sizes designed to consider the relationship of psychiatric symptoms to challenging behaviours in adults with ID. The development of standardized rating instruments such as the PAS-ADD (Moss *et al.*, 1993) and the DASH-II (Matson, 1995) now allows better comparison between such studies. However, the DASH-II is the only well validated psychopathology-rating instrument designed for people with severe and profound ID. (See also Chapter 2 by Mohr & Costello.)

Moss *et al.* (2000) used the PAS-ADD Checklist to estimate the prevalence of different psychiatric symptoms in 320 people with all levels of ID. They were also rated for challenging behaviours (when present) using a 'more demanding'/'less demanding' dichotomy. The majority of people with challenging behaviours had no psychiatric symptoms. However, the numbers of psychiatric symptoms were increased significantly in those subjects with both 'more demanding' and 'less demanding' challenging behaviours compared to the control group. For 23 out of the 26 items rated by the PAS-ADD Checklist, the prevalence was highest in the group with 'more demanding' challenging behaviours. Diagnostic categories were then derived from the PAS-ADD Checklist scores, although these did not correspond with ICD-10 diagnostic criteria. Their results suggested that the prevalence of their own defined psychiatric 'disorders', especially 'depression' and 'hypomania', was highest in the group of subjects with more demanding behaviours.

Holden and Gitleson (2003) also used the PAS-ADD Checklist in a sample of 165 adults with all levels of ID to show that challenging behaviours were associated with an increased prevalence of psychiatric symptoms. Of the 28 psychiatric symptoms, eight were significantly associated with challenging behaviours. In total, four 'diagnostic categories' were derived from the PAS-ADD Checklist, but again these did not correspond to standard diagnoses. Unlike that of Moss *et al.* (2000), this study found that 'anxiety' and 'psychosis' were the diagnoses most commonly associated with challenging behaviours. The sub-sample who showed challenging behaviours had a higher proportion of individuals with severe and profound ID.

Rojahn *et al.* (2004) studied 180 adults with severe and profound ID who were assessed with the Behaviour Problems Inventory (BPI) and the DASH-II. Those with SIB, aggressive/destructive or stereotyped behaviours had generally higher levels of psychopathology. Relationships between behaviour problems and psychiatric conditions were select and differential. Factor analysis revealed that a 'self-injury/aggression/destruction' factor was related to impulse control and conduct problems, but not to depression or mania nor stereotyped behaviours. A 'stereotyped behaviour' factor was linked to pervasive developmental disorder and somewhat less so to schizophrenia and was independent of the 'self-injury/aggression/destruction' factor. It was concluded that behaviour problems among individuals with predominantly severe to profound ID are related to certain psychiatric conditions. However, the moderate strengths of these associations suggested to the authors that behaviour problems are not generally atypical manifestations of psychiatric disorders.

Hemmings *et al.* (2006) carried out a cross-sectional survey using the PAS-ADD Checklist and the Disability Assessment Schedule (DAS) in a sample of 214 adults with all levels of ID. They found that self-injurious and, to a lesser extent, aggressive problem behaviours were most associated with affective-type symptoms. Screaming and destructive behaviours tended to be more associated with autism-related social impairment rather than conventional psychiatric symptoms. Aggressive and self-injurious behaviours were not associated with severity of ID in this study. Having more severe ID but without either autism-related social impairment and/or psychiatric symptoms was only associated with two problem behaviours: difficult or objectionable personal habits and tantrums.

(iii) Intervention studies

Intervention studies have also been used to look at possible links between psychiatric symptoms and problem behaviours in people with ID. For example, Perry *et al.* (2001) used antidepressant treatment to see which symptoms of depression and associated behaviours improved in adults with autism and moderate or severe ID. Of the seven individuals whose depressive symptoms responded to antidepressants, five also showed improvement in SIB while two showed improvement in aggression. However, studies using medication to diagnose retrospectively are problematic as medications are not specific in their actions. Similar psychological treatment studies following relationships between psychiatric symptoms and challenging behaviours have not been done, although Allen (1989) reported two case studies in which the frequency of aggressive behaviour and SIB in two individuals (one with profound ID) was reduced by anxiety management.

(iv) Factor/cluster analytic studies

The preceding approaches have used standard or modified diagnostic criteria. A radically different approach has been to attempt to identify 'behavioural syndromes' de novo using factor or cluster analysis. This 'bottom-up' approach allows fewer assumptions about psychopathology in adults with severe ID than the 'top-down' approach of applying standard or modified diagnostic criteria. It investigates whether the individual behavioural and emotional changes described group into clinically meaningful syndromes or disorders.

For example, Matson *et al.* (1991) used a factor analysis of data derived from the DASH in 506 adults with severe and profound ID to suggest that there were six dimensions of behaviour, including antisocial behaviour, emotional lability, language disorder, eating disorder, sleep disorder and social withdrawal/stereotypy. However, challenging or problem behaviours such as SIB tended to load on multiple factors. Einfield and Aman (1995) listed six general categories that seemed to form a pattern of behavioural disorders in this population: 'aggressive/antisocial/self-injurious', 'withdrawal', 'stereotyped behaviour', 'hyperactivity', 'repetitive verbalizations' and 'anxious, fearful and tense'. They noted that aggressive and impulsive behaviour, or anxiety symptoms and SIB, accompanied emotional lability.

How should future research proceed?

Stronger evidence for accepting challenging behaviours as atypical psychiatric symptoms in some individuals could be gained from longitudinal studies rather than from cross-sectional studies. Longitudinal studies may be able to show whether or not, as psychiatric symptoms change over time, challenging behaviours fluctuate in a similar and closely related manner. There have been only a few case reports and small study samples that have followed up a cohort of adults with ID. These include the two longitudinal case studies of Lowry and Sovner (1992), and Sovner *et al.* (1993) described above. These two particular studies are also notable for their (rare) collaboration between the psychopathology and behavioural approaches. Somewhat surprisingly there have been no studies published that have built on these case reports, using a behavioural monitoring system similar to that developed by Sovner and Lowry (1990). Larger intervention studies are also eventually needed, but these must be carefully based on existing evidence in order to increase validity.

Without clear-cut biological markers to 'anchor' research, the understanding of challenging behaviours in people with more severe ID using standard psychiatric diagnostic categories is always limited to some extent. In these circumstances it can be easy to devalue 'checklist' type research. But such biological markers in general are not yet available; there have been many 'false dawns' in biologically orientated research and so phenomenological investigations also need to continue. Much research has been at the syndromal level but a symptomatic approach to the classification of psychiatric symptoms and problem behaviours may be more relevant to adults with severe ID (Deb *et al.*, 2001). The factor analysis approach described above may yield diagnostic categories with more validity in this group. Another approach could be to use the diagnostic categories of childhood mental disorders. The whole concept of behavioural equivalents of psychiatric symptoms in adults with developmental delay is also supported by the findings that conduct disorders and behavioural problems such as aggression often coexist with childhood depression (Reiss and Rojahn, 1994). It may be that diagnoses of childhood mental disorders, such as attention deficit (Fox and Wade, 1998) and attachment disorders (Janssen, *et al.*, 2002), could sometimes be more appropriate diagnoses for adults with more severe ID and challenging behaviours than those used in adults with typical intelligence or at the milder end of the ID spectrum.

However using new or different classification systems for more severe ID would make evidence from studies in mild ID difficult to compare, including that of treatments. As with the entire field of mental health in ID, future research needs to aim to converge on terminology, rating instruments and diagnostic criteria as much as possible. In particular, Lowry (1997) has recommended the establishment of operationalized criteria for each individual challenging behaviour to increase the objectivity of monitoring. Future studies could thus look more closely at associations of psychiatric symptoms with individual challenging behaviours, instead of with the presence of challenging behaviours overall. Indeed, the umbrella term 'challenging behaviours' itself remains a problem; it is too vague, being simultaneously over-inclusive of a range of problem behaviours yet generally excluding of other serious problems for the individual such as social withdrawal and loss of skills. Existing rating instruments also are not always sensitive enough to examine the inter-relationships between psychiatric symptoms and challenging behaviours adequately. One particular problem is that instruments such as the PAS-ADD Checklist usually do not rate recent change in frequency or severity in chronic behaviours that could be an indication of atypical psychiatric symptoms. Future rating instruments will need to be able to adequately capture such changes.

A further way in which future studies may improve our understanding would be to collect data on autism. This is particularly important when investigating individuals with depression, if flat affect and social withdrawal is always attributed to that (Ross and Oliver, 2002). Although a 'psychiatric' disorder as defined by ICD-10, autism is often not considered as such by clinicians in the ID mental health field. However, the contribution of autism to problem behaviours seems often more important than classic psychiatric diagnoses in clinical practice. A high proportion of challenging behaviours are associated with autistic traits that are in turn more prevalent in those with more severe ID (Bhaumik *et al.*, 1997).

Conclusion

The inter-relationships between ID, psychiatric diagnoses and challenging behaviours are complex. Until recently the importance of psychiatric disorders even in people with mild ID had been overlooked. Now there is also more attention towards making sure psychiatric symptoms are not similarly undetected in those with more severe ID. However no clinician or researcher seriously expects the bulk of challenging behaviours to be as a result of undetected 'classic' psychiatric disorders. Clearly not all behavioural problems are the result of a psychiatric disorder. Even when they coexist, they are not necessarily causally related. As Sturmey (1995) has noted, individual behaviours have too many causes to assign them to particular disorders. So there are no simplistic relationships between a particular behaviour and a specific disorder. For example, Gardner and Sovner (1994) argued that psychiatric symptoms were contributory to SIB but not sufficient on their own for it to occur. However, there are still good theoretical and increasingly empirical reasons to support the clinical impression that untreated psychiatric disorders may be an important or even primary contributory factor to some challenging behaviours.

This area of research is not just crucial for clinical practice; it also has major implications for service delivery. While much of the assessment and diagnosis of psychiatric disorders in mild ID is broadly similar to that of the general population, that of people with more severe ID is yet more complex and controversial. The skills required to assess, diagnose and treat psychiatric disorders in people with more severe ID are a major reason why specialist mental health professionals are necessary for work with people with ID. The currently practising clinician must attempt to make the most accurate diagnosis possible whenever appropriate rather than use the vague label of 'challenging behaviours'. Reiss (1994) has stated useful guidelines for the practising clinician. He or she must assess whether or not there has been a clear change in behaviour from baseline levels of fluctuation. They must then consider whether any behaviour disturbance may be part of a symptom pattern that corresponds to a psychiatric disorder. They should remember that there is always the possibility that challenging behaviours may be exacerbating a coexisting psychiatric disorder, as well as the fact that psychiatric disorders can manifest as new or increased challenging behaviours. It must be accepted that the cause of the behaviours may ultimately be ambiguous; in severe ID, psychiatric diagnoses are generally tentative, often to be treated more like hypotheses (Reiss, 1994). Finally, in practice, as well as in research, efforts must continue to try to integrate all approaches in a multimodal approach (e.g. Gardner and Griffiths, 1997) to the diagnosis and treatment of challenging behaviours in people with severe and profound ID.

Summary points

- Better understanding of the relationships of challenging behaviours with psychiatric symptoms should help reduce the suffering and economic burden that they cause.
- Challenging behaviours have multiple causes. Some however may be atypical presentations of psychiatric symptoms in adults with ID.
- Research in this area has been hampered by lack of consistency in definitions, including the term 'challenging behaviours'.
- Recent large studies do support an association between psychiatric symptoms and challenging behaviours, but have differed in the patterns found.
- Future research should concentrate on the symptomatic level at first, given the controversies regarding classification of psychiatric disorders and behavioural problems in this population.
- Future research should also include prospective, descriptive and intervention studies.
- There are not likely to be any simple relationships between psychiatric symptoms and individual challenging behaviours. Challenging behaviours are usually multifactorial phenomena that require an integrated, multimodal approach to assessment and treatment.

REFERENCES

Allen, E. A. (1989). Behavioural treatment of anxiety and related disorders in adults with mental handicaps: a review. *Mental Handicap Research*, **22**, 47–60.

Bhaumik, S., Branford, D., McGrother, C. & Thorp, C. (1997). Autistic traits in adults with learning disabilities. *British Journal of Psychiatry*, **170**, 502–6.

Bodfish, J. W., Crawford, T. W., Powell, S. B. *et al.* (1995). Compulsions in adults with mental retardation: prevalence, phenomenology, and comorbidity with stereotypy and self-injury. *American Journal on Mental Retardation*, **100**, 183–92.

Clarke, D. J. & Gomez, G. A. (1999). Utility of modified DCR-10 criteria in the diagnosis of depression associated with intellectual disability. *Journal of Intellectual Disability Research*, **43**, 413–20.

Cooper, S.-A. & Bailey, N. M. (2001). Psychiatric disorders amongst adults with learning disabilities – prevalence and relationship to ability level. *Irish Journal of Psychological Medicine*, **18**, 45–53.

Cooper, S.-A., Melville, C. A. & Einfield, S. L. (2003). Psychiatric diagnosis, intellectual disabiliies and Diagnostic Criteria for Psychiatric Disorders for Use with Adults with Learning Disabilities/Mental Retardation (DC-LD). *Journal of Intellectual Disability Research*, **47** (Suppl. 1), 3–15.

Day, K. (1985). Psychiatric disorder in the middle aged and elderly mentally handicapped. *British Journal of Psychiatry*, **147**, 660–7.

Deb, S., Thomas, M. & Bright, C. (2001). Mental disorder in adults with intellectual disability. 1: Prevalence of functional psychiatric illness among a community-based population aged between 16 and 64 years. *Journal of Intellectual Disability Research*, **45**, 495–505.

Einfield, S. L. & Aman, M. (1995). Issues in the taxonomy of psychopathology in mental retardation. *Journal of Autism and Developmental Disorders*, **25**, 143–67.

Einfield, S. L. & Tonge, B. J. (1999). Observations on the use of the ICD-10 guide for mental retardation. *Journal of Intellectual Disability Research*, **43**, 408–12.

Emerson, E. (1995). *Challenging Behaviour: Analysis and Intervention in People with Learning Difficulties*. Cambridge: Cambridge University Press.

Emerson, E. & Bromley, J. (1995). The form and function of challenging behaviours. *Journal of Intellectual Disability Research*, **39**, 388–98.

Fox, R. A. and Wade, E. J. (1998). Attention Deficit Hyperactivity Disorder among adults with severe and profound mental retardation. *Research in Developmental Disabilities*, **19**, 275–80.

Fryers, T. & Russell, O. (2004). Applied epidemiology. In *Seminars in the Psychiatry of Learning Disabilities*, ed. Fraser, W. & Kerr, M. London: Gaskell, pp. 16–48.

Gardner, W. I. & Cole, C. L. (1990). Aggression and related difficulties. In *Handbook of Behavior Modification with the Mentally Retarded*, ed. Matson, J. L. New York, NY: Plenum, pp. 225–51.

Gardner, W. I. & Griffiths, D. (1997). Influence of psychiatric disorders on non-specific behavioural symptoms: diagnostic and treatment issues. In *Congress Proceedings: International Congress III on the Dually Diagnosed, Mental Health Aspects of Mental Retardation*, ed. Fletcher, R. J. & Dosen, A. New York, NY: National Association for the Dually Diagnosed.

Gardner, W. I. & Sovner, R. (1994). *Self-Injurious Behaviour, Diagnosis and Treatment: A Multi-Modal Functional Approach*. Willow Street, PA: Vida Publishing.

Gostason, R. (1985). Psychiatric illness among the mentally retarded: a Swedish population study. *Acta Psychiatrica Scandinavica*, **7** (Suppl. 318), 1–117.

Hemmings, C. P., Gravestock, S., Pickard, M. & Bouras, N. (2006). Psychiatric symptoms and problem behaviours in people with intellectual disabilities. *Journal of Intellectual Disabiliy Research*, **50**, 269–76.

Holden, B. & Gitleson, J. P. (2003). Prevalence of psychiatric symptoms in adults with mental retardation and challenging behaviour. *Research in Development Disabilities*, **24**, 323–32.

Iverson, J. C. & Fox, R. A. (1989). Prevalence of psychopathology among mentally retarded adults. *Research in Developmental Disabilities*, **10**, 77–83.

Jacobsen, J. W. (1982). Problem behaviour and psychiatric impairment within a developmentally disabled population: I. Behaviour frequency. *Applied Research in Mental Retardation*, **3**, 121–39.

Jacobson, J. W. (1990). Do some mental disorders occur less frequently among persons with mental retardation? *American Journal on Mental Retardation*, **94**, 596–602.

Janssen, C. G. C., Schuengel, C. & Stolk, J. (2002). Understanding challenging behaviour in people with severe and profound intellectual disability: a stress-attachment model. *Journal of Intellectual Disability Research*, **46**, 445–53.

King, B. H., De Antonio, C., McCracken, J. T., Forness, S. R. & Ackerland, V. (1994). Psychiatric consultation in severe and profound mental retardation. *American Journal of Psychiatry*, **151**, 1802–8.

Lowry, M. A. (1993). A clear link between problem behaviours and mood disorders. *Habilitative Mental Healthcare Newsletter*, **12**, 105–10.

Lowry, M. A. (1997). Unmasking mood disorders: recognising and measuring symptomatic behaviours. *Habilitative Mental Healthcare Newsletter*, **16**, 1–6.

Lowry, M. A. & Sovner, R. (1992). Severe behaviour problems associated with rapid cycling bipolar disorder in two adults with profound mental retardation. *Journal of Intellectual Disability Research*, **36**, 269–81.

Lund, J. (1985). The prevalence of psychiatric morbidity in mentally retarded adults. *Acta Pychiatrica Scandinavica*, **72**, 563–70.

Marston, G. W., Perry, D. W. & Roy, A. (1997). Manifestations of depression in people with intellectual disability. *Journal of Intellectual Disability Research*, **41**, 476–80.

Matson, J. L. (1995). *The Diagnostic Assessment for the Severely Handicapped-II*. Baton-Rouge, LA: Scientific-Publishers Inc.

Matson, J. L., Coe, D. A., Gardner, W. I. & Sovner, R. (1991). A factor analytic study of the Diagnostic Assessment for the Severely Handicapped Scale. *Journal of Nervous and Mental disease*, **179**, 553–7.

Matson, J. L., Sniroldi, B. B., Hamilton, M. & Baglio, C. S. (1997). Do anxiety disorders exist in persons with severe and profound mental retardation? *Research in Developmental Disabilities*, **18**, 39–44.

McBrien, J. A. (2003). Assessment and diagnosis of depression in people with intellectual disability. *Journal of Intellectual Disability Research*, **47**, 1–13.

McClintock, K., Hall, S. & Oliver, C. (2003). Risk markers associated with challenging behaviours in people with intellectual disabilities: a meta-analytic study. *Journal of Intellectual Disability Research*, **47**, 405–16.

Meins, W. (1995). Symptoms of major depression in mentally retarded adults. *Journal of Intellectual Disability Research*, **39**, 41–5.

Moss, S. C., Emerson, E., Kiernan, C. *et al.* (2000). Psychiatric symptoms in adults with learning disability and challenging behaviour. *British Journal of Psychiatry*, **177**, 452–6.

Moss, S. Kiernan, C. & and Emerson, E. (1999). The relationship between challenging behaviours and psychiatric disorders in people with severe developmental disabilities. In *Psychiatric and Behavioural Disorders in Developmental Disabilities and Mental Retardation*, ed. Bouras, N. Cambridge: Cambridge University Press, pp 40–4.

Moss, S. Patel, P., Prosser, H. *et al.* (1993). Psychiatric morbidity in older people with moderate and severe learning disability. I: Development and reliability of the patient interview (PAS-ADD). *British Journal of Psychiatry*, **163**, 471–80.

Perry, D. W., Marston, G. M., Hinder, S. A. J., Munden, A. C. & Roy, A. (2001). The phenomenology of depressive illness in people with a learning disability and autism. *Autism*, **5**, 265–75.

Reid, A. (1972). Psychoses in adult mental defectives: II. Schizophrenic and paranoid psychoses. *British Journal of Psychiatry*, **120**, 213–18.

Reid, A. H. (1980). Psychiatric disorders in mentally handicapped children: a clinical and follow-up study. *Journal of Mental Deficiency Research*, **24**, 287–98.

Reid, A. H. (1994). Psychiatry and learning disability. *British Journal of Psychiatry*, **164**, 613–18.

Reiss, S. (1994). Psychopathology in mental retardation. In *Mental Health in Mental Retardation: Recent Advances in Practice*, ed. Bouras, N. Cambridge: Cambridge University Press, pp. 67–78.

Reiss, S. & Rojahn, J. (1994). Joint occurrence of depression and aggression in children and adults with mental retardation. *Journal of Intellectual Disability Research*, **37**, 287–94.

Rojahn, J. (1994). Epidemiology and topographic taxonomy of self-injurious behaviour. In *Destructive Behaviour in Developmental Disabilities: Diagnosis and Treatment*, ed. Thompson, T. & Gray, D. B. Thousand Oaks, CA: Sage Publications Inc., pp. 49–67.

Rojahn, J., Matson, J., Naglieri, J. A. & Mayville, E. (2004). Relationships between psychiatric conditions and behavior problems among adults with mental retardation. *American Journal on Mental Retardation*, **109**, 21–33.

Ross, E. & Oliver, C. (2002). The relationship between levels of mood, interest and pleasure and 'challenging behaviour' in adults with severe and profound intellectual disability. *Journal of Intellectual Disability Research*, **46**, 191–7.

Sovner, R., Fox, C. J., Lowry, M. J. & Lowry, M. A. (1993). Fluoxetine treatment of depression and associated injury in two adults with mental retardation. *Journal of Intellectual Disability Research*, **37**, 301–11.

Sovner, R. & Hurley, A. D. (1999). Facts and fictions concerning mental illness in people with mental retardation and developmental disabilities. In *Challenging Behavior of Persons with Mental Health Disorders and Severe Developmental Disabilities*, ed. Weisler, N. A. & Hanson, R. H., Washington, DC: American Association on Mental Retardation, pp. 89–99.

Sovner, R. & Lowry, M. A. (1990). A behavioural methodology for diagnosing affective disorders in individuals with mental retardation. *Habilitative Mental Healthcare Newsletter*, **9**, 55–61.

Sturmey, P. (1995). Diagnostic-based pharmacological treatment of behaviour disorders in persons with developmental disabilities: A review and decision-making typology. *Research in Developmental Disabilities*, **16**, 235–52.

Tsiouris, J. A., Mann, R., Patti, P. J. & Sturmey, P. (2003). Challenging behaviours should not be considered as depressive equivalents in individuals with intellectual disability. *Journal of Intellectual Disability Research*, **47**, 14–21.

5

The interface between medical and psychiatric disorders in people with intellectual disabilities

Nick Lennox

Introduction

This chapter will discuss the interface between medical and psychiatric disorders in people with intellectual disabilities (ID). The Oxford Modern Australian Dictionary, 1998, defines interface as 'a place where interaction occurs between two processes'. To fully understand this interaction we will need a broad framework that accounts for the underlying influences on the clinical presentation of medical and psychiatric conditions. A proposed framework, which can assist in understanding the individual and the nature of the influences on health, will be presented and discussed. Then the evidence for the poor health status of people with ID will be presented along with reasons why this situation may currently exist. The high levels of morbidity and psychosocial neglect experienced by this population highlight the importance of this interface. Finally, commonly encountered conditions, and an approach to their clinical features, are discussed.

Conceptual framework

A conceptual framework is helpful in describing the complex interaction between psychiatric and physical disorders. This framework may also be useful for the broader conceptualization of the constructs and also during the consultative process.

The framework in Table 5.1, adapted from Professor Tony Holland's model (personal communication), and extended to incorporate more recent findings and trends, is a simple four-by-four table. According to this model, each dimension along the x-axis, from biological to spiritual, can contribute to our understanding of an individual's current presentation. These dimensions can have varying degrees of influence on the person's health and well-being. The degree of influence,

Psychiatric and Behavioural Disorders in Intellectual and Developmental Disabilities, ed. Nick Bouras and Geraldine Holt. Published by Cambridge University Press. © Cambridge University Press 2007.

Table 5.1 Conceptual framework.

	Domains (or x-axis)			
Degree of influence of domains (or y-axis)	Biological	Psychological	Social	Spiritual
Predict				
Predispose				
Precipitate				
Perpetuate				

or y-axis, can predict, predispose, precipitate or perpetuate the problem for the individual.

While it is common practice to classify using the bio-psycho-social framework, there is increasing interest in the literature about spiritual beliefs and the consequence of these beliefs on health and well-being (Gaventa, 2003; Peach, 2003). Some may prefer to omit the spiritual domain; however, even without this domain the framework is a useful mechanism to describe the interaction between psychiatric and physical disorders and the complex interplay of social and psychological factors with biology.

One example, using this table, is that of an individual with Down syndrome, who will be predisposed to developing Alzheimer's-type dementia, but recognition of the condition may be precipitated by social factors such as change of residence. Another example is an individual with a moderate ID who develops a psychotic episode (for which their disability may have been a predisposing factor, but which may actually have been precipitated by a psychological or social event), and is treated with an antipsychotic medication. The person develops tardive dyskinesia, which continues after the medication is stopped. In this case, a drug side effect (biological factor) has caused perpetuation of this condition.

Bio-psycho-socio-spiritual influences on medical and psychiatric disorders

This section will give some examples of the interactions between bio-psycho-socio-spiritual influences and medical and psychiatric disorders, starting with the more clear-cut biological influences and moving to incorporate more complex situations that involve psychological, social and/or spiritual factors.

There is an increased understanding of the consequences of underlying genotype, not only on the individual's physical characteristics, or phenotype, but on their behaviour, called the behaviour phenotype (O'Brien & Yule, 1995). For some disorders the biological genotype predicts the development of a physical disease or psychiatric disorder. In some cases, this can be predicted to occur in all people with the same genetic deficit. For example in Prader–Willi syndrome (PWS), the

30% of people who inherit the disorder via a mechanism called uniparental disomy will all develop a psychotic disorder by the age of 28 years (Boer, *et al.*, 2002). This supports the notion that certain biology can predict the development of a psychiatric disorder. As increasingly sophisticated techniques are available to define the specific genotype and the associated morbidity, more examples will emerge.

In a similar way, people with fragile X syndrome are predisposed to develop attention deficit hyperactivity disorder (ADHD), aggression and/or complex partial epilepsy. These conditions do not occur in all individuals but are associated with the underlying genetic disorder and are commonly seen in people with this syndrome (Hagerman & Cronister, 1996). This predisposition may be modified by other factors, such as adequate sleep; loving, predictable and accepting home and school environments that minimize stress and maximize communication; and/or access to respite services (see also Chapter 12 by Hodapp and Dykens).

Psychological, social and spiritual factors, as above, can influence the expression of biological predispositions, and the converse is also true. For example, the development of Alzheimer's-type dementia will have profound psycho-socio-spiritual consequences for any individual, and especially for those predisposed by their biology, such as individuals with trisomy 21 or another ID.

The examples used above are clearly delineated and common in clinical practice. However it is also common for people with ID to present with a more complex interplay between psychosocial, biological and spiritual factors and their physical and mental health. For example, psychological, social or sexual abuse is more common in people with ID and such abuse can cause psychological, as well as physical trauma. Furthermore, such abuse may establish abnormal behaviours that perpetuate the cycle of victimization and abuse (Sobsey, 1994; Sobsey & Doe, 1991).

A more subtle influence is the increased risk of physical and psychiatric morbidity and mortality that is associated with the lower socio-economic status that is often endured by people with ID (Emerson, 2003). Researchers in this area have identified that increased control over one's life circumstances is associated with better health outcomes (Griffin, 2003). People with ID do not usually experience a high degree of control over their life circumstances.

These examples illustrate a few relatively simple relationships between medical and psychiatric disorders and bio-psycho-socio-spiritual factors. However, it is not uncommon clinically to see cases that involve interactions between many more factors. For example Mr John C. is a 39-year-old man with Down syndrome who lives with, and requires support from, Mrs May C., his 80-year-old mother. They live alone in the family home, supported by pensions since the death of Mr Alan C., who died 12 months ago. Mr John C. attends a day service four days a week, while Mrs C. has set activities 2 days a week. Although restricted by her osteoarthritis and optic atrophy, Mrs C. still drives a car in the local area.

These circumstances may remain stable, although relatively fragile, for some time, but changes in the health, social circumstance or psychological well-being of mother or son could precipitate a breakdown in the structures that have been supporting their ongoing well-being. Such a breakdown could be prevented or ameliorated with greater personal or social resources, be they financial, health, social, spiritual or psychological. For example, if Mrs C. required hospitalization this would precipitate an accommodation crisis for Mr John C., but this crisis could be addressed on a psycho-social level, by providing alternative accommodation and support for him. Without this intervention, Mr John C. would be at risk of psychological and physical problems.

These examples emphasize the complex and dynamic interplay of influences on physical and psychiatric health and well-being for people with ID. Some factors can have a major influence, such as uniparental disomy in PWS, but more commonly many factors interact to affect the person's well-being or presentation for clinical assessment. The model described may be helpful in understanding the individual, and in ensuring that a wide and comprehensive approach is taken.

Health status: mortality and morbidity

The health status of people with ID is generally poor. This is perhaps most clearly indicated by the significant reduction in life expectancy for people with ID compared to the general population (Bittles, *et al.*, 2002; Durvasula *et al.*, 2002; Eyman, *et al.*, 1988). One recent, high-quality study found median life expectancies of 74.0, 67.6, and 58.6 years respectively, for people with mild, moderate, and severe levels of disability and an overall median life expectance of 68.7 years. In comparison, median life expectancy in the general population was 75.6 in males and 81.2 in females in this study (Bittles, *et al.*, 2002). Where a known genetic cause is identified, or the person has difficulties with mobility and/or ability to feed themselves, the risk of premature death is increased even further (Eyman *et al.*, 1988; Eyman *et al.*, 1993; Janicki *et al.*, 1999).

It is also clear that people with ID experience high levels of unrecognized or poorly managed physical co-morbidity (Howells, 1986; Wilson & Haire, 1990). This was initially documented in institutional populations, but has recently been reported in studies of community or combined community-institution populations (Beange *et al.*, 1995; Decker, *et al.*, 1968; Nelson & Crocker, 1978).

Perhaps the most compelling population study was performed on a representative sample of 202 adults with ID who were examined, and their health compared to the general population in the same area (Beange *et al.*, 1995). On average 5.4 conditions were found per person with ID, with a mean of 2.3 conditions being unrecognized prior to the assessment and 2.7 considered unmanaged. Major problems accounted for a mean of 2.5 conditions per person. Specialist care was considered necessary for a total of 819 conditions, which was 74% of the total conditions that were found. Comparing this data with that from the general population, it was found that blindness, deafness, epilepsy, thyroid disease and psychosis were significantly more common in people with ID than those without ID (Beange *et al.*, 1995).

The authors of a large Dutch study were able to make a direct comparison of health problems between people with and without ID, using the register of Network Family Practices of Maastricht University (van Schrojenstein Lantman-de Valk, *et al.*, 2000). In total 318 people with ID were compared to 48 459 people without ID. Within the ID group, 12% had no health problems as compared to 21% of people without ID. The ID group were 2.5 times more likely to have one or more health problems, with largest Odds Ratios of 3.5, 3.5 1.9, 2.0 and 2.0 for neurological, psychological, ear and eye problems and a group comprising endocrine, metabolic and nutritional problems. It is likely that this study under-ascertained the extent of the difficulties, as a specialist practitioner with an interest in people with ID had not examined the participants, as in the Beange *et al.* (1995) or Wilson and Haire (1990) studies.

Other studies that have ascertained the levels of specific morbidities within the population of people with ID are summarized below in Table 5.2.

Psychiatric morbidity

In probably the most succinct review of the evidence about psychiatric disorders in adults with ID, Deb *et al.* (2001) conclude 'It appears that if diagnoses like behavioural disorder, personality disorders, autism, and ADHD are excluded, the overall rate of psychiatric illness in adults with ID does not differ significantly from that in the non-intellectually disabled general population'. This is then qualified, as the authors suggest higher rates of schizophrenia among adults who have mild to moderate ID and note that the commonest cause for psychiatric referral is behavioural problems.

The diagnosis of psychiatric disorders often depends on a clear description of the person's subjective experience of psychological well-being; when the person has a diminished ability to communicate this experience, an accurate diagnosis becomes difficult. This not only makes diagnosis problematic in some individuals, but also means that diagnosis is often not made until late in the development of the disorder when profound changes in observable symptoms become apparent.

Furthermore psychiatric problems can, and often do, influence or cause physical health problems. Depression and psychotic disorders can lead to non-compliance with diabetic diets and medication, while chronic mental disorders are known to be associated with poor physical health and healthcare.

Table 5.2 Studies of specific co-morbidity.

Condition	Reference
Vision impairments 10–44%	(Beange et al., 1995; Evenhuis, 1995a; Janicki & Dalton, 1998; van Schrojenstein Lantman-de Valk et al., 1997; Warburg, 1994; Warburg, 2001)
Hearing impairments 10–28%	(Beange et al., 1995; Evenhuis, 1995b; van Schrojenstein Lantman-de Valk et al., 1997; Wilson & Haire, 1990)
Obesity 9.8–40%	(Robertson et al., 2000; Marshall et al., 2003; van Schrojenstein Lantman-de Valk et al., 1997; Wells et al., 1997; Beange et al., 1995; Wilson & Haire, 1990)
Dental pathology < 20–29%	(Cumella et al., 2000; Cathels & Reddihough, 1993; Jurek & Reid, 1994)
Inadequate review of medications: polypharmacy	(van Schrojenstein Lantman-de Valk et al., 1997; Parker, 1991; Wilson & Haire, 1990; Gowdey et al., 1987)
Epilepsy 14–44%	(Hand, 1994; Forsgren et al., 1996; Wilson & Haire, 1990; Bowley & Kerr, 2000; Morgan et al., 2003)
Osteoporosis	(Centre & McElduft, 1998; Centre et al., 1994; Tohill, 1997; Tyler, 1997)
Reflux oesophagitis	(Bohmer et al., 1997b)
Helicobacter pylori	(Wallace et al., 2002; Bohmer et al., 1997a)
Constipation and bowel obstruction	(Bohmer, 2001; Jancar, 1984)
Atherosclerotic heart disease	(Beange et al., 1995)
Infectious diseases e.g. hepatitis B	(Stehr Green et al., 1991; Cunningham, 1994)
Accidental injury	(Sherrard et al., 2001)

In conclusion some medical and psychiatric morbidities are not only more common, but are often unrecognized; recognized late in the disease process; and/or poorly managed in people with ID, compared to those without ID.

Barriers to recognition of medical and psychiatric disorders

Medical and psychiatric disorders are under-diagnosed because of a number of factors that include: difficulties that staff may have in recognizing an illness; systemic and structural barriers to high quality care; lack of health and disability professional support and training; the pervasive devaluing of people with ID; and communication difficulties (McDermott, 1997; Lennox & Diggens, 1999; Lennox & Chaplin, 1996; Lennox et al., 1997; Lennox et al., 2000). The effects of devaluing have been described extensively in the qualitative literature; however, one of the clearest quantitative examples is the large increase in life expectancy that has occurred for children with Down syndrome since the introduction of cardiac surgery (Yang et al., 2002).

This had been available, but not performed, on infants with Down syndrome until the 1970s, and its increasing use has contributed significantly to a rise in median age at death for people with Down syndrome from 25 years in 1983 to 49 years in 1997 (Yang *et al.*, 2002).

Another factor contributing to under-diagnosis is diagnostic overshadowing. This was first described by Reiss *et al.* (1982), and refers to a situation where, in the assessment of a clinician, the person's emotional problems are attributed to, or overshadowed by, the person's ID. This bias by clinicians has been consistently found across studies and continues to be a significant factor, more than 20 years later (White *et al.*, 1995).

It is estimated that, for people with any chronic physical illness, the lifetime prevalence of mental illness, particularly substance abuse, mood and anxiety disorders, is over 40% (Kaplan & Sadock, 2003). These figures may well apply to adults with ID.

Syndrome specific associations

As in the general population, a person can present with a psychiatric disorder or psychiatric symptoms which have an underlying physical cause. These include less common conditions such as Cushing's disease causing depressive symptoms and multiple sclerosis causing mania, as well as conditions that are more common in people with ID, such as thyroid disease in people with Down syndrome, seizure disorders, inter-ictal auditory hallucinations or post-ictal confusion (Kaplan & Sadock, 2003).

Medical and psychiatric conditions that are more commonly encountered

There are a number of medical disorders, which, although relatively common, are often overlooked, especially when the person with the disability has difficulty with communication. These disorders should also be considered when a person with ID presents with challenging behaviour (see also Chapter 17 by Reese *et al.*).
Unrecognized presentations include:
(1) Unrecognized pain from a variety of conditions:
    (a) Acute onset – injury, acute dental pathology, unrecognized disease including reflux oesophagitis or constipation.
    (b) Chronic onset – musculo-skeletal injury or disease, dental pathology, osteoporosis, reflux oesophagitis and constipation.
(2) Unrecognized medication side effects (see also Chapter 19 by King).
    (a) Diplopia, headache and/or nausea associated with many of the anticonvulsants (Harrison's Principles of Internal Medicine, 2005).

    (b) Restlessness and challenging behaviour in a person taking major tranquillizers and experiencing akathisia. This may be misinterpreted as an agitated depression (Sachdev & Longragan, 1991).

    (c) Depression associated with some hormonal contraceptives and anticonvulsants (Harrision's Principles of Internal Medicine. 2005).

(3) Delirium. 'Delirium is characterised by disturbance ("clouding") of the conscious state with reduced ability to focus, sustain or shift attention, and impairment of cognition (especially of orientation and memory)' (eTG, 2004). Although episodes usually present over hours to days, delirium can last for weeks if unrecognized and even, in some cases, when recognized and treated. Delirium usually indicates the presence of major underlying disease.

    Causes for delirium that are of particular importance in this population include (Harrision's Principles of Internal Medicine, 2005):

    (a) Infection – commonly pneumonia, urinary tract infection and ear infection.

    (b) Electrolyte disturbance – especially hyponatraemia (common with carbamazepine) and dehydration.

    (c) Faecal impaction or urinary retention.

    (d) Medications – especially antipsychotics (during withdrawal and normal use), anticonvulsants and other drugs with anticholinergic action.

    (e) Acute psychiatric disorder.

    (f) Cardiovascular disorder – cardiac failure or infarction.

    (g) Undiagnosed fracture.

(4) Dementia or depression presenting with anhedonia, decreased motivation and deterioration in self-care (see also Chapter 10 by Cooper and Holland).

(5) Post-traumatic stress disorder. Always consider the possibility of abuse presenting as challenging behaviour (see also Chapter by 7 Stavrakaki and Lunsky).

Clinical presentation

While it is not possible to describe all the clinical features which may alert the clinician to an unrecognized condition, there are often clues in the history. A detailed account of the person's current and past medical and psychiatric history, including a developmental and drug history, is recommended. Although essential, the history is often only available if a variety of sources are consulted, including parents, paid daytime and home support staff and a thorough examination of any records (Lennox *et al.*, 2000; Lennox & Eastgate, 2004). When the clinician has a long-term relationship with the person, history taking becomes easier and more efficient.

Once the history is gathered, a complete examination of the person is essential. This examination should include examination of the whole body to exclude trauma or other significant findings, such as undescended testes, unrecognized skin disorders or signs of a progressive neurological disorder (Beange *et al.*, 1995; Sherrard *et al.*, 2001).

When history and examination are completed, a review of common underlying psychiatric and physical causes for the presentation is useful. It is also important to carefully consider the temporal relationship of presenting symptoms. Key questions may include (see also chapter 17 by Reese *et al.*):

(1) Is this an acute, acute on chronic, chronic or fluctuating course?
(2) What major events occurred at or around this time that these symptoms or behaviours arose?
(3) Was this person being abused or neglected?
(4) Are these presenting symptoms proxies for more familiar presentations, such as head banging secondary to headaches or agitation/aggression, indicating pain or psychological distress?
(5) Am I missing one of the commonly overlooked conditions in this population?
(6) Are there useful insights that other health professionals may contribute to increase my understanding?

Investigations will be directed by the history and examination, but may also need to cover commonly missed conditions. A full blood count, ESR, urea and electrolytes, blood glucose, plain abdominal x-ray, thyroid function tests, tests for *Helicobacter pylori*, B12 and folate, Vitamin D, prolactin, mid-stream urine, MRI or CT scan of the brain, bone mineral densitometry and endoscopy, may all reveal clues to the underlying cause of the presentation and/or previously missed problems. Given the frequency of under- or misdiagnosis in this population it would seem appropriate to have a relatively low threshold for investigation, while always considering any risks of the investigation.

In addition to the above, health checks for vision and hearing impairment, dental review, and a review of health promotion and disease prevention activities is important and often overlooked (Lennox & Eastgate, 2004). The evidence strongly suggests that a comprehensive review of the person will improve their health outcomes (Lennox *et al.*, 2004).

Conclusion

Clearly, if we wish to assist any individual, a broad understanding of the biological, psychological, social, and possibly the spiritual circumstances of the person are crucial. This is of particular importance for people with ID as they have numerous social and environmental vulnerabilities and often experience multiple physical and psychiatric conditions. Such conditions are frequently identified late in the presentation, may remain unrecognized and/or may mimic other conditions. In any assessment, a broad understanding will add to the clinicians' ability to understand the whole person and to contribute positively to their physical and psychiatric well-being.

Summary points

- People with impaired communication are at risk of unrecognized psychiatric or medical disorders.
- Changes in behaviour may result from remediable physical or psychiatric pathology, and/or other bio-psycho-socio-spiritual factors.
- People often present with a complex interplay of bio-psycho-socio-spiritual factors.
- Detailed psychiatric and physical assessment is essential.

REFERENCES

Beange, H., McElduff, A. & Baker, W. (1995). Medical disorders of adults with mental retardation: a population study. *American Journal of Mental Retardation*, **99**, 595–604.

Bittles, A. H., Petterson, B. A., Sullivan, S. G. *et al.* (2002). The influence of intellectual disability on life expectancy. *Journals of Gerontology*, **57A**, 470–2.

Boer, H., Holland, A., Whittington, J. *et al.* (2002). Psychotic illness in people with Prader–Willi syndrome due to chromosome 15 maternal uniparental disomy. *Lancet*, **359**, 135–6.

Bohmer, C., Klinkenberg Knol, E., Kuipers, E. *et al.* (1997b). The prevalence of Helicobacter pylori infection among inhabitants and healthy employees of institutes for the intellectually disabled. *American Joural of Gastroenterology*, **92**, 1000–4.

Bohmer, C., Klinkenberg Knol, E., Niezen de Boer, R. *et al.* (1997a). The prevalence of gastro-oesophageal reflux disease based on non-specific symptoms in institutionalized, intellectually disabled individuals. *European Journal of Gastroenterology and Hepatology*, **9**, 187–90.

Bohmer, C. J., Taminiau, J. A., Klinkenberg Knol, E. C. *et al.* (2001). The prevalence of constipation in institutionalized people with intellectual disability. *Journal of Intellectual Disability Research*, **45**, 212–18.

Bowley, C. & Kerr, M. (2000). Epilepsy and intellectual disability. *Journal of Intellectual Disability Research*, **44**, 529–43.

Cathels, B. & Reddihough, D. (1993). The health care of young adults with cerebral palsy. *The Medical Journal of Australia*, **159**, 444–6.

Centre, J., Beange, H. & McElduff, A. (1998). People with mental retardation have an increased prevalence of osteoporosis: A population study. *American Journal of Mental Retardation*, **103**, 19–28.

Centre, J., McElduff, A. & Beange, H. (1994). Osteoporosis in groups with intellectual disability. *Australia and New Zealand Journal of Developmental Disabilities*, **19**, 251–8.

Cumella, S., Ransford, N., Lyons, J. M. & Burnham, H. (2000). Needs for oral care among people with intellectual disability not in contact with community dental services. *Journal of Intellectual Disability Research*, **44**, 45–52.

Cunningham, S., Cunningham, R., Izmeth, M. *et al.* (1994). Seroprevalence of hepatitis B and C in a Merseyside hospital for the mentally handicapped. *Epidemiology and Infection*, **112**, 195–200.

Deb, S., Thomas, M. & Bright, C. (2001). Mental disorder in adults with intellectual disability. 1: Prevalence of functional psychiatric illness among a community-based population aged between 16 and 64 years. *Journal of Intellectual Disability Research*, **45**, 495–505.

Decker, H. A., Herberg, E. N., Haythornthwaite, M. S. *et al.* (1968). Provision of health care for institutionalized retarded children. *American Journal of Mental Deficiency*, **33**, 283–93.

Durvasula, S., Beange, H. & Baker, W. (2002). Mortality of people with intellectual disability in northern Sydney. *Journal of Intellectual & Developmental Disability*, **27**, 255–64.

Emerson, E. (2003). Mothers of children and adolescents with intellectual disability: social and economic situation, mental health status, and the self-assessed social and psychological impact of the child's difficulties. *Journal of Intellectual Disability Research*, **47**, 385–99.

eTG complete. (2004). Therapeutic guidelines; see www.tg.com.au, accessed 25 May 2006.

Evenhuis, H. (1995a). Medical aspects of ageing in a population with intellectual disability: I. Visual impairment. *Journal of Intellectual Disability Research*, **39**, 19–25.

Evenhuis, H. (1995b). Medical aspects of ageing in a population with intellectual disability: II. Hearing impairment. *Journal of Intellectual Disability Research*, **39**, 27–33.

Eyman, R. K., Borthwick Duffy, S. A., Call, T. L. *et al.* (1988). Prediction of mortality in community and institutional settings. *Journal of Mental Deficency Research*, **32**, 203–13.

Eyman, R. K., Grossman, H. J., Chaney, R. H. *et al.* (1993). Survival of profoundly disabled people with severe mental retardation. *American Journal of Diseases of Children*, **147**, 329–36.

Forsgren, L., Edvinsson, S. O., Nystrom, L. *et al.* (1996). Influence of epilepsy on mortality in mental retardation: an epidemiologic study. *Epilepsia*, **37**, 956–63.

Gaventa, W. C. (2003). *Journal of Intellectual Disability Research*, **47**, 565–7.

Gowdey, C. W., Zarfas, D. E. & Phipps, S. (1987). Audit psychoactive drug prescriptions in group homes. *Mental Retardation*, **25**, 331–4.

Griffin, J. M., Fuhrer, R., Stansfeld, S. A. and Marmot, M. (2003). The importance of low control at work and home on depression and anxiety: Do these effects vary by gender and social class? In *Social and Economic Patterning of Health among Women/Les Facteurs Sociaux et Économiques de la Santé des Femmes*, Arber, S. and Khlat, M. (eds.), Paris: CICRED, 2003, pp. 297–330.

Hagerman, R. J. & Cronister, A. (eds.) (1996). *Fragile X Syndrome: Diagnosis, Treatment, and Research* (second edn). Baltimore & London: The Johns Hopkins University Press.

Hand, J. E. (1994). Report of a national survey of older people with lifelong intellectual handicap in New Zealand. *Journal of Intellectual Disability Research*, **38**, 275–87.

Harrison's Principles of Internal Medicine (2005). The McGraw-Hill Companies; Electronic version, accessed 25 May 2006.

Howells, G. (1986). Are the medical needs of mentally handicapped adults being met? *Journal of the Royal College of General Practitioners*, **36**, 449–53.

Jancar, C., Eastham, R. & Carter, G. (1984). Hypocholesterolaemia in cancer and other causes of death in mentally handicapped. *British Journal of Psychiatry*, **145**, 59–61.

Janicki, M. & Dalton, A. (1998). Sensory impairments among older adults with intellectual disability. *Journal of Intellectual and Developmental Disability*, **23**, 3–11.

Janicki, M., Dalton, A., Henderson, C. *et al.* (1999). Mortality and morbidity among older adults with intellectual disability: health services considerations. *Disability and Rehabilitation*, **21**, 284–94.

Jurek, G. & Reid, W. (1994). Oral health of institutionalized individuals with mental retardation. *American Journal of Mental Retardation*, **98**, 656–60.

Kaplan, B. & Sadock, V. (2003). *Kaplan & Sadock's Synopsis of Psychiatry, Behavioural Sciences/Clinical Psychiatry* (ninth edn). New York, NY: Lippincott Williams & Wilkins.

Lennox, N., Beange, H. & Edwards, N. (2000). The health needs of people with intellectual disability. *Medical Journal of Australia.*, **173**, 328–30.

Lennox, N. & Chaplin, R. (1996). The psychiatric care of people with intellectual disabilities: the perceptions of consultant psychiatrists in Victoria. *The Australian and New Zealand Journal of Psychiatry*, **30**(6), 774–80.

Lennox, N. & Diggens, J. (1999). Medical education and intellectual disability: A survey of Australian medical schools. *Journal of Intellectual & Developmental Disability*, **24**, 333–40.

Lennox, N., Diggens, J. & Ugoni, A. (1997). The general practice care of people with an intellectual disability: barriers and solutions. *Journal of Intellectual Disability Research*, **4**, 380–90.

Lennox, N. & Eastgate, G. (2004). Adults with intellectual disability and the GP. *Australian Family Physician*, **33**, 601–6.

Lennox, N. G., Rey-Conde, T., Bain, C. *et al.* (2004). The evidence for better health from health assessments: A large clustered randomised controlled trial. *Journal of Intellectual Disability Research*, **48**, 342.

Marshall, D., McConkey, R. & Moore, G. (2003). Obesity in people with intellectual disabilities: the impact of nurse-led health screenings and health promotion activities. *Journal of Advanced Nursing*, **41**, 147–53.

McDermott, S., Platt, T. & Krishnaswami, S. (1997). Are individuals with mental retardation at high risk for chronic disease? *Family Medicine*, **29**, 429–34.

Morgan, C. L., Baxter, H. & Kerr, A. M. (2003). Prevelence of epilepsy and associated health service utilization and mortality among patients with intellectual disability. *American Journal of Mental Retardation*, **108**, 293–300.

Nelson, R. & Crocker, A. (1978). The medical care of mentally retarded persons in public residential facilities. *The New England Journal of Medicine*, **299**, 1039–44.

O'Brien, G. & Yule, W. (eds.) (1995). *Behavioural Phenotypes* (first edn). London: MacKeith Press.

Parker, G. (1991). Developmentally disabled, doubly disadvantaged. *The Medical Journal of Australia*, **155**, 68–71.

Peach, H. G. (2003). Religion, spirituality and health. *The Medical Journal of Australia*, **178**, 415–16.

Reiss, S., Levitan, G. & Szyszko, J. (1982). Emotional disturbance and mental retardation: diagnostic overshadowing. *American Journal of Mental Deficiency*, **87**, 567–74.

Robertson, J., Emerson, E., Gregory, N. *et al.* (2000). Lifestyle related risk factors for poor health in residential settings for people with intellectual disabilies. *Research in Developmental Disabilities*, **21**(6): 469–86.

Sachdev, P. & Longragan, C. (1991). The present status of akathisia. *The Journal of Nervous and Mental Disease*, **179**, 381–91.

Sherrard, J., Tonge, B. J. & Ozanne Smith, J. (2001). Injury in young people with intellectual disability: descriptive epidemiology. *Injury Prevention Journal of the International Society for Child and Adolescent Injury Prevention*, **7**, 56–61.

Sobsey, D. (1994). *Violence and Abuse in the Lives of People with Disabilities: The End of Silent Acceptance?* Baltimore, MD: Paul H. Brookes Publishing Co.

Sobsey, D. & Doe, T. (1991). Patterns of sexual abuse and assault. *Sexuality and Disability*, **9**, 243–59.

Stehr Green, P., Wilson, N., Miller, J. *et al.* (1991). Risk factors for hepatitis B at a residential institution for intellectually handicapped persons. *New Zealand Medical Journal*, **104**, 514–16.

Tohill, C. (1997). A study into the possible link between anti-epileptic drugs and the risk of fractures in Muckamore Abbey Hospital. *Journal of Intellectual and Developmental Disability*, **22**, 281–92.

Tyler, C. V., Jr. & Bourguet, C. (2000). Primary care of adults with mental retardation. *Journal of Family Practice*, **44**, 487–94.

van Schrojenstein Lantman-de Valk, H. M. J., Akker, M. v. d., Maaskant, M. *et al.* (1997). Prevalence and incidence of health problems in people with intellectual disability. *Journal of Intellectual Disability Research*, **41**, 42–51.

van Schrojenstein Lantman-de Valk, H. M., Metsemakers, J. F., Haveman, M. J. *et al.* (2000). Health problems in people with intellectual disability in general practice: a comparative study. *Family Practice*, **17**, 405–7.

Wallace, R. A., Webb, P. M. & Schluter, P. J. (2002). Environmental, medical, behavioural and disability factors associated with Helicobacter pylori infection in adults with intellectual disability. *Journal of Intellectual Disability Research*, **46**, 51–60.

Warburg, M. (1994). Visual impairment among people with developmental delay. *Journal of Intellectual Disability Research*, **38**, 423–32.

Warburg, M. (2001). Visual impairment in adult people with intellectual disability: literature review. *Journal of Intellectual Disability Research*, **45**, 424–38.

Wells, M. B., Turner, S., Martin, D. M. *et al.* (1997). Health gain through screening – a coronary heart disease and stroke: Developing primary health care services for people with intellectual disability. *Journal of Intellectual and Developmental Disability*, **22**, 251–63.

White, M. J. N., Cassandra, N., Cook, R. S. *et al.* (1995). Diagnostic overshadowing and mental retardation: A meta-analysis. *American Journal on Mental Retardation*, **100**, 293–8.

Wilson, D. & Haire, A. (1990). Health care screening for people with mental handicap living in the community. *British Medical Journal*, **301**, 1379–81.

Yang, Q., Rasmussen, S. A. & Friedman, J. M. (2002). Mortality associated with Down's syndrome in the USA from 1983 to 1997: a population-based study. *Lancet*, **359**, 1019–25.

Part II

Psychopathology and special topics

6

The psychopathology of children with intellectual disabilities

Bruce Tonge

Introduction

There is no doubt that emotional and behavioural problems are a significant extra dimension that burdens the lives of many children with intellectual disabilities (ID) and their families and carers. Young people with ID have about three times as much psychiatric disturbance as children of average intelligence. Rutter *et al.* (1970), in their Isle of Wight population study, found that 50 per cent of children with ID with an IQ below 70 had a psychiatric disorder, compared with 6.8 per cent of children with an IQ above 70. Corbett (1979), in a study of the urban area of south-east London, found a prevalence rate of psychiatric disorder of 47 per cent in children aged up to 15 years of IQ below 50.

An epidemiological study of Australian children with ID aged between 4 and 18 years found that 41 per cent had a clinically significant emotional or behavioural disorder (Einfeld & Tonge, 1996). The study also found that disruptive and antisocial behaviours were more common in young people with mild ID but self-absorbed and social relating problem behaviours were more common in young people with more severe ID. In contrast to general childhood psychopathology, age and sex did not affect prevalence. Of concern was that fewer than 10 per cent of these children with ID had received any specialist mental health services.

A recent epidemiological study of a national survey of mental health information on more than 10 000 children aged 5 to 15 years in Great Britain revealed that 39 per cent of children with ID met DSM-IV and ICD-10 criteria for at least one psychiatric disorder, compared with 8.1 per cent of children without ID (Emerson, 2003).

Phenomenology

Children with ID can suffer from the full range of psychopathological disorders experienced by children of normal intelligence. Although the diagnosis of

Psychiatric and Behavioural Disorders in Intellectual and Developmental Disabilities, ed. Nick Bouras and Geraldine Holt. Published by Cambridge University Press. © Cambridge University Press 2007.

psychiatric disorders is unlikely in preschool children, there is evidence that by age 3 developmentally delayed children are three times more likely to have a clinically significant level of emotional and behavioural disturbance which persists to age 4 (Baker *et al.*, 2002, Baker *et al.*, 2003). Anxiety disorders, depression and bipolar affective disorders, attention deficit hyperactivity disorder (ADHD), schizophrenia and psychotic disorders have all been described in young people with ID (Matson & Barrett, 1982). Children with ID, compared with children without ID, are at greater risk for ADHD, conduct disorders, depression, anxiety disorders (including separation anxiety and phobias) and autistic disorder (Emerson, 2003; Tonge & Einfeld, 2003; Stromme & Diseth, 2000). ID is present in at least 70 per cent of cases of autism (Prior & Tonge, 1990). There is not yet an international agreement on a common approach to the classification and diagnosis of the range of disturbed emotions and behaviours exhibited. There are some patterns of disturbed emotions and behaviours in young people with ID that cannot be adequately described by current psychiatric diagnostic systems such as the ICD-10 (World Health Organization, 1992) and the DSM-IV (American Psychiatric Association, 1994) (see also Chapter 1 by Sturmey). The validity of these two major systems of psychiatric diagnosis is yet to be demonstrated when applied to young people with ID.

The types of psychopathological disorders in children with mild ID are more likely to resemble those found in the general population. It is increasingly difficult for the clinician to apply the criteria of existing diagnostic classifications in individuals with more severe levels of ID who do not have the ability to share with others the content of their thinking and emotional experience. In these circumstances a diagnosis must be made on the basis of observed behaviours and change in patterns of behaviour, daily living skills, interests, social interaction and interpersonal relationships.

A supplement to the ICD-10, *The ICD-10 Guide for Mental Retardation* (World Health Organization, 1996), is an important attempt to approach this issue. This guide has some applicability to the psychiatric assessment of children with ID (Einfeld & Tonge, 2000). Further research is required in order to establish if certain behavioural problems are more common, or even unique, in people with ID. The development of a new taxonomy of psychiatric syndromes or disorders is required that takes into account symptoms specific to persons with ID and the limitations that impaired communication ability places on the assessment of diagnostic criteria (McLean, 1990; Rutter, 1991). An example of such a new psychopathological disorder specific to ID, which is included in ICD-10, is 'over active disorder associated with mental retardation and stereotype movements' (World Health Organization, 1992). The Royal College of Psychiatrists (2001) has produced diagnostic criteria for psychiatric disorders in adults with ID, the DC-LD, which relates to ICD-10 and DSM-IV classification systems. Although designed for use in adults, the

DC-LD does provide criteria for some disorders first manifest in children: specifically, Pervasive and Specific Developmental Disorders and Hyperkinetic Disorders, as well as some Problem Behaviours such as oppositional behaviour (see also Chapter 1 by Sturmey).

Another approach to the description of emotional and behavioural problems is the quantitative taxonometric model based on the statistical analysis of symptom questionnaires collected on defined populations of individuals with ID. A review of six rating scales used to describe psychopathology in persons with ID identified six similar groupings of disturbance derived by factor analysis related to aggression – antisocial behaviour, disruptive-hyperactive behaviour, repetitive communication disturbance, anxiety-fearfulness and social withdrawal (Aman, 1991). These factors describe common dimensions or syndromes of disturbance and therefore have clinical utility but the checklist approach is less likely to detect uncommon disorders.

An example of this approach in children are studies using the Developmental Behaviour Checklist (DBC), a reliable and valid 96-item questionnaire of emotional and behavioural problems in young people with ID that is completed by parents, or carers, or teachers (Einfeld & Tonge, 2002) (see also Chapter 2 by Mohr & Costello). These studies have followed the mental health of a representative sample of young people aged 4–18 years with ID over the past 14 years, which initially included a sub-sample of 309 children aged 4–12 years (Tonge *et al.* 1996, Tonge & Einfeld, 2003). At the beginning of this study, 45 per cent of the children had clinically significant levels of emotional and behavioural disorder. Symptoms of ADHD, manifest as poor concentration, distractibility, impulsiveness and hyperactivity, were present in 32 per cent of the children. The symptoms were not related to gender – in contrast to the general population, where ADHD is more prevalent in males. The prevalence of ADHD symptoms significantly reduced to 14 per cent over 14 years as the young people moved into late adolescence and early adult life, suggesting a maturational effect. This happened at a faster rate for girls (decreasing to 9 per cent) than for boys (decreasing to 17 per cent). A total of 9 per cent of the children were reported by their parents to have persistent symptoms of depression, tearfulness, irritability and low self-esteem. This prevalence of depression did not change over 14 years and was not related to gender – in contrast to the general population, where depression increases through adolescence and is more common in females. These symptoms of depression were less prevalent (3 per cent) among those with severe or profound ID.

There were 8 per cent of children who suffered from anxiety and phobias. The prevalence of anxiety disorders did not change over 14 years among boys, but increased among girls (to 20 per cent), though initially there was no significant gender difference. In the general population of young people, females are twice as likely as males to suffer from anxiety disorders (Tonge, 1988). Those with severe or profound ID had a lower prevalence of anxiety disorders. These findings indicate that specific psychopathological disorders of childhood such as ADHD, depression and anxiety are at least four to five times more prevalent in children with ID than in other children. Co-morbidity is also common, with 19 per cent of the children with ADHD also suffering from depression and 12 per cent from anxiety. For children with depression 70 per cent also have ADHD and 30 per cent have anxiety. The burden of specific psychopathological disorders in young people with ID highlights the imperative for better assessment and treatment services for this at risk group of children.

Clinical assessment

The clinical interview is the essential component in diagnosis and assessment and is therefore necessary in the process of deciding on a rational management and treatment plan. The presence and severity of ID in the child necessitates some modification of a routine child psychiatric assessment and mental state examination. Information from the parents or carers and direct observation of the child, preferably in a variety of settings such as at school as well as at the clinician's office, are essential.

Cox and Rutter (1985) have demonstrated that the combined use of non-directive interview techniques together with more directive and structured questions, supplemented by parent and teacher completed checklists, provides the most comprehensive information and significantly improves assessment and diagnosis. This combined, unstructured and structured approach is still effective in promoting rapport and the expression of affect.

This work has been replicated in an analysis of 70 psychiatric assessments of children with ID (Einfeld & Tonge, 2002). The non-directive interview component of the assessment revealed parental concern regarding an average of nine symptoms; compared to an average of 35 symptoms scored by the parents on a DBC they had previously completed (Einfeld & Tonge, 2002). The use of a parent or carer completed checklist such as the DBC clearly enriches the clinical assessment process, and parents reported that they felt the problems they faced had been fully explored and understood.

A framework for the clinical assessment is presented in Table 6.1.

It is useful during part of the assessment to interview the parents or carers and the child, together, and if the child can manage the separation, it is essential to see the child individually. Information from others, such as teachers, provides a broader perspective as well as information on contextual elements of the child's emotional or behavioural problems, and more resilient and adaptive behaviour. A comprehensive cognitive assessment is also necessary in order to place the child's

Table 6.1 Clinical assessment.

Interview with parent(s)/carers
Presenting problems: detailed description, antecedents, context, consequences
Mental state: anxieties and worries, fears, mood, anger and aggression, perceptual disturbances and
  sensitivities
Behavioural review: appetite and eating, sleep, bowel and bladder control, play and interests, family/carer/
  sibling attachment, socialization and friendships, activity level, learning and school adjustment,
  concentration and impulsiveness, behavioural control, disruptiveness and compliance, repetitive and
  compulsive behaviour, response to change, motor skills and co-ordination, sexual behaviours,
  episodic/cyclical phenomena
Developmental history: pregnancy, birth, attachment behaviour and separations, milestones, cognitive and
  learning, medical illnesses/treatment, communication and socialization, abuse/neglect and alternative care
Family history: (best completed during the family meeting), genogram, parental health, mental health and
  relationship, family illnesses, mental illness, learning problems, genetic disorders, siblings, social and
  cultural context, support and adversity
Parent/carer-completed questionnaires (e.g. DBC)

Interview with child
Rapport-building discussion, play
School experience: friends, learning, play, teasing
Mental state: observation, worries/anxieties, fears, mood, anger, perceptual disturbance (e.g. hallucinations,
  delusions)
Play: free and structured (e.g. form boards), drawing (squiggle, draw a person, draw a dream), motor skills
  (catching, hopping, pencil grip)
Medical/neurological examination

Other investigations (as indicated)
Teacher's reports
Psychological/cognitive assessment
Medical investigations (e.g. EEG, chromosome analysis, metabolic studies)
Multidisciplinary case conference

Complete multiaxial diagnosis

DSM-IV-TR (APA, 2000)	ICD-10 (WHO, 1996)	DC-LD (RC Psych, 2001)
Axis I	Axis I	Axis I
Clinical disorders	Severity of retardation and problem behaviours	Severity of LD
Axis II	Axis II	Axis II
Personality disorder	Associated medical	Causes of LD
Mental retardation	conditions	
Axis III	Axis III	Axis III
General medical conditions	Associated psychiatric disorders	A. Developmental disorders
		B. Psychiatric illness
Axis IV	Axis IV	C. Personality disorders
Psychosocial and	Global assessment of	D. Problem behaviours
environmental problems	psychosocial disability	E. Other disorders
Axis V	Axis V	Appendices
Global assessment of	Associated abnormal	• ID behavioural phenotypes
functioning	psychosocial	• Medical conditions
	situations	• Factors influencing health status

behaviour into a developmental perspective and to understand the influence and impact of any cognitive impairments or specific pattern of cognitive performance on behaviour, communication and comprehension. For example, children with autism usually have better visual and performance skills than verbal and social comprehension skills, which can account for some of their frustration and difficult behaviour and has implications for education and management.

Assessments of communication and motor skills can also add considerable information to the overall picture. To date, there are no standardized general psychiatric assessment interviews validated for use with young people with ID. The parent's version of the Anxiety Disorders Interview Schedule (Albano & Silverman, 1996), which provides an algorithm for DSM-IV diagnoses, is being used in some clinical studies of anxiety disorders in children with moderate or less severe levels of ID. In the specific area of autism spectrum disorders, Lord *et al.* (1994) have developed the Autism Diagnostic Instrument (ADI), which comprises a structured parental interview. The ADI is supplemented by a clinician-led, structured play task interaction with the child: the Autism Diagnostic Observation Schedule (ADOS) (Lord *et al.*, 1999). The ADI/ADOS provides a reliable and valid diagnosis of pervasive developmental disorders. It requires a skilled clinician to administer and is appropriately time consuming, given the complexity and the serious implications of this diagnosis.

The application of current psychiatric classification becomes more difficult as the severity of ID increases. At profound levels of ID, a form of organic brain syndrome is the only diagnosis that is likely to be made with any reliability.

It is evident that the psychiatric assessment of young people with ID is complex, and requires information from all those involved in their care, as well as detailed mental state, psychological, developmental and physical assessment of the child. This process is usually of necessity a multidisciplinary one, requiring contributions from psychiatrists, psychologists, paediatricians and, when appropriate, others such as speech pathologists, occupational therapists, physiotherapists and special teachers. To be effective, this multidisciplinary assessment requires co-ordination, usually through a case conference in which one of the specialist clinicians is designated as the case manager.

Assessment issues

There is usually a range of contextual problems and factors that influence and complicate the presentation of emotional and behavioural problems in young people with ID, which need to be taken into account in order to achieve a satisfactory assessment, diagnosis and a rational treatment plan (Tonge & Einfeld, 1991).

Developmental level and cognitive ability

The diagnosis of many psychiatric disorders requires an assessment of the person's thought processes and content. This may be possible in a child with mild ID and some communication skills, but becomes progressively more difficult as the level of disability becomes more severe. Costello (1982) argues that it is impossible to diagnose schizophrenia in people with an IQ under 45 because their lack of cognitive and verbal ability makes it virtually impossible for thought disorder, delusional thinking, and for any perceptual abnormality such as auditory hallucinations to be assessed. The development of persistent disorganized behaviour has been suggested as a behavioural equivalent of psychosis in individuals with more severe levels of ID who are unable to communicate perceptual phenomena (Hardy-Bayle *et al.*, 2003, Cherry *et al.*, 2000). However there is still no reliable and valid method to diagnose psychosis purely on the basis of observed behaviour (see also Chapter 8 by Clarke). Similar problems apply to the diagnosis of affective disorder, for which impaired communication skill and concrete thinking, even in the more able, makes it difficult, if not impossible, for young people with ID to describe their feelings. The clinician must often rely on observation of behaviour and signs such as changes in appetite, sleep and activity level, as well as observed mood, to make a presumptive diagnosis of affective disorder (Costello, 1982; Sovner, 1986) (see also Chapters 3 by O'Hara and 4 by Hemmings). The developmental level of a child must also be taken into account when assessing the significance of problem behaviours. Normal behaviours in young children, such as separation anxiety or short attention span, may be seen in a much older child with ID who is still functioning at that younger developmental level. This is recognized by some of the diagnostic categories in DSM-IV-TR (Text Revision) (APA, 2000) and ICD-10 (World Health Organization, 1992) such as autistic disorder and attention deficit hyperactivity disorder, which indicate that the criteria for these disorders are only met if the behaviour is abnormal for a person of the same mental age and developmental level. The assessment of antisocial, aggressive and defiant behaviour should take into account the child's developmental level when making a diagnosis of conduct disorder. The capacity of the child to understand social rules and right from wrong usually excludes children with autism or more severe levels of ID from the diagnosis of conduct disorder. In some children, organic deterioration of cognitive ability, or behavioural consequences of puberty and hormones may also cause psychopathological symptoms and complicate or alter response to treatment.

Multiple disabilities and medical illness

Children and adolescents with ID are more likely than the general population to have a range of physical and sensory impairments and medical illness that handicap their lives and complicate the assessment of emotional and behavioural problems (Sovner & Hurley, 1989). For example, deafness may lead to behaviour that is seen in autistic children or children with conduct disorder. Hearing impairment may also aggravate psychiatric disorders such as separation anxiety. Children with ID are much more likely to have medical illnesses or abnormalities of the brain such as epilepsy. Children in the general population with chronic illness that affects the brain have a higher prevalence of associated psychiatric disorder (Tonge, 1991). Epilepsy can cause disturbed behaviour and aggravate existing emotional and behavioural problems, particularly if the epilepsy is poorly controlled (Lewis *et al.*, 2000). Down syndrome is associated with oppositional, defiant behaviour in childhood, then an earlier adult onset of Alzheimer's dementia (Rubin, 1987). The onset of depression and a loss of interest in usual activities during adolescence might herald this decline (Einfeld *et al.*, 2000). Autism is associated with a range of medical conditions such as tuberous sclerosis and other psychiatric conditions such as Tourette syndrome (Prior & Tonge, 1990). Specific patterns of behaviour are also evident as the behavioural phenotypic expression of some genetic disorders associated with ID, for example shyness in children with fragile X syndrome (Einfeld *et al.*, 1994), and insomnia, anxiety and irrepressibility in children with William's syndrome (Einfeld *et al.*, 1997). Children with Prader–Willi syndrome are likely to develop other obsessive compulsive disorder problems unrelated to food, aggressive impulsive behaviour and anxiety and depression, then psychosis as they move into adult life (Dykens, 1998; Einfeld *et al.*, 1998). Children with ID may also not be able to communicate effectively that they are suffering from pain or the symptoms of a fever or physical illness. Instead, they may exhibit disturbed behaviour such as irritability, restlessness, or withdrawal, which may be misunderstood as being caused by a psychiatric disorder.

Psychosocial and family factors

Children and adolescents with ID are more likely than the general population to experience a range of psychosocial stresses and environmental experiences that adversely affect their personality development, emotional adjustment and attachment behaviour and can result in impoverished or distorted and inappropriate social behaviour (Sovner, 1986; Aman & Schroeder, 1990). The families of children living in alternative residential care may not be available for interview to provide reliable developmental and family histories. Institutional records often give an unreliable and inadequate account of the person's history. Observation and assessment of the child's interaction with the family, or with staff and residents of the alternative care environment, are essential in order to understand the behaviour and psychosocial context and the contribution that these interactions make to the psychopathology. For example, in response to environmental stress, some children with ID may experience a regression and disintegration of their already impaired cognition, resulting in bizarre and psychotic-like behaviour that can be misdiagnosed as schizophrenia. Another child might be withdrawn, listless and apathetic in response to parental overprotection and lack of stimulation. Environmental deprivation and abuse, and a lack of stimulation and opportunity for play, activity and socialization, aggravate ID, prevent children from reaching their full potential, and lead to a range of attachment, personality, emotional and behavioural problems and handicaps.

Caring for a child with ID is also associated with an increased risk that the parents may suffer from mental health problems and stress particularly when the child also has emotional and behavioural problems (Baker *et al.*, 2003). Therefore the effective management of emotional and behavioural disorder in a child with ID may also require parent education, support and management of any parent mental health problems such as maternal depression or paternal alcohol abuse.

Management principles

Successful management begins with the establishment of a positive relationship with the parents and carers and, if possible, the child during the assessment process. A working diagnosis that takes into account the biological, psychological and social contributing factors and context, provides the key to a rational management plan. Treatment is usually multimodal, requiring a combination of parent support and skills training, behavioural interventions, modifications to the social and educational environment, modified psychological treatments and, as a second line of treatment in combination with psychological and supported management, the use of psychoactive medication when indicated (Table 6.2).

Some young people with moderate or less severe level of ID have sufficient communication skills and understanding of consequences to be able to benefit from a modified form of cognitive behaviour therapy. This involves a combination of relaxation training, modelling and reinforcement of confident and prosocial behaviours, formulating positive self-thoughts and statements instead of negative attributions, and providing a structured experience of rewarding educational and social activities and skills.

There is no evidence that family therapy has a direct effect, but it does reduce family dysfunction and conflict and modify problematic family interactional patterns, such as parental overprotection, which contribute to psychopathology in the child. The provision to the parents of educational information on ID in general, and on the nature of the ID and the psychopathological disorder in their child in particular, helps the parents generate their own adaptive responses and co-operate as partners with a range of services in the management of their child. A co-operative working relationship with the parents does make it more likely that they will feel encouraged to share their grief regarding their child's disability, and this in itself is

Table 6.2 Approaches to management.

Assessment and diagnosis

Behaviour analysis and management

Cognitive-behavioural therapy modified according to level of intellectual disability (e.g.
    relaxation, modelling, behavioural reinforcement, positive statements, social skills,
    including social stories and role play; schedule activities of interest, reward achievement,
    promote self esteem)

Communication, motor, sensory-integrative skills training

Special education

Parent education, support and skills training

Family therapy

Social support (e.g. respite care, home help)

Psychotropic drugs, judicious selection, follow-up to monitor compliance, side-effects and
    response

Consultation and case conferencing with parents, carers and other professionals

also therapeutic. Counselling and the provision of psychological and educational interventions for siblings may also be necessary to promote family functioning.

Behaviour management using operant conditioning techniques can be an effective strategy for managing difficult behaviours. The design of an effective behaviour-modification programme requires a detailed behavioural analysis regarding the context, the communication intent of the behaviour, consequences that reinforce the behaviour, i.e. the response by others to the behaviour, and the longer-term consequences of the behaviour.

There is a secondary role of drug treatment, but it should form part of a broader psychotherapeutic and supportive management plan. Most research on the use of pharmacotherapy in children with ID is focused on aggression and self-injurious behaviours (see also Chapter 19 by King). Controlled trials of haloperidol and more recently risperidone have shown that they are effective in the treatment of aggression, hyperactivity and stereotypic behaviours, particularly in children with ID and autism; although these drugs, particularly haloperidol, are associated with dystonic reaction and other troublesome side effects (Campbell *et al.*, 1993; Lindsay & Aman, 2003). Lithium, carbamazepine, beta-blockers such as propranolol and the alpha-2 antagonist clonidine, have been shown (mostly in open trials) to reduce aggressive, disruptive and agitated behaviour. Opiate agonists and antagonists (e.g. naloxone and naltrexone) may have some role in reducing self-injurious behaviours (Botteron & Geller, 1993). Stimulant drugs such as dexamphetamine and methylphenidate may be useful in the treatment of unequivocal attention deficit and hyperactivity symptoms (Birmaher *et al.*, 1988; Dulcan, 1990), but the efficacy of the more recent atomoxetine in children with ID has not been established.

A favourable response to stimulant medication in children with ID and those with autism who also have attention deficit hyperactivity disorder may not be as marked as in children with attention deficit hyperactivity disorder who do not have ID. In young people with more severe ID, stimulant drugs may even exacerbate stereotypic and disturbed behaviour. Anxious and obsessional behaviour in young people with ID, particularly those with autism, may respond to treatment with selective serotonin reuptake inhibitors such as fluoxetine, and the older tricyclic antidepressants such as clomipramine and imipramine, but firm evidence from controlled trials is still required, and it is not clear if these reported therapeutic effects are caused by specific effects on serotonin metabolism. Drug treatment requires regular follow-up and monitoring for compliance, the development of side effects and therapeutic response. It is preferable to document the therapeutic response through the use of behavioural observations and a symptom checklist.

Case examples

The application of the clinical principles outlined in this chapter is highlighted in the following four case studies.

1. Susan, aged seven years

Susan was reported by the school psychologist to have a severe degree of ID and little functional language. She was integrated into a rural primary school. She did not participate in educational or social activities, and sat at the back of the class on a rubber mat because she was incontinent. Susan spent most of her time rocking, being withdrawn and 'nodding off to sleep'. Both the teacher and the school psychologist were concerned that she might have autism or a degenerative condition. Her parents reported that her behaviour was similar at home. Her birth was a complicated forceps delivery caused by failure to progress in labour, and there was associated perinatal cerebral anoxia. She was an irritable baby with delayed developmental milestones, but did form a reciprocal attachment with her parents and showed emerging play and social skills. She had a series of grand mal epileptic seizures between 18 months and two years of age, and was placed on anticonvulsant medication. The family then moved to a small country town, and although she remained on a low dose of anticonvulsant medication, a specialist neurologist did not review her epilepsy again. When this was finally reviewed as part of this assessment, it was found on EEG that she was having frequent epileptic activity and complex partial seizures, which were associated with incontinence, cognitive impairment and behavioural withdrawal and disturbance. The re-introduction of a therapeutic level of anticonvulsant medication produced a dramatic therapeutic response, with improvements in her cognitive ability, communication and social skills, mood and behaviour, and capacity to enjoy life. Her teacher even jokingly complained that she had become assertive in pushing to join in all the classroom activities. Subsequent cognitive assessment revealed that the level of her ID was in the moderate range.

The next two examples are teenage boys who were referred with the same problem behaviour: that of masturbating in public.

2. Bill, aged 13 years

Bill had a moderate degree of ID, with some basic language skills, and attended a special school. He lived with his mother and father and two younger siblings. The cause of his ID was not known, although he had some dysmorphic features and was a tall, ungainly and clumsy boy for his age. The school and his parents referred him because he was masturbating in public. This activity was solitary and in the context of general social withdrawal, but occurred in public places, such as an isolated corner of the school grounds and the back corner of a supermarket.

The parents completed the DBC, which provided a score of 44 with 38 problem items checked. These comprised 22 emotional disturbance items (internalizing symptoms), 1 social relating problem item and 14 disturbed behaviour items (externalizing problems). The items that were noted by the parents as being 'very true or often true' about Bill were: appears depressed and unhappy, cries easily, irritable, lacks self-confidence, poor self-esteem, and loss of appetite (with weight loss of around 2 kg over the past six months). Bill also had frequent temper tantrums and the questionnaire revealed that he was generally distressed and anxious, had some nightmares, and had become fearful about going to school and leaving the house and becoming separated from his mother. These behaviours had been getting worse over the preceding 12 months.

Bill presented as a dejected and depressed-looking boy, who was listless and appeared to have no energy. He was generally withdrawn and showed no interest in toys or play activity. He became distressed and anxious when separated from his parents and spent some time crying. His parents claimed that he had told them he wished he was dead, although it was not possible during the assessment to get him to communicate verbally, other than with some occasional monosyllabic answers.

His symptoms and presentation fulfilled the DSM-IV diagnostic criteria for a dysthymic disorder. There were some contributing family factors. His paternal grandmother and a paternal uncle had both been treated for depressive illness. Bill's emotional disorder began about 18 months earlier, at about the time of onset of puberty. Growth and hormonal changes of puberty may have contributed to his depression, but at that time his parents also began to have increasing unresolved parental conflict about a number of interpersonal and financial problems. This marital conflict had led to brief marital separation on two occasions. Therefore,

Bill's depressive illness and anxiety had occurred in the context of a probable genetic predisposition, but was also influenced by the biological and psychological impact of puberty and significant interactional distress, consequent upon parental marital conflict.

Treatment involved the use of a tricyclic antidepressant (imipramine) chosen also for its anxiolytic effects, participation in a social skills training group, and a behavioural programme at school and at home aimed at building self-esteem through setting achievable tasks and rewarding and positively commenting on all achievements, no matter how small. The parents were also keen to seek help for their marital difficulties and were able to resolve these after a few sessions of marital therapy. Bill made a good response to these treatments and within four weeks was more cheerful and positive, had regained his appetite and was sleeping well, had more energy and was interested in social relationships. He no longer engaged in self-preoccupied masturbation in public.

3. Brian, aged 15 years

Brian had a moderate level of ID and simple language skills. He lived with his parents and attended a special school. His mother suffered toxaemia during the pregnancy. His birth was prolonged and complicated and he may have suffered some degree of cerebral anoxia.

His parents completed the DBC, which revealed a total score of 62. A total of 35 behavioural problems (externalizing) were identified, and 2 emotional problems (internalizing) and 8 social-relating problem behaviours were described. Most of the disturbed behaviour items related to disruptive overactive behaviour with associated distractibility and limited attention span. He was noisy and boisterous, particularly in the family meeting, interrupting his parents with a mixture of sounds and simple phrases. He was also aggressive, uncooperative and generally very difficult to manage by both his parents and teachers. His masturbatory behaviour, which led to the referral, was not frequent but occurred as a provocative and threatening act towards his female teacher and also a party of young girls having a picnic in a park near the family home, from which he had run away. Both the parents and the school believed that it might be better for Brian to be cared for in a community residential unit. Brian presented as a wiry boy for his age, who acted as if he was driven by a motor. He could not sit still and focus on any task, particularly when he was together with his parents in a room that contained many toys and other items of interest. In a small, confined room, bare except for table and chairs, he was able to focus better on items such as a form board when these were individually shown to him, although he generally remained easily distracted. Neurological examination revealed some soft neurological signs and clumsiness, more marked on the right side of his body. Further detailed neurological assessment failed to find any specific neurological disorder. He had entered puberty 9–12 months earlier.

Brian was the youngest child in the family, with two older brothers in their early twenties who had not experienced any developmental difficulty. There was no family history of any physical or psychiatric illnesses. His parents had a good and effective relationship and there were no significant interactional difficulties in the family. Brian had always been an overactive and easily distracted boy, but since entering puberty this behaviour had become significantly worse and, with his larger body size, he was more difficult to manage.

Taking his moderate degree of ID into account, his symptoms were still excessive for a child of his mental age, and therefore a DSM-IV diagnosis of attention deficit hyperactivity disorder could be made. It is possible that hormonal and other biological changes of puberty had produced a worsening of his behaviour. Increase in body size and new behavioural problems of a sexual nature made him more difficult to manage at home and school, and created anxiety for both parents and teachers, who had previously been able to contain and manage him. On the basis of this assessment, he received a trial of a stimulant medication (methylphenidate), which produced a rapid and dramatic improvement in his behaviour. He became less active and his attention span improved, particularly in one-to-one or small-group teaching situations in which there was a focused activity and no distractions in the surrounding environment. A behaviour modification programme, based on a combination of reducing environmental stimulation and providing a range of separate enjoyable tasks for which his performance was rewarded, was instituted. His father also involved Brian in a daily exercise programme of swimming in a private pool, where there were no other distractions, and bicycle riding in a quiet park. These activities were undertaken in consultation with a physiotherapist, who also provided a remedial gymnasium programme at the school. All of these interventions combined to create a significant improvement in Brian's behaviour, which could be contained by his parents and teachers. The use of stimulant medication was kept under review and its effectiveness was tested by occasional periods off the medication.

4. Darren, aged 16 years

Darren was referred because of disruptive behaviour, particularly in the environment of the residential unit in which he lived. Over the past year, he increasingly had arguments with the other residents and, when reprimanded by the staff and put into his bedroom for time out, he would become angry and lose control, smashing furniture, breaking windows, kicking doors and walls. After up to an hour of rage, he would calm down and then usually become remorseful and emotionally upset about the episode. He had a mild degree of ID and attended a special school. His educational progress was not as good as might be expected, given his relatively mild degree of ID documented on psychological assessment. He was socially confident, at times beyond the level of his social competence and skill, and this led to problems. For example, he would abscond and take public transport, claiming he was looking for a relative, but end up getting lost. His father and three younger siblings lived in another state.

The care staff of the residential unit completed the DBC. This revealed a score of 39, with 15 problems in the emotional (internalizing) problem area and 18 items of disturbed behaviour (externalizing) being identified. The major behaviours identified were that he was often downcast and unhappy, with poor self-esteem, and showed frequent mood changes, and that he also frequently had tempers and was irritable. Staff had heard him talk on several occasions about killing himself, after angry outbursts. He was reported to make up stories about what he had been doing and was regarded as untrustworthy by the staff. The record of his past history was inadequate. The record revealed that he had a mild degree of developmental delay and was rather overactive during childhood, but was otherwise no problem for his parents. His mother died in a motor-car accident when Darren was aged nine. His behaviour began to deteriorate in early secondary school and his father requested alternative care for Darren when he was 13. At that time he was reported to be irritable and aggressive, frequently absconded from home and was threatening towards the young children of the woman with whom his father was living and subsequently married. His father, stepmother and all the other children in the family moved to another state shortly after Darren was placed in a residential unit. Since then, he had only occasional contact with his father and had not been given his telephone number or address.

Darren presented as a tall, rather thin young man. He was initially inappropriately overfriendly, demonstrating clumsy social skills. He embellished accounts of events and it was obvious that at times he made up stories to put himself in a favourable light. He had few, if any, friends, although he was very keen to visit places where young people gathered, such as a local shopping centre, and observe and try to participate in the activities of these young people. He became upset when talking of his father and it became clear that he could not understand why his father had gone to live in another state without taking him with the family. When asked to draw a picture of a bad dream (Tonge, 1982), he produced the drawing in Figure 6.1. He said 'I'm in mum's car on the way from her work. A truck was out of the lane. There was crash. Mum died.' He spoke with increasing distress about the accident in which his mother died. He was also in the car, but was lucky to escape uninjured. He observed his mother being covered by a sheet and taken away in the ambulance, never to see her again. He was not allowed to go to the funeral. He claimed that often he would go out to try to look for the cemetery where his mother is buried,

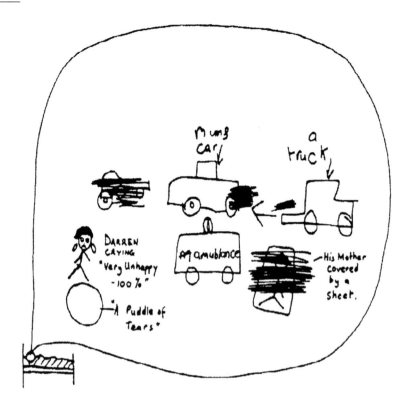

Fig. 6.1   Darren's dream drawing.

although he had no idea where that is. He was asked to draw a picture of himself, showing how he still felt about his mother's death. He drew a picture of himself crying, with a puddle of tears at his feet, saying that he was 'very unhappy 100 per cent'.

Darren presented with a depressive disorder that fulfilled the DSM-IV criteria for dysthymia. This was in the setting of prolonged psychosocial stress, beginning with the death of his mother. He had not been able to resolve his loss satisfactorily and the process of grief and mourning had been further complicated by rejection from his family and his placement in a residential unit that had frequently changing staff. A number of different treatment approaches was needed in order to help him recover from this complex psychological disorder, from which he had suffered for seven years of his life. A morning dose of a selective serotonin reuptake inhibitor (SSRI) antidepressant (fluoxetine) was prescribed. A behavioural programme was provided that focused on relaxation skills and training for anger management, which included some aspects of cognitive therapy that taught him to say positive things about himself. It was realized that Darren's superficial social confidence covered some significant deficits in social skills, so arrangements were made for him to attend a social skills training group at his school. He attended fortnightly for some brief psychotherapy aimed at helping him ventilate his grief, anger and distress about events in his life such as his mother's death and his father moving away. Arrangements were made for him to visit his mother's grave. The supervisor of the residential unit went to considerable effort to contact the father and, after some initial difficulty, managed to get the father to contact Darren on a regular basis by telephone. Finally, regular holidays with his father were arranged. This treatment process took about 12 months, but at the end of that time Darren had become a co-operative and helpful member of the residential unit, was making significant educational progress at school, and was exhibiting social behaviour more appropriate to a young adolescent.

Conclusion

There is no doubt that psychiatric disorder is a major source of distress, extra handicap and burden for young people with ID and their families, carers and teachers. Considerable research is required to understand further the epidemiology, phenomenology, classification, aetiology and treatment of this psychopathology. However, by taking a comprehensive bio-psycho-social approach to the assessment of these often complex emotional and behavioural problems, a diagnosis and multidimensional formulation become possible, which then provide the basis for a rational treatment and management plan.

Summary points

- Children with ID have 3–4 times the prevalence of psychopathology than other children. Co-morbidity is common.
- Assessment comprises a combined non-directive and structured interview of parents and child together and separately, supplemented by questionnaires competed by parents and teachers.
- Diagnosis is more difficult in children with more severe ID but a combination of categorical diagnosis (ICD or DSM) together with a quantitative checklist description of symptoms provides a useful formulation on which to base a treatment plan.
- The presenting mental state of the child is influenced by intellectual level and profile of cognitive skills; the presence of physical disabilities and medical illness; parental mental health; family function and social context.
- Treatment is usually multimodal and family focused, including parent education and skills training, special education, behaviour management, modified cognitive behavioural therapy and psychotherapy and, if indicated, pharmacotherapy targeted at specific symptoms or diagnoses for which there is evidence of efficacy.
- Follow up of response to treatment facilitated by a symptom checklist is necessary.

REFERENCES

Albano, A. M. & Silverman, W. K. (1996). *Anxiety Disorders Interview Schedule for DSM4V. Clinicians Manual.* San Antonio IX: The Psychological Corporation, Harcourt Brace & Company.

Aman, M. G. (1991). Review and evaluation of instruments for assessing emotional and behavioural disorders. *Australian and New Zealand Journal of Developmental Disabilities,* **17,** 127–45.

Aman, M. G. & Schroeder, S. R. (1990). Specific learning disorders and mental retardation. In *Handbook of Studies on Child Psychiatry,* ed. B. J. Tonge, G. D. Burrows & J. Werry, pp. 209–24. Amsterdam: Elsevier.

American Psychiatric Association (1994). *Diagnostic and Statistical Manual of Mental Disorders,* 4th edn. Washington, DC: American Psychiatric Association.

American Psychiatric Association (2000). *Diagnostic and Statistical Manual of Mental Disorders,* 4th edn, text revision. Washington, DC: American Psychiatric Association.

Baker, B. L., Blacker, J., Crnic, K. A. & Edelbrock, C. (2002). Behaviour problems and parenting stress in families of three-year-old children with and without developmental delay. *American Journal on Mental Retardation,* **107,** 433–44.

Baker, B. L., McIntyre, L. L., Blacker, J. *et al.* (2003). Preschool children with and without developmental delay: Behaviour problems and parenting stress over time. *Journal of Intellectual Disability Research,* **47,** 217–30.

Birmaher, B., Quintana, H. & Greenville, L. L. (1988). Methylphenidate treatment of hyperactive autistic children. *Journal of the American Academy of Child and Adolescent Psychiatry,* **27,** 248–51.

Botteron, K. & Geller, B. (1993). Disorders, symptoms and their pharmacotherapy. In *Practitioner's Guide to Psychoactive Drugs for Children and Adolescents,* ed. J. Werry & M. Aman, pp. 179–201. New York, NY: Plenum Medical.

Campbell, N., Gonzales, N. M., Bernst N., Silva R. R. & Werry J. S. (1993). Antipsychotics (neuroleptics). In *Practitioners' Guide to Psychoactive Drugs for Children and Adolescents,* ed. J. Werry & M. Aman, pp. 269–96. New York, NY: Plenum Medical.

Cherry, K. E., Penny, D., Matson, J. L. & Bamburg, J. W. (2000). Characteristics of schizophrenia among persons with severe or profound mental retardation. *Psychiatric Services,* **51,** 7–17.

Corbett, J. A. (1979). Psychiatric morbidity and mental retardation. In *Psychotherapy in the Mentally Retarded,* ed. F. E. James & R. P. Snaith, pp. 28–45. New York, NY: Grune and Stratton.

Costello, A. (1982). Assessment and diagnosis of psychopathology. In *Psychopathology in the Mentally Retarded,* ed. J. L. Matson & R. P. Barrett, pp. 37–52. New York, NY: Grune and Stratton.

Cox, A. & Rutter, M. (1985). Diagnostic appraisal and interviewing. In *Child and Adolescent Psychiatry: Modern Approaches,* 2nd edn, ed. M. Rutter & L. Hersov, pp. 233–47. Oxford: Blackwell Scientific Publications.

Dulcan, M. K. (1990). Using psycho-stimulants to treat behavioural disorders of children and adolescents. *Journal of Child and Adolescent Psychopharmacology,* **1,** 7–20.

Dykens, E. M. (1998). Maladaptive behaviour and dual diagnosis in persons with genetic syndromes. In *Handbook of Mental Retardation and Development*, ed. J. A. Burak, R. M. Hodapp & E. Zigler, pp. 542–62. Cambridge: Cambridge University Press.

Einfeld, S. L., Smith, A., Durvasula, S., Florio, T. & Tonge, B. J. (1998). Behavioural and emotional disturbance in Prader–Willi Syndrome. *American Journal of Medical Genetics*, **82**, 123–7.

Einfeld, S. L. & Tonge, B. J. (1996). Population prevalence of behavioural and emotional disturbance in children and adolescents with mental retardation: II. Epidemiological findings. *Journal of Intellectual Disability Research*, **40**(2), 99–109.

Einfeld, S. L. & Tonge, B. J. (2000). Observations on the use of the ICD-10 guide for mental retardation. *Journal of Intellectual Disability Research*, **44**(3–4), 273.

Einfeld, S. L. & Tonge, B. J. (2002). Manual for the Developmental Behaviour Checklist (2nd edn). Melbourne: Centre for Developmental Psychiatry & Psychology, Monash University.

Einfeld, S. L., Tonge, B. J. & Florio, T. (1994). Behavioural and emotional disturbance in fragile X syndrome. *American Journal of Medical Genetics*, **51**, 386–91.

Einfeld, S. L., Tonge, B. J. & Florio, T. (1997). Behavioural and emotional disturbance in individuals with Williams syndrome. *American Journal on Mental Retardation*, **102**(1), 45–53.

Einfeld, S. L., Tonge, B. J., Turner, G., Parmenter, T. & Smith, A. (2000). Longitudinal course of behavioural and emotional problems of young persons with Prader–Willi, Fragile-X, Williams and Down syndromes. *Journal of Intellectual Disability Research*, **44**(3–4), 273.

Emerson, E. (2003). Prevalence of psychiatric disorders in children and adolescents with and without intellectual disability. *Journal of Intellectual Disability Research* **47**, 51–8.

Hardy-Bayle, M., Sarfati, Y. & Passerieux, C. (2003). The cognitive basis of disorganization in schizophrenia and its clinical correlates: toward a pathogenic approach to disorganization. *Schizophrenia Bulletin*. **29**, 459–71.

Lewis, J. N., Tonge, B. J., Mowat, D. R. *et al.* (2000). Epilepsy and associated psychopathology in young people with intellectual disability. *Journal of Paediatrics and Child Health*, **36**(2), 172–5.

Lindsay, R. L. & Aman, M. G. (2003) Pharmacologic therapies aid treatment for autism. *Paediatric Annals*, **32**(10):671–6.

Lord, C., Rutter, M., DiLavore, P. & Risi, S. (1999). Autism Diagnostic Observation Schedule (ADOS) manual. Los Angeles, CA: Western Psychological Services.

Lord, C., Rutter, M. & Le Couteur, A. (1994). Autism Diagnostic Interview – Revised: a revised version of a diagnostic interview for caregivers of individuals with possible pervasive developmental disorders. *Journal of Autism and Developmental Disorders*, **24**(5), 659–85.

Matson, J. & Barrett, R. P. (eds.) (1982). *Psychopathology in the Mentally Retarded*. New York, NY: Grune and Stratton.

McLean, W. E. Jr (1990). Issues in the assessment of aberrant behaviour among persons with mental retardation. In *Assessment of Behavior Problems in Persons with Mental Retardation Living in the Community*, ed. E. Dibble & D. B. Gray, pp. 135–45. Rockville, MD: National Institute for Mental Health.

Prior, M. & Tonge, B. J. (1990). Pervasive developmental disorders. In *Handbook of Studies on Child Psychiatry*, ed. B. J. Tonge, G. D. Burrows & J. S. Werry, pp. 193–208. Amsterdam: Elsevier.

Royal College of Psychiatrists (2001). *DC-LD (Diagnostic Criteria for Psychiatric Disorders for Use with Adults with Learning Disabilities/Mental Retardation)*. London: Gaskell.

Rubin, L. I. (1987). Health care needs of adults with mental retardation. *Mental Retardation*, **25**, 201–6.

Rutter, M. (1991). Annotation: child psychiatric disorders in ICD-10. *Journal of Child Psychology and Psychiatry*, **30**, 499–513.

Rutter, M., Tizard, J. & Whitmore, K. (1970). *Education Health and Behaviour*. London: Longman.

Sovner, R. (1986). Limiting factors in the use of DSM-III criteria with mentally ill/mentally retarded persons. *Psychopharmacology Bulletin*, **22**, 1055–9.

Sovner, R. & Hurley, A. D. (1989). Ten diagnostic principles for recognizing psychiatric disorder in mentally retarded persons. *Psychiatric Aspects of Mental Retardation Reviews*, **8**, 9–13.

Stromme, P. & Diseth, T. H. (2000). Prevalence of psychiatric diagnoses in children with mental retardation: data from a population-based study. *Developmental Medicine and Child Neurology*, **42**, 266–70.

Tonge, B. J. (1982). Draw a dream: an intervention promoting change in families in conflict. In *The International Book of Family Therapy*, ed. E. W. Kaslow, pp. 212–26. New York, NY: Brunnel/Mazel.

Tonge, B. J. (1988). Anxiety in adolescence. In *Handbook of Anxiety Vol. 2. Classification, Etiological Factors and Associated Disturbances*, ed. R. Noyes, M. Roth & G. D. Burrows, pp. 269–88. Amsterdam: Elsevier.

Tonge, B. J. (1991). Children with physical impairments. In *Handbook of Studies on General Hospital Psychiatry*, ed. F. K. Judd, G. D. Burrows & D. R. Lipsitt, pp. 195–206. Amsterdam: Elsevier.

Tonge, B. J. & Einfeld, S. (1991). Intellectual disability and psychopathology in Australian children. *Australia and New Zealand Journal of Developmental Disabilities*, **17**, (2) 155–67.

Tonge, B. J. & Einfeld, S. L. (2003). Psychopathology and intellectual disability: The Australian child to adult longitudinal study. In L. M. Glidden (ed.), *International Review of Research in Mental Retardation*, **27**, 61–91. San Diego, CA: Academic Press.

Tonge, B. J., Einfeld, S. L., Krupinski, J. *et al.* (1996). The use of factor analysis for ascertaining patterns of psychopathology in children with intellectual disability. *Journal of Intellectual Disability Research*, **40**(3), 198–207.

World Health Organization (1992). *The 1CD-10 Classification of Mental and Behavioural Disorders*. Geneva: World Health Organization.

World Health Organization (1996). *The ICD-10 Guide for Mental Retardation*. Geneva: World Health Organization.

7

Depression, anxiety and adjustment disorders in people with intellectual disabilities

Chrissoula Stavrakaki and Yona Lunsky

Introduction

Depression, anxiety and adjustment disorders are particularly more prevalent amongst people with intellectual disabilities (ID) than in the general population (Richards *et al.*, 2001; Tu & Zellweger, 1965). This is the case for most psychiatric disorders (Einfeld, 1992; Gitta & Goldberg, 1995; King *et al.*, 1994; Singh, *et al.*, 1991; Sovner and Horley, 1989; Stavrakaki and Mintsioulis, 1997; Vitello and Behar, 1992). King *et al.* (1994) found that the most common diagnoses in individuals with ID at the Landerman Developmental Center in California were impulse control disorders, stereotypical/habit disorders, anxiety disorders and mood disorders. In a similar study in Canada, Gitta (1995) concluded that co-existence of anxiety disorders, adjustment disorders and depression was high in people with ID.

This chapter describes the main clinical aspects of depression, anxiety and adjustment disorders and considers the similarities and differences of the three conditions in people with ID.

Depression

The current American classification system for mental diseases (DSM-IV-TR, (*Diagnostic and Statistical Manual of Mental Disorders*, Amercian Psychiatric Association, 1994; *Diagnostic and Statistical Manual of Mental Disorders*, American Psychiatric Association 2000)), includes two types of depressive disorders:
(a) major depressive disorders, and
(b) dysthymic disorders.

Major depressive disorder is characterized by one or more major depressive episodes (i.e. at least two weeks of depressed mood or loss of interest). According to this classification, five or more of the following symptoms of depression must

Psychiatric and Behavioural Disorders in Intellectual and Developmental Disabilities, ed. Nick Bouras and Geraldine Holt. Published by Cambridge University Press. © Cambridge University Press 2007.

be present during the same two-week period for a diagnosis of major depressive disorder to be made:

- depressed mood most of the day
- markedly diminished interest or pleasure in all activities
- considerable weight loss or gain
- insomnia or hypersomnia
- psychomotor agitation or retardation
- fatigue or loss of energy
- feelings of worthlessness
- diminished ability to think or concentrate
- recurrent thoughts of death

Dysthymic disorder is characterized by at least two years of depressed mood for more days than not, accompanied by additional depressive symptoms that do not meet the criteria for a major depressive episode. The DSM-IV-TR criteria for dysthymic disorder require that depressed mood should be present for most of the day, more days than not, for at least two years. The presence of two or more of the following symptoms is necessary for the diagnosis of dysthymic disorder to be made:

- poor appetite or overeating
- insomnia or hypersomnia
- low energy or fatigue
- low self-esteem
- poor concentration
- feelings of worthlessness

Although people with all levels of ID have been described as suffering from mood disorders, systematic, prospective, well-controlled studies with reliable means of assessing the presence of these disorders, have not been conducted with representative samples of persons with ID. However, there is a general consensus that the diagnostic criteria for depressive disorders in DSM-IV-TR apply to people with ID, especially in the higher levels of cognitive functioning. One of the main problems in diagnosing these disorders in persons with severe and profound ID is that people with such disabilities have either limited or non-verbal communication, cannot express subjective feelings such as lack of pleasure, or material which is primarily 'internal' (Einfeld & Tonge, 1999). Another factor that imposes a challenge in the diagnosis of these disorders in this population is that persons with ID are a highly heterogeneous group (Harris, 1998). Thus, great variations exist in the levels of cognitive and social skills amongst individuals within the same level of functioning, as well as at the different cognitive levels (mild to profound). Therefore, there has been concern that depressive disorders are not properly recognized in this population and remain under-diagnosed. Studies such as King et al. (1994) and Gitta

(1995) emphasized the apparent high incidence of depressive disorders in people with ID. Other studies have described single case studies or have focused on specific subpopulations, i.e. those with pervasive developmental disorder (Ghaziuddin & Tsai, 1991) or Down syndrome (Cooper & Collacott, 1994; Stavrakaki *et al.*, 2004c).

Most recent studies have shown that persons with ID do present with symptoms of depression, including mood symptoms (Clarke & Gomez, 1999; Tsiouris, *et al.*, 2003). The prevalence of major depressive episodes in the general population has been estimated to be from 10 to 25% for women and from 5 to 12% for men. The prevalence of dysthymic disorder has been found to be approximately 8 % for both sexes. Several recent studies have reported point prevalence rates of depressive episodes in adults with ID at about 4% (Meins, 1995; Patel *et al.*, 1993; Deb, 2001). These may be underestimates, however. In a study of adults with ID attending a psychiatric out-patient clinic, 26 people (9.1%) of a total sample of 285 were found to have a depressive or dysthymic disorder (Stavrakaki & Mintsioulis, 1997). Fewer studies have examined prevalence rates in children. A recent study reported a depression rate of 1.5% in a child/adolescent community sample (Emerson, 2003), whereas a similar study reported a rate of 4.4% (Dekker & Koot, 2003). Masi *et al.* (1999) estimated, based on their small sample study of dysthymic disorder in adolescents, that rates of dysthymic disorder in adolescents with ID could be higher than 20%.

Aetiology

The causes of depressive disorders in people with ID are similar to the causes of these disorders in the general population. Although the latter have been extensively studied in recent years, there is a paucity of research for people with ID. Collacott *et al.* (1992) examined 378 adults with Down syndrome and compared them with an almost equal number of adults with ID caused by other pathologies. They concluded that patients with Down syndrome were more likely to have been diagnosed as having depression with dementia (see also Chapter 10 by Cooper and Holland). Several studies have reported that depressive disorders, similar to the general population, are more common in women than men with ID (Lunsky & Canrinus, 2005), but it is not clear whether these higher rates are owing to biological or psychosocial influences.

Biological and genetic factors have been identified as causing depression in people with Down syndrome (Collacott *et al.*, 1992; Stavrakaki *et al.*, 2004c; Tu & Zellweger, 1965). Similar factors may be responsible for the higher incidence of depressive disorders in people with pervasive developmental disorders (Davis *et al.*, 1997; Ghaziuddin & Tsai, 1991). Genetic syndromes such as fragile X syndrome, Down syndrome, fetal alcohol syndrome and Williams syndrome have also been linked with mood disorders (Einfeld *et al.*, 2001).

The relationship between stressful life events and depressive disorders has been of long-standing interest for clinicians and researchers. This is particularly important for people with ID whose lives may be characterized by frequent major adverse life events such as separation from caregivers, and other traumatic events (Stavrakaki & Mintsioulis, 1997). In a recent study of adults with ID diagnosed as having depressive disorders, there was a high frequency of life events occurring one to three months prior to the onset of depression. Major depressive disorder was associated with sexual assault, physical assault, parental loss and parental separation.

Dysthymic disorder was linked with parental illness, parental separation, divorce and change of residence. Two more recent studies found an association between life events and the affective disorders – Hastings, *et al.*, 2004; Owen *et al.*, 2004 – with the latter study reporting that exposure to one or more life events in the previous 12 months significantly increased the odds of affective disorder (OR = 2.23). Important risk factors for depression, in addition to major life events such as abuse or loss, include a lack of social support, daily hassles and negative social interactions (Lunsky, 2003; Lunsky & Benson, 2001).

Symptom presentation

The use of strict criteria for the diagnosis of depressive disorders in people with ID may exclude potential cases and lead to the under-representation of the problem. Recent research has focused on the presentation of symptoms as they appear in depressed people to ensure a more accurate diagnosis, particularly for those with severe ID.

Meins (1995), in his study of 32 adults with ID, found that those with severe disabilities presented more atypical symptoms such as irritability, psychomotor agitation, increased behaviour problems and, rarely, a loss of adaptive behaviour. Those with mild disabilities were diagnosed successfully by using the DSM-III-R (revised) diagnostic criteria.

Marston *et al.* (1997) found common and distinct symptoms in the presentation of the depressive disorders in people with ID based on their degree of disability. The common symptoms were depressed affect and sleep disturbance. The distinct symptoms, based on the degree of disability were:

For mild ID

- tearfulness
- diurnal mood variation
- loss of energy
- loss of interest
- low self-esteem

For moderate ID
- social isolation
- self-injurious behaviour
- weight loss

For severe/profound ID
- screaming
- aggression
- self-injurious behaviour

It appears from the existing literature that depressive symptoms in adults with ID vary according to the degree of their disability: the higher their intellectual ability, the closer their symptoms of depression are to those of the general population. In people with severe disability, depression seems to be presented with atypical symptoms or 'behavioural equivalents'.

Not everyone agrees on 'atypical symptoms of depression' reported by individuals such as Marston *et al.* (1997), however. For example, a recent study by Tsiouris and colleagues failed to replicate Marston's findings that self-injury, screaming and aggression were equivalents to depressive symptoms in individuals with severe to profound ID (Tsiouris *et al.*, 2003). To understand the complex relationship between challenging behaviour and depression level of ID, the type of aggression may be relevant (Lunsky & Palucka, 2004).

Assessment

Depressive disorders are easier to diagnose in people with mild and moderate ID than in those whose disabilities are severe and profound (Gitta & Goldberg, 1995; Marston *et al.*, 1997; Stavrakaki & Mintsioulis, 1997). Modified ICD-10 and DSM-IV-TR diagnostic criteria have been used to diagnose depression in people with ID. Two recent examples of standardized criteria are the Diagnostic Manual of Mental Disorders in Persons with ID, a compendium to the DSM-IV-TR, with criteria specifically addressing mental disorders with persons in ID (DSM-IV-ID, in press) and the Diagnostic Criteria for Learning Disability (DC-LD) (Royal College of Psychiatrists, 2001).

In addition to utilizing diagnostic criteria developed for the ID population, several assessment tools have been developed in recent years. These tools may be self-report for more verbal individuals, caregiver ratings, or observation schedules. Examples of self-report scales include modifications of the Children's Depression Inventory (CDI) (Meins, 1995), the Reynolds Depressive Symptoms Questionnaire (Reynolds & Baker, 1988), the Beck Depression Inventory (Powell, 2003), the Birleson Depression Questionnaire (Benson & Ivins, 1992; Lunsky, 2003), or the Glasgow Depression Scale (Cuthill *et al.*, 2003). The Glasgow Depression Scale is unique in that it was developed especially to target the unique symptoms of depression in ID, in language most easily understood. It has good reliability and criterion validity, along with suggested clinical cut-offs and a parallel informant measure (Lunsky & Palucka, 2004). Informant ratings are more popular because they can be completed by caregivers regardless of the cogntive ability of those under their care. Examples of informant measures include a modified CDI, in an informant-rating version (Meins, 1996), the depression subscale of the Comprehensive Psychopathological Rating Scale (CPRS) (Meins, 1995) a nine-item scale that can be used for almost all people with varying degrees of ID, including the severely and profoundly disabled; a checklist of 30 symptoms developed by Marston *et al.* (1997), derived from the ICD-10 diagnostic criteria (World Health Organization, 1992), and the depressed mood subscale of the ADAMS (Esbensen *et al.*, 2003). The ADAMS is a 28-item measure whose items were empirically derived as opposed to clinically selected.

The diagnosis of depressive disorders in people with ID needs further systematic research in order to develop standardized assessment and diagnostic instruments specifically for this population. The Psychiatric Assessment Schedule for Adults with Developmental Disability (Moss *et al.*, 1993) is a promising development in this respect. Conceptual issues about the assessment and diagnosis of mental health problems including depression are also described in Chapters 2 and 3.

Anxiety disorders

Anxiety disorders, as defined in DSM-IV-TR (1994), are clinically significant, unpleasant emotions that have the quality of fear, dread and alarm in the presence or absence of an identifiable psychosocial stressor or stresses. The following conditions are described as anxiety disorders in DSM-IV-TR:

- panic disorder with agoraphobia
- panic disorder without agoraphobia
- agoraphobia without panic disorder
- specific phobias
- social phobias
- obsessive-compulsive disorder (OCD)
- post-traumatic stress disorder
- acute stress disorder
- generalized anxiety disorder.

Anxiety disorders are one of the commonest catagories of mental disorders reported in the general population but also in persons with ID (DSM-IV-TR 2000; DSM-ID, in press). The diagnostic criteria of ICD-10 and DSM-IV-TR can apply to persons with mild and moderate degrees of ID when speech and communication are reasonable. In persons with severe and profound levels of ID, as well as other individuals, with limiting or non-existent language skills, the diagnotic criteria have to be adjusted and can rely heavily on observations or informant reports. The DC-LD (Royal College of Psychiatrists, 2001) allows individuals to describe their fear/anxiety, or their 'expression or behaviour may demonstrate anxiety or fear'. For specific disorders (panic disorder, phobias, and generalized anxiety disorder), irritability owing to anxiety/fear is considered an observable symptom. In OCD, the DC-LD considers anger/aggression, when an attempt is made by others to prevent a compulsion, to be an observable symptom.

Anxiety disorders are reported to be as common or even more common in persons with ID (Deb, 2001; King *et al.*, 1994) although most studies focus on anxious symptoms as opposed to the prevalence of anxiety disorders. A recent epidemiological study of children and adolescents reported a prevalence rate of 8.7%, such that anxiety disorders were 2.5 times more common in those with ID versus children without disabilities (Emerson, 2003). Despite the recent reports, anxiety disorders may still be under-diagnosed in this population (Veernhoven & Tuinier, 1997).

Aetiology

Various theories have been put forward concerning the aetiology of anxiety disorders in people with ID (Gitta & Goldberg, 1995; King *et al.*, 1994; Ryan, 1994; Stavrakaki & Mintsioulis, 1997). Recent literature suggest a relationship between anxiety disorders and the underlying pathology responsible for the ID, such as genetic syndromes of fragile X, Rubenstein–Tabyi, Williams syndrome, Prader–Willi and Cornelia de Lange syndrome. Stavrakaki *et al.* (2004c) found that persons with Down syndrome are more prone to anxiety and OCD following traumatic events. Charlot *et al.* (2002) noted obsessional slowness, a variant of OCD, in adults with Down syndrome.

Others have pointed to environmental factors such as physical illness, trauma and abuse to explain the higher incidence of anxiety disorders amongst these people (Ryan, 1994; Stavrakaki *et al.*, 2004c). With regard to simple phobias, Pickersgill *et al.* (1994) suggest that communication impairments make it challenging to explain or dismiss fears when they arise and lead to over-generalization. In addition, overprotection from caregivers can lead to learned dependence and avoidance of feared stimuli.

Prior to the recognition that post-traumatic stress disorder (PTSD) can occur in ID, post-traumatic stress in people with ID was attributed to a number of other psychiatric diagnoses. Common diagnoses included autism and intermittent explosive disorder, and less common diagnoses included affective disorders, personality disorders and adjustment. One major cause of PTSD in these individuals are high rates of physical and sexual abuse. People with ID are vulnerable to physical (Gil, 1970) and to sexual abuse (Elvik *et al.*, 1990). Their reactions may be very similar to the general population and PTSD symptoms are common (Sequeria *et al.*, 2003). Like young children, they may be unable to relate the details of the abusive event. It is, then, very difficult to assess the extent of the abuse, especially because the tools used with non-verbal sexually abused children, such as anatomically detailed dolls, developmentally targeted interviews etc., are problematic when used with people with ID (Lunsky & Benson, 2001).

Symptom presentation

A person with ID can show signs of anxiety in response to a threat in his or her own environment that do not interfere with their life activities. In some instances, however, especially when the stressors are enduring, symptoms of anxiety may interfere with the person's ability to function. Bailey and Andrews (2003) provide an excellent, detailed review of symptoms of anxiety in anxiety disorders in the ID population.

The presentation of anxiety disorders in individuals with ID is still being explored, in contrast to the vast literature that exists for the general population. This is partly because, within the anxiety disorders spectrum, there are several distinct disorders which, although they share a similar response, the behavioural manifestations of anxiety and the triggers that have caused them differ.

The most severe form of anxiety disorder perhaps is PTSD. In her study of PTSD in people with ID, Ryan (1994) examined the symptoms and reasons for psychiatric referral and found that almost all of her clients were referred for violent or disruptive behaviours.

Stavrakaki and Mintsioulis (1997) found that 70 patients out of a total of 257 (27%) with ID suffered from anxiety disorders. In relation to the symptomatology of the anxiety disorders found in this study, the prevailing common symptoms were: aggression, agitation, obsessive-compulsive phenomena, i.e. self-mutilation, obsessive fears, ritualistic behaviours and insomnia. Specific symptoms for each subcategory of anxiety were: overactivity, panic attacks, agoraphobia, sexual dysfunction, mood changes, depersonalization and derealization. Stavrakaki and Mintsioulis (1997) also summarized the life events that had preceded the onset of symptoms in the same sample of patients by three to six months. Out of 70 patients, 63 had been exposed to one or more of the following life events:

- rape/sexual assault
- physical assault
- accidents
- illness
- move
- loss of caregiver
- change in policy

Simple phobias in adults with ID may be more comparable to phobias in children as opposed to other adults. Common fears include fear of the dark, fear of dogs, fear of dentists or fear of blood.

Obsessive-compulsive disorder is the other well-studied anxiety disorder in the ID population. It is challenging to diagnose obsessions because of the difficulty people with ID have describing their thoughts. However, compulsions are readily observable, as is the mounting anxiety or tension when a compulsion is prevented or interrupted. It can also be challenging to differentiate between complusions, sterotypies and tics, all common in the ID population (Bodfish & Madison, 1993; King *et al.*, 1994). Finally, there is also some debate about the overlap between compulsive and autistic behaviour (for a good review on OCD symptomatology, see Bailey & Andrews, 2003). Several researchers have suggested that the types of compulsions evident in individuals with ID such as Down syndrome or autistic disorder differ from the compulsions most commonly seen in the general population (see Bailey & Andrews, 2003). Whether the differences are attributable to cognitive level, behaviour repertoire, or brain-based differences is unclear.

Assessment

It is difficult to assess anxiety disorders in people with ID. Criteria similar to those applied to the general population can apply, but they have to be modified and are dependent upon the ability of the individuals concerned to communicate their subjective feelings of discomfort. In studies of anxiety in the general population, people are usually asked to self-rate their anxiety on one of the standard assessment tools available for research. The problem with this method when applied to the ID group is that it is difficult for people with severe and profound ID to rate their own anxiety. Some attempts have been made by Lindsay and Michie (1988) to adapt one of the standard anxiety assessment scales for use with this group of people. The Zung Self-Rating Anxiety Scale (SAS) (Zung, 1971) has been widely used in the assessment of generalized anxiety and treatment effects because this scale can be adjusted to be more easily understood by people with ID by simply indicating presence or absence of anxiety symptoms. However, the main problem inherent in the standard presentation of the responses in the Zung SAS is the complex conceptual awareness of one's own anxiety. For individuals with ID, it is almost impossible to categorize and to rate the extent of their anxiety from 'never' to 'some of the time', 'a good part of the time', and 'most or all of the time'.

A recently standardized scale that can be easily understood with only three choices is the Glasgow Anxiety Scale for ID (Mindham & Espie, 2003). Items for this measure were derived based on direct experiences of anxious adults with ID and on clinical opinion. The 27-item scale successfully discriminated between anxious and non-anxious individuals and also correlated with a physiological measure of anxiety.

Gedye developed a compulsive behaviour checklist for people with ID in order to assess and to grade the severity of obsessions with 25 types of compulsions in five categories (Gedye, 1993). This behaviour checklist has yielded good results (Bodfish & Madison, 1993) and has been used extensively by several facilities and services. Compulsive behaviour can also be assessed with the ADAMS (discussed earlier), an informant measure.

The PAS-ADD interview (Moss, 1997) also includes an anxiety section. The clinician assesses observed tension and worries and specifies whether autonomic symptoms of anxiety relate to simple or social phobias component. The PAS-ADD allows for self-report and informant perspectives (see also Chapter 3 by O'Hara). Masi *et al.* (2000) reported some success with the K-SADS-P, a structured diagnostic interview developed for children without ID, and with adolescents with mild ID, to assess generalized anxiety disorder.

Anxiety can also be assessed through behavioural assessments, which do not require verbal ability. The behavioural approach test is a common technique where the person is observed approaching a feared stimulus and how they respond at different stages of exposure is recorded. Electrodermal and cardiac rates can also be measured objectively.

Adjustment disorders

Adjustment disorders are partially related to anxiety and partially to the depressive disorders. They are defined on DSM-IV-TR criteria as clinically significant emotional or behavioural symptoms in response to identifiable psychosocial stressors. The clinical categories of adjustment disorders are:
- depressed mood
- anxiety
- mixed anxiety and depressed mood
- mixed disturbance of emotions and conduct
- unspecified

Adjustment disorders can be seen as the precursor of anxiety and depressive disorders. In some instances it is very difficult to disentangle the symptoms associated with adjustment disorders from those of anxiety and depressive disorders. There are, however, incidents in which specific stressors can cause an adjustment disorder with its own characteristic symptomatology that will run its own course and will have a specific prognosis. In general, a stressor can be anything in the life of a person with ID, beyond the person's power to resolve it alone (Levitas & Gilson, 2001). The clinician, therefore, must be aware of the details of any changes in the lives of the clients (Casey *et al.*, 2001). The stressors may be a single event, multiple stressors and/or stressors that affect a single individual, an entire family or a large group or community (Diagnostic and Statistical Manual of Mental Disorders, 2000).

As already mentioned, the lives of the people with ID are affected by multiple traumas. As a result, the prevalence of adjustment disorders can be significantly increased (Gitta & Goldberg, 1995; Göstason, 1987; Levitas & Gilson, 2001; Ryan, 1994; Stavrakaki & Mintsioulis, 1997). The symptom presentation of adjustment disorders seems to follow patterns similar to those of anxiety disorders. However, there are common and specific presentations of the symptoms of the two disorders. Common symptoms between adjustment and anxiety disorders include disruptive behaviours, i.e. aggression, agitation, distractibility, physical and verbal abuse and self-mutilation. Specific symptoms for the adjustment disorder include somatic complaints and biological symptoms, i.e. sleep and appetite disturbance. The specific symptoms have more resemblance to the depressive disorders (Stavrakaki & Mintsioulis, 1997)

The concept of adjustment disorder is a very important one in the lives of people with ID as it, usually, indicates that removal of such challenges can ameliorate or resolve the signs and symptoms of the mental disorder, thus preventing any other major clinical entities such as anxiety or depression from occurring. As in other psychiatric disorders, adjustment disorder as a diagnosis must not only be sought for but must also be ruled out when the phenomena displayed do not meet DSM-IV-TR criteria (Levitas *et al.*, 2000).

Treatment methods

The treatment methods used for people with ID and depression, anxiety and adjustment disorders, are similar to those used in the general population and include the following.

Pharmacotherapeutic regimes

Pharmacotherapeutic regimes including antidepressants, anxiolytics, neuroleptics, mood stabilizers, anticonvulsants, beta-blockers etc. have been widely used to treat depression and anxiety disorders in people with ID over time (see Chapter 19 by King).

Pharmacotherapy should be used cautiously in the treatment of anxiety and depressive/mood disorders in this group of people because of the relatively high rate of unwanted side effects, including increased susceptibility, paradoxical and even toxic reactions (Bodfish & Madison, 1993; Ratey *et al.*, 1991; Ryan, 1994; Stavrakaki *et al.*, 2004a; Stavrakaki *et al.*, 2004b; Stavrakaki *et al.*, 2002; Stavrakaki & Mintsioulis, 1997). There has been a general agreement that the doses of medication used for the treatment of people with ID suffering from depression, anxiety and adjustment disorders should be kept lower than normal and reviewed at regular intervals (Antochi *et al.*, 2003; Stavrakaki *et al.*, 2002).

Behaviour therapies

Behaviour therapies such as progressive relaxation (Jacobson, 1938), graduated exposure and desensitization and abbreviated progressive relaxation (Bernstein & Borkovec, 1973) have been used to treat a variety of behaviour and cognitive problems, including self-injurious behaviour, inappropriate sexual responses, temper tantrums, phobic symptoms and psychomotor seizures. These techniques seem to be most successful when applied to individuals with moderate and mild levels of ID. They can also be effective with specific problems in individuals with more severe ID (Altabet, 2002; Lindsay *et al.*, 1989). Cognitive behavioural interventions have been found to be effective for treating depression in adults with mild ID (Lindsay *et al.*, 1997), simple phobias, e.g. dog phobia (Newman & Adams, 2004), dental phobia (Altabet, 2002), and PTSD (Lemmon & Mizes, 2002). Khreim and Mikkelsen (1997) provided case examples of successful combined medication/cognitive therapy treatments of generalized anxiety disorder and panic disorder in people with mild ID.

Environmental factors

Environmental changes are frequently detrimental to people with ID and anxiety disorders. Environmental triggers are very important in the development of dissociative phenomena, for example, in cases of PTSD (Ryan, 1994; Stavrakaki *et al.*, 2004c). Individuals with ID can become very anxious and feel threatened in the course of their daily activities by environmental stimuli. In most cases, these problems are preventable (Levitas & Gilson, 2001). Careful review of living conditions and daily activities of these individuals is necessary to ensure that triggers and other factors that create extensive anxiety and inordinate stress can be ameliorated. Both clients and caregivers can benefit from being taught ways to cope with anxiety when they are confronted with unavoidable stressful situations.

Staff training

Staff training has been highly recommended in the overall treatment of depression and anxiety disorders in people with ID (Ryan, 1994; Stavrakaki & Mintsioulis, 1997). More recently, structured staff training techniques have been gaining increasing interest (Bouras & Holt, 1997; Holt *et al.*, 2005). Another approach, person-centred planning, was conseptualized as a way to reorganize and reorient the service systems to achieve such goals as safe home environment, satisfying personal relationships and acceptance by the community. This approach was also brought forth in order to address the dwindling resources and increasing demands for such services (Gahan *et al.*, 2002).

Identification of physical problems

The identification of physical problems is of major importance for people with ID. Often, physical discomfort may be expressed as aggressive or agitated behaviour in these individuals. Early recognition and treatment of underlying physical problems will have an overall beneficial effect (Levitas *et al.*, 2000) (See also Chapters 5 by Lennox and 17 by Reese *et al.*).

Conclusion

Depression, anxiety and adjustment disorders are more frequent than previously accepted in people with ID. Although they are distinct clinical entities, they may also interrelate and overlap with each other. The symptom presentation of each of the three disorders in higher functioning individuals is distinct and follows the generally accepted criteria as they apply to the general population. However, in adults with severe/profound ID, the symptoms of the three disorders overlap and tend to include more behavioural disturbances such as aggression, irritability and self-injurious behaviour.

Areas of future research should address the possibility of identifying biological markers related to these disorders. Pharmacological studies including randomized samples should be specifically designed for people with ID. The early recognition and identification of depression, anxiety and adjustment disorders, together with appropriate therapeutic interventions, are necessary in order to prevent, modify and ameliorate their clinical impact. There is a great need for specialized services dealing with people with dual diagnosis and their families. These services should offer a holistic approach and address the mental health needs of these people in a manner that enhances the quality of their lives.

Summary points

- Depression, anxiety and adjustment disorders are particularly prevalent in people with ID.
- Assessment tools exist for these disorders.
- They may be under-diagnosed even though often the typical symptoms and signs are present. Atypical presentation is more common in people with severe ID.
- PTSD may be attributed incorrectly to other psychiatric disorders.

- Symptoms of PTSD commonly occur after being abused.
- Treatment methods for these disorders are similar to those used in the general population.

REFERENCES

Altabet, S. C. (2002). Decreasing dental resistance among individuals with severe and profound mental retardation. *Journal of Developmental and Physical Disabilities*, **14**, 297–305.

Antochi, R., Stavrakaki, C. & Emery, P. C. (2003). Psychopharmacological treatments in persons with dual diagnosis of psychiatric disorders and developmental disabilities. *Postgrad. Med. J.*, **79**, 139–146.

Bailey, N. M. & Andrews, T. M. (2003). Diagnostic Criteria for Psychiatric Disorders for Use with Adults with Learning Disabilities/Mental Retardation (DC-LD) and the diagnosis of anxiety disorders: a review, **47** (Suppl. 1) 50–61.

Benson, B. A. & Ivins, J. (1992). Anger, depression and self-concept in adults with mental retardation. *J. Intellect. Disabil. Res.* **36**, 169–75.

Bernstein, D. A. & Borkovec, T. D. (1973). Progressive Relaxation Training: A Manual for the Helping Profession. Champaign, IL: Research Press.

Bodfish, J. W. & Madison, J. T. (1993). Diagnosis and fluoxetine treatment of compulsive behavior disorder of adults with mental retardation. *Am J. Ment. Retard.*, **98**, 360–7.

Bouras, N. & Holt, G. (1997). Crisis in London's mental health services. Meeting the needs of people with learning disabilities would unblock acute beds. *BMJ*, **314**, 1278–9.

Casey, P., Dowrick, C. & Wilkinson, G. (2001). Adjustment disorders: fault line in the psychiatric glossary. *Br. J. Psychiatry*, **179**, 479–81.

Charlot, L., Fox, S. & Friedlander, R. (2002). Obsessional slowness in Down syndrome. *J. Intellect. Disabil. Res.*, **46**, 517–24.

Clarke, D. J. & Gomez, G. A. (1999). Utility of modified DCR-10 criteria in the diagnosis of depression associated with intellectual disability. *J. Intellect. Disabil. Res.*, **43**(Pt 5), 413–20.

Collacott, R. A., Cooper, S. A. & McGrother, C. (1992). Differential rates of psychiatric disorders in adults with Down syndrome compared with other mentally handicapped adults. *Br. J. Psychiatry*, **161**, 671–4.

Cooper, S. A. & Collacott, R. A. (1994). Clinical features and diagnostic criteria of depression in Down's syndrome. *Br. J. Psychiatry*, **165**, 399–403.

Cuthill, F. M., Espie, C. A. & Cooper, S. A. (2003). Development and psychometric properties of the Glasgow Depression Scale for people with a Learning Disability. Individual and carer supplement versions. *Br. J. Psychiatry*, **182**, 347–53.

Davis, J. P., Judd, F. K. & Herrman, H. (1997). Depression in adults with intellectual disability. Part 1: A review. *Aust. N. Z. J. Psychiatry*, **31**, 232–42.

Deb., S. (2001). *Epidemiology of Psychiatric Illness in Adults with Intellectual Disability*. L. Hamilton Kirkwood, Health Evidence Bulletins – Learning Disabilities. Cardiff: Health Evidence Bulletins.

Dekker, M. C. & Koot, H. M. (2003). DSM-IV disorders in children with borderline to moderate intellectual disability. II. Child and family predictors. *J. Am. Acad. Child. Adolesc. Psychiatry*, **42**, (8) 923–31.

Diagnostic and Statistical Manual of Mental Disorders. (1994). (4th edn). Washington, DC: American Psychiatric Association.

Diagnostic and Statistical Manual of Mental Disorders. (2000). (4th edn – text revised). Washington, DC: American Psychiatric Association.

Diagnostic and Statistical Manual for Persons with Intellectual Disabilities. (DSM-IV-ID) (in press).

Einfeld, S. L. (1992). Clinical assessment of psychiatric symptoms in mentally retarded individuals. *Aust. N. Z. J. Psychiatry*, **26**, 48–63.

Einfeld, S. L. & Tonge, B. J. (1999). Observations on the use of the ICD-10 guide for mental retardation. *J. Intellect. Disabil. Res.*, **43**(Pt 5), 408–12.

Einfeld, S. L., Tonge, B. J. & Rees, V. W. (2001). Longitudinal course of behavioral and emotional problems in Williams syndrome. *Am. J. Ment. Retard.*, **106**, 73–81.

Elvik, S. L., Berkowitz, C. D., Nicholas, E., Lipman, J. L. & Inkelis, S. H. (1990). Sexual abuse in the developmentally disabled: dilemmas of diagnosis. *Child Abuse Negl.*, **14**, 497–502.

Emerson, E. (2003) Prevalence of psychiatric disorders in children and adolescents with and without intellectual disability, *J. Intellect. Disabil. Res.*, **47**, 51–8.

Esbensen, A. J., Rojahn, J. Aman, M. G. & Ruedrich, S. (2003). Reliability and validity of an assessment instrument for anxiety, depression, and mood among individuals with mental retardation, *J. Autism Dev. Disord.*, **33**, 617–29.

Gahan, S., Dykstra, L. & Summers, J. (2002). *Person-Centered Approaches to Services and Supports* (1st edn). *The Habilitative Mental Health Resource Network: Dual Diagnosis. An Introduction to the Mental Health Needs of Persons with Developmental Disabilities.* Ontario: National Association for the Dually Diagnosed.

Gedye, A. (1993). Evidence of serotonergic reduction of self-injurious movements. *The Habilitative Mental Health Care Newsletter*, **12**, 53–6.

Ghaziuddin, M. & Tsai, L. (1991). Depression in autistic disorders. *Br. J. Psychiatry*, **159**, 721–3.

Gil, D. G. (1970). *Violence Against Children: Physical Child Abuse in the United States.* Cambridge, MA: Harvard University Press.

Gitta, M. Z. & Goldberg, B. (1995). Dual diagnosis: psychiatric and physical disorders in a clinical sample, Part II. *Clinical Bulletin of Developmental Disabilities Program*, **6**, 1–2.

Göstason, R. (1987). Psychiatric illness among the mildly mentally retarded. *Upsala Journal of Medicine and Science* (Suppl.) 115–24.

Harris, J. (1998). Physical interventions. *Br. J. Psychiatry*, **173**, 442.

Hastings, R. P., Hatton, C., Taylor, J. L. & Maddison, C. (2004). Life events and psychiatric symptoms in adults with intellectual disabilities. *J. Intellect. Disabil. Res.*, **48**, 42–6.

Holt G., Hardy S. & Bouras, N. (2005). *Mental Health in Learning Disabities: A Training Resource.* Brighton: Pavilion Publishing.

Jacobson, E. (1938). *Progressive Relaxation.* Chicago, IL: University of Chicago Press.

King, B. H., Carlo DeAntonio, B. A., McCracken, J. T., Fomess, S. R. & Ackerland, V. (1994). Psychiatric consultation in severe and profound mental retardation. *Am. J. Psychiatry*, **151**, 1802–8.

Khreim, I. & Mikkelsen, E. (1997). Anxiety disorders in adults with mental retardation. *Psychiatric Annals*, **27**(3), 175–81.

Lemmon, V. A. & Mizes, J. S. (2002). Effectiveness of exposure therapy: A case study of posttraumatic stress disorder and mental retardation. *Cognitive Behavioral Practice*, **9**, 317–23.

Levitas A. & Gilson, S. F. (2001). Predictable crises in the lives of persons with mental retardation. *Mental Health Aspects of Developmental Disabilities*, **4**, 89–100.

Levitas, A., Hurley, A. & Pary, R. (2000). Mental status examination of persons with intellectual disability. *Mental Health Aspects of Developmental Disabilities*, **4**, 2–16.

Lindsay, W., Neilson, C. & Lawrenson, H. (1997). Cognitive-behaviour therapy for anxiety in people with learning disabilities. In B. S. Kroese, D. Dagnan & K. Loumidis (eds.), *Cognitive-Behaviour Therapy for People with Learning Disabilities* (pp. 124–40). London: Routledge.

Lindsay, W. R., Baty, F. J., Michie, A. M. & Richardson, I. (1989). A comparison of anxiety treatments with adults who have moderate and severe mental retardation. *Res. Dev. Disabil.*, **10**, 129–40.

Lindsay, W. R. & Michie, A. M. (1988). Adaptation of the Zung self-rating anxiety scale for people with a mental handicap. *J. Ment. Defic. Res.*, **32**(Pt 6), 485–90.

Lunsky, Y. (2003). Depressive symptoms in intellectual disability: does gender play a role? *J. Intellect. Disabil. Res.*, **47**, 417–27.

Lunsky, Y. & Benson, B. A. (2001). Association between perceived social support and strain, and positive and negative outcome for adults with mild intellectual disability. *J. Intellect. Disabil. Res.*, **45**, 106–14.

Lunsky, Y. & Canrinus, M. (2005). Gender issues, mental retardation and depression. In *Mood Disorders in People with Mental Retardation*. (pp. 113–29). Kingston, NY: National Association for the Dually Diagnosed Press.

Lunsky, Y. & Palucka, A. (2004). Depression in intellectual disability. *Current Opinion in Psychiatry*, **17**, 359–63.

Marston, G. M., Perry, D. W. & Roy, A. (1997). Manifestations of depression in people with intellectual disability. *J. Intellect. Disabil. Res.*, **41**(Pt 6), 476–80.

Masi, G., Favilla, L. & Mucci, M. (2000). Generalized anxiety disorder in adolescents and young adults with mild mental retardation. *Psychiatry*, **63**, 54–64.

Masi, G., Mucci, M., Favilla, L. & Poli, P. (1999). Dysthymic disorder in adolescents with intellectual disability. *J. Intellect. Disabil. Res.*, **43**, 80–7.

Meins, W. (1995). Symptoms of major depression in mentally retarded adults. *J. Intellect. Disabil. Res.*, **39**(Pt 1), 41–5.

Meins, W. (1996). A new depression scale designed for use with adults with mental retardation. *Journal of Intellectual Disability Research*, **40**(3), 222–6.

Mindham, J. & Espie, C. A. (2003). Glasgow Anxiety Scale for people with an Intellectual Disability (GAS-ID): development and psychometric properties of a new measure for use with people with mild intellectual disability. *J. Intellect. Disabil. Res.*, **47**, 22–30.

Moss, S. C. (1997). Manchester: Hester Adrian Research Centre, PAS-ADD Checklist.

Moss, S., Goldberg, D., Patel, P. & Wilkin, D. (1993). Physical morbidity in older people with moderate, severe and profound mental handicap, and its relation to psychiatric morbidity. *Soc. Psychiatry. Psychiatr. Epidemiol.*, **28**, 32–9.

Newman, C. & Adams, K. (2004). Dog gone good: managing dog phobia in a teenage boy with a learning disability. *British Journal of Learning Disabilities*, **32**, 35–8.

Owen, D. M., Hastings, R. P., Noone, S. J. *et al.* (2004). Life events as correlates of problem behavior and mental health in a residential population of adults with developmental disabilities. *Res. Dev. Disabil.*, **25**, 309–20.

Patel, P. Goldberg, D. & Moss, S. (1993). Psychiatric morbidity in older people with moderate and severe learning disability. II: The prevalence study. *Br. J. Psychiatry*, **163**, 481–91.

Pickersgill, M. J., Valentine, J. D., May, R. & Brewin, C. R. (1994) Fears in mental retardation: I. Types of fears reported by men and women with and without mental retardation. *Advances in Behavior Research & Therapy*, **16**(4), 277–96.

Powell, R. (2003). Psychometric properties of the Beck depression inventory and the Zung self rating depression scale in adults with mental retardation. *Mental Retardation*, **41**, 88–95.

Ratey, J., Sovner, R., Parks, A. & Rogentine, K. (1991). Buspirone treatment of aggression and anxiety in mentally retarded patients: a multiple-baseline, placebo lead-in study. *Journal Clinical Psychiatry*, **52**, 159–62.

Reynolds, W. M. & Baker, J. A. (1988). Assessment of depression in persons with mental retardation. *American Journal on Mental Retardation*, **93**(1), 93–103.

Richards, M., Maughan, B., Hardy, R. *et al.* (2001). Long-term affective disorder in people with mild learning disability. *Br. J. Psychiatry*, **179**, 523–7.

Royal College of Psychiatrists (2001). Diagnostic Criteria for Psychiatric Disorders for Use with Adults with Learning Disabilities/Mental Retardation (DC-LD). London: Royal College of Psychiatrists.

Ryan, R. (1994). Posttraumatic stress disorder in persons with developmental disabilities. *Networker*, 1–5.

Sequeria, H., Howlin, P. & Hollins, S. (2003). Psychological disturbance associated with sexual abuse in people with learning disabilities: case control study. *Br. J. Psychiatry*, **183**, 451–6.

Singh, N. N., Sood, A., Sonenklar, N. & Ellis, C. R. (1991). Assessment and diagnosis of mental illness in persons with mental retardation. Methods and measures. *Behav. Modif.*, **15**, 419–43.

Sovner, R. H. & Hurley A. D. (1989). Ten diagnostic principles for recognising psychiatric disorders in mentally retarded persons. *Psychiatric Aspects of Mental Retardation Reviews*, 9–14.

Stavrakaki, C., Antochi, R. & Emery, P. C. (2004a). Olanzapine in the treatment of pervasive developmental disorders: a case series analysis. *J. Psychiatry. Neurosci.*, **29**, 57–60.

Stavrakaki, C., Antochi, R. & Emery, P. (2004b). Pharmacological treatments for behavioural disturbances in persons with developmental disabilities. *Psych. Annals*, **34**, 205–11.

Stavrakaki, C., Antochi, R. & Emery, P. (2004c). Obsessive compulsive disorder in adults with Down syndrome and other developmental disabilities. *Psych. Annals*, **34**, 196–200.

Stavrakaki, C., Antochi, R., Summers, J. & Adamson, J. (2002). *Psychopharmacological Treatment in Persons with Developmental Disabilities*. The Habilitative Mental Health Resource Network: Dual Diagnosis – an Introduction to the Mental Health Needs of Persons with Developmental Disabilities.

Stavrakaki, C. & Mintsioulis, G. (1997). Implications of a clinical study of anxiety disorders in persons with mental retardation. *Psych. Annals*, **27**, 182–9.

Tsiouris, J. A., Cohen, I. L., Patti, P. J. & Korosh, W. M. (2003). Treatment of previously undiagnosed psychiatric disorders in persons with developmental disabilities decreased or eliminated self-injurious behavior. *J. Clin. Psychiatry*, **64** 1081–90.

Tu, J. B. & Zellweger, H. (1965). Blood-serotonin deficiency in Down's syndrome. *Lancet*, **2**, 715–16.

Veernhoven, W. & Tuinier, S. (1997). Neuropsychiatric consultations in mentally retarded patients. *European Psychiatry*, **12**, 242–8.

Vitello, B. & Behar., D. (1992). Mental retardation and psychiatric illness. *Hospital Community Psychiatry*, 494–9.

World Health Organization. (1992). *The International Classification of Mental and Behaviour Disorders – Clinical Descriptions and Diagnostic Guidelines*. Geneva: World Health Organization.

Zung, W. K. (1971). A rating instrument for anxiety disorders. *Psychosomatics*, **12**, 371–9.

8

Schizophrenia spectrum disorders in people with intellectual disabilities

David Clarke

Introduction

This chapter discusses the concept and classification of schizophrenia spectrum disorders, their diagnosis, their relationship to intellectual disabilities (ID), and services appropriate to meet the needs of people with ID who also have psychoses.

It is helpful for those who work with people with ID to have some knowledge of psychoses and their treatment. They will often be better placed than a psychiatrist to communicate with the person concerned and to notice small changes in behaviour or functioning that may indicate the presence of a psychotic disorder. They may also notice benefits from treatment or side effects produced by medication.

Psychosis

Psychosis is a form of mental illness in which contact with reality is lost or seriously impaired. Psychotic disorders are characterized by features such as delusions (false beliefs that are not the result of the person's educational, social or cultural background), hallucinations (perceptions that occur with no external stimulus, such as 'voices') and profound changes in mood.

Psychoses are conventionally divided into those for which there is an obvious organic cause (such as delirium related to an infection, or a dementing illness caused by Alzheimer's disease) and 'functional' psychoses where an organic cause is not apparent (such as schizophrenia). This distinction between organic and functional psychoses is clinically useful because the symptoms are different, and the treatment of organic psychosis is directed at the underlying cause, whereas the treatment of functional psychoses is directed towards the relief of symptoms. However, there is increasing evidence that 'functional' psychoses are associated with organic brain changes (in structure or function). The term 'functional' is therefore not entirely

Psychiatric and Behavioural Disorders in Intellectual and Developmental Disabilities, ed. Nick Bouras and Geraldine Holt. Published by Cambridge University Press. © Cambridge University Press 2007.

appropriate, but retained because of convention and in the absence of any wholly satisfactory alternative.

The nature and classification of functional psychoses

Functional psychoses have traditionally been divided into affective (mood) disorders and schizophrenia and related disorders. This dichotomy is broadly reflected in current classificatory systems such as the Classification of Mental and Behavioural Disorders within the 10th Revision of the International Classification of Diseases (ICD-10; World Health Organization, 1992). However, some psychoses may encompass symptoms suggestive of both affective and schizophrenic psychoses, and others may involve only one or two symptoms (such as isolated delusions or hallucinations).

Research has failed to support fully the notion that affective and schizophrenic psychoses are entirely distinct and separate disorders. Some psychiatrists view them as poles on a continuum. Others have argued that the concept of 'schizophrenia' lacks any single defining principle, and is best regarded as a label for a syndrome reflecting a pattern of brain dysfunction that may have many causes. Because they are used widely, and are of help in predicting treatment response, this chapter will describe some of the categories of psychosis (including schizophrenia and related disorders) listed in ICD-10, and will refer to the additional guidance about diagnosis and classification given in DC-LD (Royal College of Psychiatrists, 2001) (see also Chapter 1 by Sturmey).

There is increasing evidence that genetic predisposition, resulting from the interplay of several different genes, combines with environmental and social factors to make some people more prone to psychotic symptoms than others. The significance attached to external events (and their likelihood of leading to firmly held beliefs that may be erroneous) appears to be mediated by dopamine dependent neural networks, and over-activity in such pathways may lead to psychosis (Kumar, 2003).

Affective disorders

Affective (mood) disorders include states of abnormally low mood (depressive disorders) and states where mood is abnormally elevated (manic states). These disorders differ from ordinary unhappiness or euphoria because the mood state is persistently abnormal, and accompanied by other characteristic features. The term bipolar affective disorder is used to describe recurrent psychoses (two or more episodes, at least one of which was manic). The term recurrent depressive disorder is used to delineate multiple (two or more) episodes of depression. In hypomanic states, mood is abnormally and persistently elevated, and accompanied by features such as increased activity, restlessness, increased talkativeness, distractibility, decreased need for sleep, increased sexual energy, over-spending or other irresponsible behaviour, disinhibition and over-familiarity. When severe (a manic, as opposed to hypomanic state), other features occur, such as flight of ideas (where thoughts race from one topic to another, reflected in the person's speech), abnormally increased self-esteem or grandiosity, and reckless behaviour. Delusions and hallucinations are not uncommonly associated with severe manic states. These are usually mood-congruent (consistent with the mood abnormality, such as voices announcing that the person has won a large prize, or the belief that the person has special powers). Depressive disorders are characterized by low mood, reduced energy and activity, anhedonia (loss of enjoyment and satisfaction), reduced appetite and libido, sleep abnormalities (typically with early-morning waking), and ideas of guilt or worthlessness that may be delusional.

Schizophrenia and schizophrenia spectrum disorders

Schizophrenia is characterized by fundamental and characteristic distortions of thinking and perception, and mood states that are inappropriate to the social context or that are flat and unchanging. Typical clinical features ('positive' symptoms) are listed in Table 8.1, with brief descriptions and examples of the experiences as perceived by the patient. Negative symptoms include social withdrawal, blunting of affect and problems with attention.

Schizophrenic disorders can be either continuous or episodic (with a progressive or stable pattern of deficits), or there may be one or more episodes with complete or incomplete remission. Schizophrenia should not be diagnosed during states of drug intoxication or withdrawal, or 'in the presence of overt brain disease' (ICD-10).

The ICD-10 groups schizo-affective disorders (episodic psychoses in which both affective and schizophrenic symptoms are prominent) with schizophrenia, while noting that their relationship to schizophrenia and the affective disorders remains to be clarified. Other schizophrenia spectrum disorders include delusional disorders characterized solely or predominantly by abnormal beliefs such as the conviction that small louse-like insects have infested the head. Cycloid psychoses, or acute and transient psychotic disorders, are characterized by a sudden onset and a shifting, polymorphous pattern of symptoms including agitation, anxiety and mood and schizophrenic symptoms.

Psychoses are not uncommon among the general population. About 1% will have one or more episodes of schizophrenia in their life and a similar proportion (0.6–1%) will experience bipolar affective disorder. Less severe forms of depression are much commoner, and more common in women than men.

Table 8.1 Clinical features occurring in schizophrenia spectrum disorders.

Clinical feature	Description
Thought echo	Thoughts are repeated in audible form (occasionally, thoughts are anticipated rather than repeated).
Thought insertion	Thoughts are suddenly put into the mind, disrupting the train of thought.
Thought withdrawal	Thoughts are suddenly withdrawn from the mind, disrupting the train of thought.
Thought broadcasting	Thoughts are apparent to others as soon as they occur. The patient may have an 'explanation' such as telepathy or a mind-reading machine.
Delusional perception	An ordinary stimulus (seeing a fir tree in a garden), leads suddenly to a delusion that is unconnected (the person is going to be assassinated by an occult organization).
Delusions of control or influence, or passivity experiences	Delusional beliefs that the patient's body or mind are controlled by some external force. An 'explanation' may be linked to other psychopathology ('the BBC make my mind go blank using a transmitter').
Auditory hallucinations	The 'voices' are usually of a characteristic nature in schizophrenia; they are often derogatory and may comment on the person in the third person, or make other remarks ('She's turned the tap on. Stupid isn't she?') or argue with each other.
Thought disorder	Used to describe disordered speech reflecting underlying thought disorganization. Neologisms (non-existent words) may be used ('I never eat sphericks'.)

Among people with ID, the pooled results of studies suggest rates of between 2% and 6% for schizophrenia (usually only diagnosed among people with mild ID) and between 3 and 8% for affective disorders. These prevalence rates are about four times higher than for the general population.

Schizophrenia and intellectual functioning

There is increasing evidence that neurocognitive deficits are present in people with schizophrenic psychoses who do not have an ID (MacCabe & Murray, 2004). These deficits are mild, compared with those characteristic of ID, and occur in all domains. Schizophrenic disorders are now regarded as disorders of neurodevelopmental origin, in which environmental factors operating in utero disrupt cortical development and predispose to psychosis. Precipitating factors operating in adolescence and early adult life then lead to manifest psychotic illness. The neuropsychological deficits associated with schizophrenia appear to be relatively stable during the early course of the illness, but may worsen later in life (possibly as a result of a neurodegen-erative process). Greenwood *et al.* (2004) noted a familial association between ID and schizophrenia, and suggested that this lent support to the neurodevelopmental hypothesis of the causation of psychoses. Hucker *et al.* (1979) studied people with ID and schizophrenia, and made comparisons with people with ID alone. There were higher proportions of people with impaired hearing, gestation below 36 weeks and low birth weight in the group with schizophrenia. O'Dwyer (1997) reported higher rates of obstetric complications among people with ID and schizophrenia than among controls matched for age, sex, severity of ID and presence or absence of epilepsy. Further evidence for brain dysfunction associated with schizophrenia comes from neuroimaging studies (Hill *et al.*, 2004) and from the finding that transcranial magnetic stimulation can be used both as a diagnostic aid and as a treatment for schizophrenia spectrum disorders (Haroldsson *et al.*, 2004). More is becoming known about the interplay between genetic factors and abnormalities in neurotransmitter systems in psychoses, and several genes thought to increase risk for schizophrenia have been identified (Harrison & Weinberg, 2004).

Psychosocial factors also impact on the prevalence of schizophrenia associated with ID. People with such disabilities are at greater risk for adverse life experiences such as physical and sexual abuse and bullying. They may have lower self-esteem and lead to less well-developed social networks, in turn leading to isolation and lack of support. Research suggests an association between social isolation and increased risk for schizophrenia spectrum disorders (Van Os *et al.*, 2000).

Recent evidence suggests that antipsychotic medication use does not result in appreciable cognitive deficits, and newer 'atypical' antipsychotics may improve cognitive functioning (Weiss *et al.*, 2002).

Clinical features, assessment and diagnosis

The diagnosis of psychoses among people with mild ID is not usually problematic for an experienced clinician, although more weight may have to be given to non-verbal clinical features and accounts from carers. If the person has a moderate, severe or profound ID, the diagnosis of schizophrenia or related psychoses may be impossible (because of severely impaired communication). This reflects the extraordinary nature of the complex subjective experiences involved (see Table 8.1) and the difficulty people have in conveying these experiences to others. In addition to the positive features of psychosis described in Table 8.1, negative symptoms such as social withdrawal, apathy, impaired emotional responses and problems with attention can have a major impact on quality of life for affected people.

A presumptive diagnosis of a non-organic psychotic disorder can sometimes be made on the basis of observable features. These may include behaviour strongly suggestive of auditory hallucinations (such as shouting 'back' at people not present), social withdrawal, blunted or inappropriate affect and suspiciousness not previously evident in the person's personality. Diagnostic instruments have been of limited use, because they usually rely on a 'snap shot' of the person in the form of lists of clinical features that have to be rated by a carer. This can cause diagnostic confusion (such as confusing autism with chronic schizophrenia), but may be useful as a screening technique for research purposes. Newer instruments such as the Psychopathology Assessment Schedule for Adults with Developmental Disability (PAS-ADD) (Moss et al., 1993) appear to have fewer limitations (see also Chapter 2 by Mohr and Costello). The use of instruments in the assessment of psychiatric and behavioural abnormalities has been reviewed by Sturmey et al. (1991). Hucker et al. (1979) used Research Diagnostic Criteria developed by Feighner et al. (1972) with a group of people with ID, and concluded that it was relatively easy to develop criteria for the diagnosis of affective disorders, whereas the criteria for schizophrenia were more problematic and controversial. Brugha et al. (1988) used draft ICD-10 criteria, and found that people with mild ID had little difficulty in reporting symptoms such as delusions and hallucinations. Clarke et al. (1994) used draft Diagnostic Criteria for Research linked to ICD-10, and found these to be relatively easy to apply to populations of people with ID with psychiatric and behavioural disorders, with the exception of schizophrenia. The Royal College of Psychiatrists in the UK has published DC-LD (Royal College of Psychiatrists, 2001) to aid in the diagnosis of psychotic disorders associated with ID (see also Chapter 1 by Sturmey). Melville (2003) provided a critique of the DC-LD section on non-affective psychoses, and pointed to possible problems with reliability, validity and utility.

Psychoses represent a *change* in mental functioning, and this can be helpful to distinguish them from disorders such as autism if the change is recent. Much care is needed to differentiate functional psychoses from other emotional and behavioural abnormalities seen in association with ID, such as stereotyped movements related to a syndrome such as Rett syndrome or an autistic disorder. Apparently incongruous affect may result from distractibility or a disorder such as Angelman syndrome (see also Chapter 12 by Hodapp and Dykens). Unusual preoccupations associated with autistic disorders may be difficult to differentiate from delusions. 'Practice' repetitive vocalizations, or talking to an imaginary friend, may lead to a suspicion of auditory hallucinations (see also Chapter 13 by Saulnier and Volkmar). The difficulties of establishing accurate diagnoses for young people with ID who have psychotic symptoms have been discussed by Friedlander and Donnelly (2004). These authors have also given information about prognosis for the group of 21 young people with ID and early-onset psychoses that they studied (see also Chapter 6 by Tonge). The assessment of possible psychotic disorders has been discussed by Vanstraelen et al. (2003) who noted the need for attention to the person's communicatory ability, information from informants, direct observation, an assessment of the presenting problem over time, the developmental history and the medical history and presence of other disabilities or sensory impairments. Meadows *et al.* (1991) studied 25 people with ID and schizophrenia and 26 controls without ID. The symptomatology of the two groups was very similar, the commonest features being delusions and hallucinations. Little support was found for the view that psychotic disorders occurring in association with ID are characterized by atypical symptoms and much behavioural 'overlay'. Bouras *et al.* (2004) reported differences in the clinical characteristics of people with schizophrenia spectrum disorders associated with ID, compared with a control group with schizophrenia but without ID. The group with ID was found to have more obviously observable psychopathology, more negative symptoms and greater functional impairments. These authors also found no significant differences in associated behavioural disorder between the groups with and without ID.

Disorders resulting in an association between intellectual disabilities and psychosis (see also Chapter 12 by Hodapp and Dykens)

Usher's syndrome

Sensory impairments are more common among people with ID. There is a specific association with psychosis in some cases of Usher's syndrome, which consists of retinitis pigmentosa, congenital deafness, vestibulo-cerebellar ataxia, ID (in about 23%) and psychosis (usually schizophrenia) in about 15% of cases (Hallgren, 1959).

Velo-cardio-facial syndrome

The report of Goldberg *et al.* (1993) suggested that velo-cardio-facial syndrome (VCFS) might be associated with a relatively high prevalence of severe psychiatric disorder. Subsequent, more methodologically sound studies have confirmed an association with disorders variously described as schizophrenia, schizophrenia with some atypical features, and bipolar affective disorder. An overview of the psychiatric, behavioural and neuropsychological complications of VCFS has been provided by Murphy (2004).

Prader–Willi syndrome

Clarke (1993) reported cases of psychosis with affective symptoms associated with Prader–Willi syndrome (PWS), and noted other reports in the literature. Subsequent population-based research has demonstrated that PWS caused by maternal uniparental disomy is associated with a risk of psychosis with affective symptoms that approaches 100% by the age of 30 years (Boer *et al.*, 2002).

General principles of treatment

Pharmacological treatments

The pharmacological treatment of psychoses is discussed in Chapter 19. Psychoses associated with ID are treated in the same way as psychoses affecting other groups of people, but drug treatments have to be tailored to the individual and the particular problems they have. This may mean using drugs with a particular adverse effect profile to minimize the effect on, for example, a concurrent seizure disorder or motor problem.

Non-pharmacological treatments

Non-pharmacological treatments may be used in combination with medication or, more rarely, alone. As with medication, most of the research into non-pharmacological approaches to treating functional psychoses has been carried out on study samples of people without ID. Such interventions include cognitive techniques to address maladaptive assumptions that may maintain depressive states (Blackburn et al., 1981), the use of distraction or masking techniques to treat auditory hallucinations (Nelson et al., 1991), and interventions to reduce expressed emotion and help prevent relapse of schizophrenic psychoses (Anderson & Adams, 1996). Some of these techniques are used in clinical practice with people with ID, but systematic evaluations are rarely published (see also Chapter 20 by Dagnan). The teaching of techniques to aid anxiety or anger management (Rose, 1996) may also be of help to prevent symptoms emerging through heightened anxiety and to lessen their impact on quality of life. Techniques to reduce the impact of auditory hallucinations by masking may be helpful for some people with ID, if they are able to tolerate an ear-plug or can comply with techniques such as sub-vocal counting.

Programmes to reduce expressed emotion focus primarily on family members or others in regular face-to-face contact with the person who has a psychotic disorder. Where a person with ID is living in a group home, the standard techniques of working with families may have to be modified to take account of other residents' difficulties with language or with the understanding of concepts such as 'hostility'. A community nurse or psychologist may be able to work with residents and staff members to reduce criticism of the person concerned, but input may have to consist of relatively short discussions spread over a long time period, with 'refresher' visits as necessary.

Services for people with intellectual disabilities and psychoses

The components of a psychiatric service for people with ID and psychoses will depend to some extent on local expertise and the availability of resources. A hospital admission service will be necessary to assess and treat people detained using mental health legislation. A home treatment or intensive support service may reduce the need for such admissions, and offers a form of assessment that may be more informative than admission in some circumstances (because changes consequent on alterations in the living environment are reduced). For some people, home treatment is not an option (for example, where the person has delusions concerning family members, and may be at risk of acting on the delusions). Most people with psychoses can be managed as outpatients or on a domiciliary basis. Adequate outpatient facilities, expertise within community teams, and mechanisms to facilitate liaison with other statutory and voluntary organizations should be in place (see also Chapter 23 by Davidson and O'Hara).

An effective day, respite and home treatment service will reduce (but not eliminate) the need for inpatient facilities, and staff training will reduce exclusions from non-specialist day and residential settings. Bouras and Holt (1997), and Holt *et al.* (2005) have developed training packages for people working with mentally ill people with ID.

Conclusion

Schizophrenia spectrum disorders are more common among people with ID than in the general population. They can adversely affect quality of life. Diagnosis can be problematic. Treatment can improve quality of life. Pharmacological treatments should be monitored to ensure the best risk/benefit ratio for the individual. A range of services is needed to meet the needs of this client group. Further research is needed, especially into associations with genetic causes of ID and differential responses to treatment.

Summary points

- Schizophrenia spectrum disorders are more common among people with ID than in the general population.
- Schizophrenia and related disorders arise through genetic predisposition, probably mediated through early neurodevelopmental abnormalities.
- Overt psychosis may be triggered by environmental factors, often acting in adolescence or early in adult life.
- Research investigating groups of people with increased risk or atypical symptomatology, including people with velo-cardio-facial syndrome and Prader–Willi syndrome, has proved fruitful.
- The features of psychotic disorders are often distressing and may lead to behaviours such as self-harm, social withdrawal or aggression.

- The diagnosis of psychosis associated with intellectual disability requires special expertise.
- Recent studies have identified differences between people with schizophrenia spectrum disorders who have intellectual disabilities, and those who do not have ID.
- Treatments usually involve the prescription of psychoactive medications. These are usually effective in relieving positive symptoms of psychosis, and do not cause further cognitive impairment.
- Non-drug treatments, such as interventions to reduce expressed emotion, may be appropriate for some people.
- The psychiatrist's role involves a careful balancing of potential risks and benefits from treatment, bearing in mind the presence of other illnesses or disabilities.
- A comprehensive range of community and inpatient services is necessary to meet the needs of people with ID and schizophrenia spectrum disorders.

REFERENCES

Anderson, J. & Adams, C. (1996). Family interventions in schizophrenia: an effective but under-used treatment. *British Medical Journal*, **313**, 505–6.

Blackburn, I. M., Bishop, S., Glen, A. I. M., Whalley, L. J. & Christie, J. E. (1981). The efficacy of cognitive therapy on depression: a treatment trial using cognitive therapy and pharmacotherapy, each alone and in combination. *British Journal of Psychiatry*, **139**, 181–9.

Boer, H., Holland, A., Whittington, J. *et al.* (2002). Psychotic illness in people with Prader–Willi syndrome due to chromosome 15 maternal uniparental disomy. *Lancet*, **359**, 135–6.

Bouras, N. & Holt, G. (1997). *Mental Health and Learning Disabilities Training Package*, 2nd Edn. Brighton: Pavilion Press.

Bouras, N., Martin, G., Leese, M. *et al.* (2004). Schizophrenia-spectrum psychoses in people with and without intellectual disability. *Journal of Intellectual Disability Research*, **48**, 548–55.

Brugha, T. S., Collacot, R., Warrington, J., Deb, S. & Bruce, J. (1988). Eliciting and reliably rating delusions and hallucinations in the mildly retarded. Paper read at: *Eighth Congress of the International Association for the Scientific Study of Mental Deficiency*, August 1988, Dublin, Eire.

Clarke, D. J. (1993). Prader–Willi syndrome and psychoses. *British Journal of Psychiatry*, **163**, 680–4.

Clarke, D., Cumella, S., Corbett, J. *et al.* (1994). Use of ICD-10 research diagnostic criteria to categorise psychiatric and behavioural abnormalities among people with learning disabilities: The West Midlands field trial. *Mental Handicap Research*, **7**, 273–85.

Feighner, J. P., Robins, E., Guze, S. B. *et al.* (1972). Diagnostic criteria for use in psychiatric research. *Archives of General Psychiatry*, **26**, 57–63.

Friedlander, R. I. & Donnelly, T. (2004). Early-onset psychosis in youth with intellectual disability. *Journal of Intellectual Disability Research*, **48**, 540–7.

Goldberg, R., Motzkin, B., Marion, R., Scambler, P. J. & Shprintzen, R. J. (1993). Velo cardio facial syndrome: A review of 120 patients. *American Journal of Medical Genetics*, **45**, 313–19.

Greenwood, C. M. T., Husted, J., Bomba, M. D., Hodgkinson, K. A. & Bassett, A. S. (2004). Elevated rates of schizophrenia in a familial sample wth mental illness and intellectual disability. *Journal of Intellectual Disability Research*, **48**, 531–9.

Hallgren, B. (1959). Retinitis pigmentosa combined with congenital deafness; with vestibulo-cerebellar ataxia and mental abnormality in a proportion of cases. A clinical and genetico-statistical study. *Acta Psychiatrica Neurologica Scandinavica*, **24** (Suppl. 138), 1–101.

Haroldsson, H. M., Ferrarelli, F., Kalin, N. H. & Tononi, G. (2004). Transcranial magnetic stimulation in the investigation and treatment of schizophrenia: a review. *Schizophrenia Research*, **71**, 1–16.

Harrison, P. J. & Weinberger, D. R. (2004). Schizophrenia genes, gene expression, and neuropathology: on the matter of their convergence. *Molecular Psychiatry*, advance online publication, 20 July 2004, doi: 10.1038/sj.mp.4001558.

Hill, K., Mann, L., Laws, K. R. *et al.* (2004). Hypofrontality in schizophrenia: a meta-analysis of functional imaging studies. *Acta Psychiatrica Scandinavica*, **110**, 243–56.

Holt, G., Hardy, S. & Bouras, N (2005). *Mental Health in Learning Disabilities: A Training Resource.* Brighton: Pavilion Publishing.

Hucker, S. J., Day, K. E., George, S. & Roth, M. (1979). Psychosis in mentally handicapped adults. In P. Snaith & P. E. James (eds.), *Psychiatric Illness and Mental Handicap.* London: Gaskell.

Kumar, S. (2003). Psychosis as a state of aberrant salience: a framework linking biology, phenomenology, and pharmacology in schizophrenia. *American Journal of Psychiatry*, **160**, 13–23.

MacCabe, J. H. & Murray, R. M. (2004). Intellectual functioning in schizophrenia: a marker of neurodevelopmental damage? *Journal of Intellectual Disability Research*, **48**, 519–23.

Meadows, G., Turner, T., Campbell, L. *et al.* (1991). Assessing schizophrenia in adults with mental retardation: a comparative study. *British Journal of Psychiatry*, **158**, 103–5.

Melville, C. (2003). A critique of the Diagnostic Criteria for Psychiatric Disorders for Use with Adults with Learning Disabilities/Mental Retardation (DC-LD) chapter on non-affective psychotic disorders. *Journal of Intellectual Disability Research*, **47** (Suppl. 1), 16–25.

Moss, S., Patel, P., Prosser, H. *et al.* (1993). Psychiatric morbidity in older people with moderate and severe learning disability. I: Development and reliability of the patient interview (PAS-ADD). *British Journal of Psychiatry*, **163**, 471–80.

Murphy, K. C. (2004). The behavioural phenotype in velo-cardio-facial syndrome. *Journal of Intellectual Disability Research*, **48**, 524–30.

Nelson, H. E., Thrasher, S. & Barnes, T. R. E. (1991). Practical ways of alleviating auditory hallucinations. *British Medical Journal*, **302**: 327.

O'Dwyer, J. (1997). Schizophrenia in people with intellectual disability: the role of pregnancy and birth complications. *Journal of Intellectual Disability Research*, **41**, 238–51.

Rose, J. (1996). Anger management: a group treatment programme for people with mental retardation. *Journal of Developmental and Physical Disabilities*, **8**, 133–49.

Royal College of Psychiatrists (2001). *Diagnostic Criteria for Psychiatric Disorders for Use with Adults with Learning Disabilities/Mental Retardation (DC-LD).* London: Gaskell.

Sturmey, P., Reed, J. & Corbett, J. (1991). Psychometric assessment of psychiatric disorders in people with learning disabilities (mental handicap): a review of measures. *Psychological Medicine*, **21**, 143–55.

Van Os, J., Driessen, G., Gunther, N. & Delespaul, P. (2000). Neighbourhood variation in incidence of schizophrenia. Evidence for person-environment interaction. *British Journal of Psychiatry*, **176**, 243–8.

Vanstraelen, M., Holt, G. & Bouras, N. (2003). Adults with learning disabilities and psychiatric problems. In Fraser, W. & Kerr, M. (eds.), *Seminars in The Psychiatry of Learning Disabilities*, 2nd edn. London: Gaskell.

Weiss, E. M., Bilder, R. M. & Fleischbacker, W. W. (2002). The effects of second-generation antipsychotics on cognitive functioning and psychosocial outcome in schizophrenia. *Psychopharmacology*, **162**, 11–17.

World Health Organization (1992). *The ICD-10 Classification of Mental and Behavioural Disorders: Clinical Descriptions and Diagnostic Guidelines*. World Health Organization: Geneva.

9

Personality disorder

William R. Lindsay

Introduction

Both DSM-IV and ICD-10 have classifications for a range of personality disorders (PD). Both have a categorical structure to classification and have the same strengths and weaknesses. The research covered in this chapter will allude primarily to DSM-IV-TR classifications but is directly relevant to considerations on ICD-10 classification. It should be noted that there has recently been a review of ICD-10 classifications, that takes account of an intellectual disabilities (ID) perspective, DC-LD (Royal College of Psychiatrists, 2001). From the viewpoint of PD there are interesting basic alterations in DC-LD. Firstly, it recommends that, because of developmental delay in these individuals, diagnosis should not be made until at least 21 years of age. In addition, DC-LD requires the initial confirmation of PD unspecified, before progressing to more general diagnoses of PD. Personality disorder unspecified requires that the characteristics must not be a direct consequence of the person's ID and also states specifically that there must be associated significant problems in occupational and/or social functioning. Therefore, the impact of personality on the person's general social and occupational function is explicitly considered as a requirement for diagnosis (see also Chapter 1 by Sturmey).

The DSM-IV-TR (American Psychiatric Association, 2000) has extensive trait descriptions for ten specific PDs in three clusters. Cluster A includes paranoid PD (suspiciousness and distrust); schizoid PD (detachment from social relationships, a restricted range of emotional expression); and schizotypal PD (acute discomfort in close relationships, eccentricities of behaviour including magical control and idiosyncratic speech). Cluster B includes antisocial personality disorder (lack of empathy, callousness, contempt for the rights of others); borderline personality disorder (instability of interpersonal relationships, impulsivity); histrionic personality disorder (excessive emotionality, attention seeking, shallow and shifting emotion);

Psychiatric and Behavioural Disorders in Intellectual and Developmental Disabilities, ed. Nick Bouras and Geraldine Holt. Published by Cambridge University Press. © Cambridge University Press 2007.

and narcissistic PD (grandiosity, arrogance, lack of empathy, exploitation). Cluster C includes avoidant PD (social avoidance, preoccupation with rejection); dependent PD (fear of separation, need for reassurance, need for others to assume responsibility); and obsessive-compulsive PD (preoccupation with perfectionism, over conscientious, stubborn). Personality disorder not otherwise specified is a final category in which there may be a number of features of more than one PD but not enough to meet the full criteria for a specific disorder.

Recent commentators have drawn attention to the growing body of studies recording problems in the classification of personality disorder (Blackburn, 2000, Livesley, 2002). With both DSM-IV and ICD-10 classifications, the diagnosis of personality disorder has low reliability. Reliability increases if two assessors use the same structured diagnostic instrument but decreases once again if different diagnostic instruments are employed. Co-morbidity of two or more PD is common, indicating that each disorder is not at all discrete and personality traits are not unique to particular PDs. The internal integrity of certain disorders has also been questioned. For example, positive and negative dimensions of schizotypal PD have been shown to be differentially prevalent in different groups (Blackburn, 2000). Finally, there is the fundamental criticism that the categorical nature of PD classification is not consistent with knowledge on the nature of personality, which organizes personality factors, e.g. extraversion or neuroticism, along dimensions from very little of the characteristic to excessive amounts of the characteristic.

Somewhat paradoxically, commentators also point out that the establishment of DSM diagnostic categories of PD has stimulated large amounts of research which has subsequently reinforced the importance of the concept of PD in relation to service planning, management and treatment for a range of individuals including psychiatric patients, offenders and people with ID.

The main findings from research have been interesting and, if replicated, may be extremely important for the development of assessment and treatment research and implementation of social policy. High levels of certain PDs have been associated with poorer treatment outcomes (Tyrer & Simmonds, 2003). Hembree *et al.* (2004) in a study of 75 adult women with post-traumatic stress disorder (PTSD), found that there was no difference between those participants with and without PD on prevalence of PTSD at the end of treatment. However, participants with a PD were significantly less likely to attain good end-state functioning following treatment. In a different area, Seto and Barbaree (1999) studied the relationship between psychopathy, treatment compliance and treatment outcome in 244 sex offenders. They found that those individuals with higher psychopathy ratings and good treatment compliance had higher recidivism rates. On the other hand, Skeem *et al.* (2002) in a study of 871 psychiatric patients, found that traits of psychopathy did not affect engagement with treatment for violence and were not associated with violence reduction. Authors reviewing these fields have noted this lack of consistent findings in relation to outcome for anxiety treatment (Dreessen & Arntz, 1998) and offender treatment (D'Silva *et al.*, 2004). If there are circumstances in which PD diminishes the potency of treatment, a further avenue for research is to investigate treatment alternatives, which might counteract negative effects of PD on treatment progress.

A second crucial finding is that Cluster B PD and especially antisocial PD are reasonable predictors of future aggression and are significantly more prevalent among inmates of correctional settings (Fazel & Danesh, 2002). In addition, psychopathy as measured by the Psychopathy Checklist – Revised (PCL-R: Hare, 1991) is related to Cluster B PDs (Blackburn, 2000) and also successfully predicts future aggression in a range of populations of criminals (Grettan *et al.*, 2001, Hill *et al.*, 2004). A final important finding is that antisocial PD and the PCL-R make significant contributions to the prediction of recidivism in a range of offences (Harris *et al.*, 2003). Therefore, from a number of points of view, research on PD has been shown to produce extremely important findings in relation to the planning and development of services and treatment.

Personality disorder and intellectual disabilities

There has been a slow but steady flow of research on ID and PD from early idiosyncratic writings, which focused on personality characteristics such as weakness, simplicity, immaturity, and instability to more recent perceptive analyses and scientific work based on recognized diagnostic classifications (Alexander & Cooray, 2003, Reid *et al.*, 2004). The first systematic investigation into PD in adults with ID was conducted by Corbett (1979) when he reported a prevalence rate of PD of 25% in a large community sample of 402 persons. Of those diagnosed with PD the categories were as follows: 4% paranoid, 2% schizoid, 15% impulsive, 47.5% immature/unstable, 22.5% anxious and 9% explosive. Over the following 10 years, others found similar, relatively high rates of PD in this population. For example, Reid and Ballinger (1987) found a rate of severe personality disorder of 22% in a general, institutionalized population of people with ID. They found a predominance of explosive personality disorder in males, cyclothymic personality disorder in females and an approximately equal distribution of hysterical personality disorder between males and females. These authors, among others, were of the view that the diagnostic criteria for PD did not apply to people with severe or profound ID but rather should be confined to those individuals with mild or moderate ID.

This latter point has been reiterated more recently with respect to DSM-IV classification (Lindsay *et al.*, in press, a). Individuals with severe or profound ID may have such severe communication and language difficulties, lack of understanding of the

laws and mores of society and such profound developmental delay that consideration of personality and subsequently personality disorder in a normal, mainstream
context is inappropriate. Therefore, these earlier authors were already pointing out
some of the difficulties in the judgement of PD in this client group. Separating an
immature personality from the ID itself is likely to be problematic. Early writing
mentions weakness, simplicity and immaturity, while Corbett (1979) found that
almost half of those diagnosed with PD were classified as immature/unstable. It
might be considered that diagnosis of PD in this client group might result in an
over preponderance of classifications such as dependant PD, which might simply
be a reflection of the necessary requirements of ID. In addition, a high rate of anger
and aggression has been reported across a number of samples in this client group
(Novaco & Taylor, 2004) but the link between high rates of aggression and underlying personality structures of explosive, impulsive or antisocial traits or disorders
remains uninvestigated.

More recent work has produced more fluctuating figures with regard to prevalence of personality disorder. Reviewing this literature, Alexander and Cooray
(2003) comment on the lack of reliable diagnostic instruments, difference between
ICD-10 and DSM-IV diagnostic systems, confusion of definition and personality
theory, and the difficulties of distinguishing personality disorder from other problems integral to ID, e.g. communication problems, sensory disorders and developmental delay. They conclude 'the variation in the co-occurrence of personality
disorder in *(intellectual disability)* with prevalence rates ranging from 1% to 91% ...
is too large to be explained by real differences' (p. 528). They recommend tighter
diagnostic criteria, greater use of behavioural observation and increased use of
informant information.

Personality and personality disorder

The extensive research on personality (in contrast to personality disorder) has not
extended to the field of ID. Blackburn (2000) notes that a five-factor model has
emerged from a wealth of research investigating personality structure, with the
'big five' factors represented by extraversion, neuroticism, openness, agreeableness
and conscientiousness. This five-factor solution has been replicated on numerous
occasions (although it is not without its critics) and Costa and McCrae (1985)
have employed the model to develop the NEO Personality Inventory (NEO-PI)
to assess these factors along five dimensions. However, in ID the most prominent
group working in this field have developed personality assessment from a completely different perspective to that of mainstream researchers. Over the course of
40 years, Zigler and his colleagues (Zigler *et al.*, 2002) have conducted extensive
research into personality and ID. Zigler's early work demonstrated that, although

children with cultural–familial developmental disabilities appeared to pass through the same developmental stages as other children, their experience of development was significantly different from other children. Specifically, he hypothesized that their repeated experience of failure on academic and other tasks changed their style of problem solving. This led them to avoid novel challenging tasks, expecting to fail, and to look to others for cues as to how to solve these tasks. This series of studies led Zigler *et al.* (2002) to hypothesize seven personality dimensions along which people with ID varied as follows: *positive reaction tendency* (a heightened motivation . . . to both interact with, and be dependent upon, a supportive adult); *negative reaction tendency* (initial wariness shown . . . when interacting with strange adults); *expectancy of success* (the degree to which one expects to succeed or fail when presented a new task); *outer directedness* (tendency . . . to look to others for the cues to solutions for difficult or ambiguous tasks); *efficacy motivation* (the pleasure derived from tackling and solving difficult problems); *obedience; curiosity/creativity*. It is immediately noticeable that these personality traits bear little resemblance to the 'big five'. It would appear that none of Zigler's factors is related to mood or emotion, which is one of the most enduring factors in personality research.

Reid *et al.* (2004) report on the adaptation and use of the NEO-PI on six individuals with ID. The 240 individual items required considerable simplification both in their presentation and in their response formats in order that participants with ID could respond during interview to the self-report inventory. The NEO-PI has an informant version and these authors found that the self-report and informant results were broadly in agreement across the five personality factors for all six participants. Taking all 30 personality factors rated (six participants × five factors), 50% were in exact agreement on dimensional bands (very low, low, average, high, very high), and 90% were within one band of disagreement. This last study is the only piece of work reporting on the use of a standard, mainstream personality inventory with people with ID. This is perhaps because it takes so long to administer the large number of items. The adapted NEO-PI with 240 items takes up to four hours, with breaks, to administer.

Major technical advances have been made in the development of self-report instruments for this client group (Finlay & Lyons, 2001). Several authors have demonstrated the reliability of alternative administration procedures for assessments and that, given reliable administration and responding, results parallel those found in mainstream populations (Lindsay & Taylor, 2005). It would certainly be expedient for these recent advances now to extend to inventories of personality and personality disorder.

This work is mentioned to point out the impoverished state of personality research on this client group. In mainstream research (e.g. Livesley, 2002; Blackburn, 2000) there has been extensive work on the integration of research on personality and PD. Livesley (2002) has written, 'empirical evaluations of the category-dimension distinction suggest that an empirically based classification should adopt a dimensional approach or at least incorporate a dimensional scheme to describe individual differences in personality pathology' (p.164). He reports studies which consistently identify a four-factor structure underlying personality disorder criteria and traits, which are represented by: neuroticism; psychoticism/antisocial; obsessive-compulsive; and suspicious avoidance/intraversion. Clearly much work is required on the integration of personality and personality disorder theory and research in the field of ID and these authors provide directional indicators for those of us embarking on this work.

Diagnosis of personality disorder in people with ID

Taking this work into consideration, Lindsay *et al.* (2005) have made several recommendations for the careful consideration of PD in this client group. They reiterate the recommendations of Alexander and Cooray (2003) that classification requires greater use of behavioural observation and increased use of informant information. In addition, they note a number of cultural factors that must be taken into account in classification. People with ID may have lived more restricted lives than those in the mainstream population and, as such, may have had less opportunity to experience a range of social and sexual relationships, which in turn may have hindered personality development. This is likely to be true for a large section of this population and, therefore, one must have knowledge of the cultural norms in this regard before making a diagnosis of PD. Similarly, they note higher levels of aggression and suggestibility, lower levels of occupational activity and higher levels of required dependency such as those individuals on guardianship or financial dependency on the state. All of these contextual issues are important when considering a PD classification. This makes diagnosis of PD particularly problematic and these authors have written

we are also aware that we run the risk of falling into the twin traps of, on the one hand declaring that persons with ID are immune from some PD or, on the other, suggesting that they present in ways grossly divergent from persons without ID . . . an unusual personal history does not exclude someone from a diagnosis of PD. The diagnosis is made, or not made, on the basis of whether the person's behaviour, cognition and attitudes meets or does not meet the criteria set

They also note that there may be a reasonable expectation that someone who has lived in a restricted or institutionalized environment might be re-socialized through combined social learning and treatment procedures. Therefore, they also recommend that individuals be reassessed annually during any treatment, habilitation or socialization process.

The Psychopathy Checklist – Revised (PCL-R)

The PCL-R is included in this chapter because it is a frequently researched personality measure, and high scores on the PCL-R are reliably related to aggression and recidivism (Hill *et al.*, 2004; Harris *et al.*, 2003). The PCL-R scores have been found to relate to Cluster B personality disorders (Blackburn, 2000). Morrissey (2003) has developed guidelines for scoring the PCL-R with offenders with ID. Reid *et al.* (2004) report on the relationship between high and low PCL-R respondents and their profile on the NEO-PI. As with mainstream research, they found that psychopathy as measured by the PCL-R had an association with low agreeableness and low conscientiousness on the 'big five' personality factors. Morrissey *et al.* (submitted for publication) have reported on the use of the PCL-R with three cohorts of offenders with ID: high security, medium/low security and those in the community. They found that average PCL-R scores for the cohorts varied as predicted, with those in high security having the highest average scores and those in the community lowest. In addition, preliminary factor analysis found a similar factor structure to that of previous authors (e.g. Cooke & Michie, 2001; Hill *et al.*, 2004). Therefore it would seem that with appropriate adaptations, PCL-R results from this client group provide broadly similar patterns to mainstream offenders.

Recent studies

Naik *et al.* (2002) report a study of 430 outpatients with ID in which they found a prevalence rate of PD of 7%. Of those individuals diagnosed with PD, 59% were classified with dissocial/antisocial PD, 28% emotionally unstable PD and 10% with both diagnoses. They found a high percentage of co-morbidity with Axis I disorders and 59% had had one or more admissions to hospital. These figures, in a heterogeneous outpatient sample, are considerably lower than those reviewed by Alexander and Cooray (2003). Lindsay *et al.* (in press, b) in a report related to that of Morrissey *et al.* (2005), mentioned above, found an overall rate of 39% of participants diagnosed as having a PD (total $n = 164$). Given that the three cohorts were administratively selected for having been referred to offender services for people with ID, this relatively high rate of diagnosis seems reasonable. By far the most prominent diagnosis in these samples was antisocial PD, with participants in the high-security setting having a significantly greater rate of diagnosis. This study took some care to address previous criticisms of PD research in that extensive training of research assistants and clinical informants was conducted, care was taken to ensure inter-rater reliability, and multiple information sources were employed including file reviews, clinical informants, carers and nursing staff. Those diagnosed with PD were found to have a significantly higher level of risk for violence, as measured by actuarial measures of risk, than those with no diagnosis of PD. However, those with a PD diagnosis did not differ from those without on actuarial measures of risk of sexual recidivism. These authors went on to combine PD classifications with PCL-R data to construct a simple dimensional system of increasing indications of PD. They found strong relationships between increasing indications of PD and actuarial measures of risk for future violence. Relationships with actuarial measures of sexual risk were significant but less strong.

Conclusion

Although the available evidence is sparse, it would suggest that the study of PD in individuals with ID is certainly no less important than in mainstream popula-tions. There are preliminary indications that measures of PD may relate to risk of recidivism and to aggression although, as yet, there is little information relating PD and response to treatment and management. Some initial work with main-stream populations suggests that, in contrast to earlier assertions, the presence of PD may not prevent therapeutic alliance and improvement. As mentioned previ-ously, Hembree *et al.* (2004) found some treatment improvement on prevalence of PTSD in participants with PD. Similarly, Greevan and De Ruiter (2004) reported on the impact of inpatient treatment on 59 participants with an initial PD diag-nosis. Following 2 years of compulsory treatment, 23 of the 59 had ceased to show clinical features sufficient to meet criteria for PD. Therefore there are indications from mainstream research that treatment can have an impact not only on clinical symptoms in the presence of PD, but also on the PD itself. In the field of ID, there has been recent work on populations that might be considered to have similar fea-tures to those populations reported in studies in mainstream research. Lindsay *et al.* (2004) and Taylor *et al.* (in press) have reported larger-scale studies on ID popu-lations that include forensic cases, detained cases, compulsory and court ordered treatment. They report considerable treatment improvement in these participant groups, that will undoubtedly contain a significant percentage of individuals who satisfy conditions for classification with PD.

Work on personality inventories, including self-report and informant inventor-ies, is at an early stage although initial evidence from Zigler *et al.* (2002) suggests that important personality constructs in this population might vary somewhat from the mainstream population. Given this possibility, it seems all the more pressing to conduct this work. However, there are clear practical difficulties since people with ID would be unable to read and complete such an inventory alone and the time requirement required to help someone fill out a 200- or 250-item inventory is considerable. Nevertheless, until such work is completed, it is difficult even to begin to embark upon a synthesis of work on the measurement of personality and the diagnosis of PD.

Summary points

- There are problems with the reliability of PD diagnosis and with the overlap of traits between categories.
- A PD may be associated with differential response to treatment and with violence.
- There have been huge variations in the prevalence of PD noted in different studies of populations with ID.
- Diagnosis should be completed with the aid of a wide range of information, including behavioural observation and informant information.
- Diagnosis of PD should not be made before the age of 21 years.
- Work is required on the integration of research on personality and personality disorder in the field of ID.

REFERENCES

Alexander, R. & Cooray, S. (2003). Diagnosis of personality disorders in learning disability. *British Journal of Psychiatry*, **182** (Suppl. 44), S28–31.

American Psychiatric Association (2000). *Diagnostic and Statistical Manual of Mental Disorders, DSM-IV-TR* (4th edn. – text revision). Washington, DC: American Psychiatric Association.

Blackburn, R. (2000). Classification and assessment of personality disorders in mentally disordered offenders: a psychological perspective. *Criminal Behaviour & Mental Health*, **10** (Suppl.), S8–32.

Cooke, D. J. & Michie, S. (2001). Refining the construct of psychopathy: towards a hierarchical model. *Psychological Assessment*, **13**, 171–88.

Corbett, J. A. (1979). *Psychiatric Illness in Mental Handicap*. London: Gaskell Press.

Costa, P. T. Jr. & McCrae, R. R. (1985). *The NEO Personality Inventory*. Odessa, FL: Psychological Assessment Resources.

Dreessen, L. & Arntz, A. (1998). The impact of personality disorders on treatment outcome of anxiety disorders: best evidence synthesis. *Behaviour Research & Therapy*, **36**, 483–504.

D'Silva, K., Duggan, C. & McCarthy, L. (2004). Does treatment really make psychopaths worse? A review of the evidence. *Journal of Personality Disorders*, **18**, 163–77.

Fazel, S. & Danesh, J. (2002). Serious mental disorder among 23,000 prisoners: systematic review of 62 surveys. *Lancet*, **16**, 545–50.

Finlay, W. M. & Lyons, E. (2001). Methodological issues in interviewing and using self-report questionnaires with people with mental retardation. *Psychological Assessment*, **13**, 319–35.

Greevan, P. G. J. & De Ruiter, C. (2004). Personality disorders in a Dutch forensic psychiatric sample: changes with treatment. *Criminal Behaviour & Mental Health*, **14**, 280–90.

Grettan, H. M., McBride, M., Hare, R. D., O'Shaughensey, R. O. & Kumka, G. (2001). Psychopathy and recidivism in adolescent sex offenders. *Criminal Justice & Behaviour*, **28**, 427–49.

Hare, R. D. (1991). *The Hare Psychopathy Checklist – Revised*. Toronto: Multi Health Systems.

Harris, G. T., Rice, M. E., Quinsey, V. L. *et al.* (2003). A multi-site comparison of actuarial risk instruments for sex offenders. *Psychological Assessment*, **15**, 413–25.

Hembree, E. A., Cahill, S. P. & Foa, E. B. (2004). Impact of PD on treatment outcome for female assault survivors with chronic PTSD. *Journal of Personality Disorder*, **18**, 117–27.

Hill, C. D., Neumann, C. S. & Rogers, R. (2004). Confirmatory factor analysis of the Psychopathy Checklist: screening version in offenders with Axis-I disorders. *Psychological Assessment*, **16**, 90–5.

Lindsay, W. R., Gabriel, S., Dana, L., Young, S. & Dosen, A. (in press, a). Personality disorders. In R. Fletcher, E. Loschen & P. Sturmey (eds.), *Diagnostic Manual of Psychiatric Disorders for Individuals with Mental Retardation*. Kingston, NY: National Association for Dual Diagnosis.

Lindsay, W. R., Hogue, T., Taylor, J. *et al.* (in press, b). Two studies on the prevalence and validity of personality disorder in three forensic intellectual disability samples. *Journal of Forensic Psychiatry and Psychology*.

Lindsay, W. R., Smith, A. H. W., Law, J. *et al.* (2004). Sexual and non-sexual offenders with intellectual and learning disabilities: a comparison of characteristics, referral patterns and outcome. *Journal of Interpersonal Violence*, **19**, 875–90.

Lindsay, W. R. & Taylor, J. L. (2005). A selective review of research on offenders with developmental disabilities: assessment and treatment. *Clinical Psychology & Psychotherapy*, **12**, 201–14.

Livesley, W. J. (2002). Diagnostic dilemmas in classifying personality disorder. In K. A. Phillips, M. B. First, and H. A. Pincus (eds.), *Advancing DSM: Dilemmas in Psychiatric Diagnosis* (pp. 153–89). Washington, DC: American Psychiatric Association.

Morrissey, C. (2003). The use of the PCL-R in forensic populations with learning disability. *The British Journal of Forensic Practice*, **5**, 20–24.

Morrissey, K., Hogue, T., Mooney, P., Lindsay, W. R. & Taylor, J. L. (submitted for publication) Uses of the PCL-R in offenders with intellectual disability.

Naik, B. I., Gangadharan, S. K. & Alexander, R. T. (2002). Personality disorders in learning disability – the clinical experience. *British Journal of Developmental Disabilities*, **48**, 95–100.

Novaco, R. W. & Taylor, J. L. (2004). Assessment of anger and aggression in male offenders with developmental disabilities. *Psychological Assessment*, **16**, 42–50

Reid, A. H. & Ballinger, B. R. (1987). Personality disorder in mental handicap. *Psychological Medicine*, **17**, 983–7.

Reid, A. H., Lindsay, W. R., Law, J. & Sturmey, P. (2004). The relationship of offending behaviour and personality disorder in people with developmental disabilities. In W. R. Lindsay, J. L. Taylor & P. Sturmey (eds.), *Offenders with Developmental Disabilities* (pp. 289–304). Chichester: John Wiley & Sons Ltd.

Royal College of Psychiatrists (2001). *DC-LD (Diagnostic Criteria for Psychiatric Disorders for use with Adults with Learning Disabilities/Mental Retardation)*. London: Gaskell.

Seto, M. C. & Barbaree, H. E. (1999). Psychopathy, treatment, behaviour and sex offender recidivism. *Journal of Interpersonal Violence*, **14**, 1235–48.

Skeem, J. L., Monahan, J. & Mulvey, E. P. (2002). Psychopathy, treatment involvement and sub-sequent violence among civil psychiatric patients. *Law & Human Behaviour*, **26**, 577–603.

Taylor, J. L., Novaco, R. W., Gillmer, B. T., Robertson, A. & Thorne, I. (in press). Individual cognitive behavioural anger treatment for people with mild–borderline intellectual disabilities and histories of aggression: a controlled trial. *British Journal of Clinical Psychology.*

Tyrer, P. & Simmonds, S. (2003). Treatment models for those with severe mental illness and comorbid personality disorder. *British Journal of Psychiatry*, **182** (Suppl. 44) S15–18.

Zigler, E., Bennett-Gates, D., Hodapp, R. & Henrich, C. C. (2002). Assessing personality traits of individuals with mental retardation. *American Journal on Mental Retardation*, **107**, 181–93.

10

Dementia and mental ill-health in older people with intellectual disabilities

Sally-Ann Cooper and Anthony J. Holland

Introduction

People with intellectual disabilities (ID) form a small proportion of the whole population but, because of special needs, require suitable services and supports. Older persons form only a small proportion of all people with ID. However, the needs of older compared with younger adults with ID do have some differences and, in many developed countries, services are only starting to recognize and adapt to meet such needs. Additionally, the number of people with ID who will reach old age is increasing.

Demography

The proportion of older people within the population is increasing. This is in part caused by changing birth rates – for example, the post-war baby boom cohort of the 1940s which affects people with ID as well as people of average ability. Additionally, life expectancy for the whole population is increasing, and although life expectancy for people with ID is still shorter than for the general population (McGuigan et al., 1995; Durvasula et al., 2002), it is increasing at a faster velocity. This is owing to more person-centred and improved quality of care and support, improved access to medical treatments such as for respiratory infections and congenital heart disease, changing attitudes and improved lifestyle opportunities, and reduced spread of infectious diseases. These factors have contributed to the increased life expectancy of people with ID at all ages and all ability levels. Hence there is a growing number of older adults with ID, and also a growing number of persons with severe and profound ID in all age cohorts, when compared with numbers in the past.

In 1929, the life expectancy for an infant born with Down syndrome was only 9 years (Penrose, 1949). For people with ID of any cause in the early 1930s the

Psychiatric and Behavioural Disorders in Intellectual and Developmental Disabilities, ed. Nick Bouras and Geraldine Holt. Published by Cambridge University Press. © Cambridge University Press 2007.

average age of death for men was 15 years and for women was 22 years (Puri *et al.*, 1995). Over the course of the twentieth century, these figures improved. Only 28% of children with ID aged 10 years were expected to survive to 60 years of age in 1932 (Dayton *et al.*, 1932), whereas 40 years later this proportion had risen to 46% (Balakrishnan and Wolf, 1976). This increase in life expectancy has been found in both institutional and community studies (Puri *et al.*, 1995; Wolf and Wright, 1987; McCurley *et al.*, 1972; Miller and Eyman, 1978; Strauss and Eyman, 1996; Bittles *et al.*, 2002; Janicki *et al.*, 1999; Patja, 2000). Many persons with ID now achieve middle and older age. This also means that there has been a gradual increase in the size of the population. In the UK, the number of people with ID increased by 53% over the 35-year period 1960–95 (McGrother *et al.*, 2001), an increase of 1.2% per annum. This is owing to increasing survival, particularly in old age.

The emerging cohort of older adults with ID do have some differences in their developmental profile, when compared with younger cohorts. This is because certain factors co-vary with significantly reduced life expectancy (more so than for the whole population with ID). Life expectancy is shortest for people with ID who have a lower ability level (Patja, 2000; Janicki *et al.*, 1999; Bittles *et al.*, 2002; Durvasula *et al.*, 2002). People with Down syndrome have a reduced life expectancy compared with people with ID of other causes (Strauss and Eyman, 1996; Janicki *et al.*, 1999), as do people with epilepsy and hearing impairment (Patja, 2000; Puri *et al.*, 1995), reduced mobility (Hollins *et al.*, 1998), tube feeding (Eyman *et al.*, 1990), and male gender.

The physical health profile of older adults with ID differs from that of the general population of older adults, particularly so for persons with a lower ability level. This includes differences in the leading causes of death (Puri *et al.*, 1995; Janicki *et al.*, 1999; Hollins *et al.*, 1998; Patja *et al.*, 2001a). In the UK general population, the leading causes of death are cancer, then ischaemic heart disease, and thirdly, cerebrovascular disease (General Register Office for Scotland, 2002). The most common cancers are of the trachea, bronchus and lung, followed by prostate in men and breast in women. In contrast, the leading cause of death for people with ID is respiratory disease (Janicki *et al.*, 1999; Durvasula *et al.*, 2002; Hollins *et al.*, 1998; Patja *et al.*, 2001a), which relates to pneumonia and aspiration, posture, swallowing and feeding problems and gastro-oesophageal reflux disorder. This is followed by cardiovascular diseases: congenital heart disease rather than ischaemia (Kapell *et al.*, 1998). Cancer is a lower-ranked cause of death, and the cancer profile also differs from the general population (Böhmer *et al.*, 1997; Cooke, 1997; Patja *et al.*, 2001b). People with ID have reduced rates of lung, prostate and urinary tract malignancies compared with the general population, but increased rates of oesophageal, stomach and gall bladder malignancies (Cooke, 1997). The differences are partly explained by lower rates of smoking and high rates of untreated gastro-oesophageal reflux disorder. These differences have important public health sequelae, as strategies and interventions implemented to improve the health and lifespan of the general population are unlikely to be equally beneficial for adults with ID – as such implementations will be targeting the most common needs of the general population, which are not the most common needs of the older population with ID.

Physical ill-health is common amongst older persons with ID, who can therefore benefit from health assessment and interventions. Some needs are related to the person's developmental disabilities; other health needs are related to ageing. Older persons with ID have a higher level of health need compared with similarly aged cohorts from the general population (Cooper, 1998a; Kapell et al., 1998; Janicki et al., 2002; van Schrojenstein Lantman-de Valk et al., 1997; Hand, 1994; Evenhuis, 1997; Evenhuis, 1995a). There are some similarities in the prevalence of hypertension, stroke and ischaemia, but a higher prevalence rate of sensory impairment (Kapell et al., 1998; van Schrojenstein Lantman-de Valk et al., 1997; Evenhuis, 1995a; Evenhuis, 1995b), thyroid disorders (Kapell et al., 1998), obesity (Janicki et al., 2002); non-atherosclerotic heart disorders (Cooper, 1998a; Kapell et al., 1998), mobility impairment (Evenhuis, 1997); osteoporosis (Janicki et al., 2002; Center et al., 1998), and respiratory problems.

The rest of this chapter focuses on older persons with ID and their experience of psychiatric, rather than physical, disorders.

Whilst the number of older persons with ID is increasing, a major service provision challenge remains, in that the overall number of such older persons is small compared with both the older general population, and the whole population with ID, yet they experience a high level of need. Older persons with ID live in a diverse range of accommodation/support settings, where they are usually a minority group. Diagnostic overshadowing can be contributory to needs not being addressed: in ID settings, additional health needs are often inappropriately accepted as just being a part of ageing; whereas in old-age settings, additional health needs are inappropriately attributed to the person's ID. Older persons with ID are unlikely to report symptoms (Evenhuis, 1997). Unlike the older general population, or younger adults with ID, the older person with ID is unlikely to have close family supports once they have lost their own parents, being unlikely to have married or had children. Service supports therefore need to be robust (Cooper, 1998b).

Dementia

Dementia is associated with older age. There are many causes of dementia, with the most common types being dementia in Alzheimer's disease and vascular dementia.

A recent analysis of all comprehensive European studies revealed the European general population prevalence rates for dementia in five-year age groups from 60–94 years as: 1.0%, 1.4%, 4.1%, 5.7%, 13.0%, 21.6% and 32.2% respectively (Hofman *et al.*, 1991). Amongst the ID population, the prevalence of dementia is considerably higher than for the age-matched general population. This is particularly true for people with Down syndrome, but also for people with ID of other causes.

Down syndrome and dementia

An association between Down syndrome and possible premature ageing has been noted for many years. Fraser and Mitchell (1876) referred to a 'precipitated senility' (by which they meant features of ageing, rather than specifically dementia). Strüwe (1929) (cited by Oliver and Holland, 1986) described neuropathological changes of Alzheimer's disease in Down syndrome, and Jervis (1948) described the clinical deterioration of three patients and demonstrated Alzheimer's disease at postmortem. Mann (1988) reviewed all published neuropathological reports amongst people with Down syndrome: of those aged over 40 years, almost 100% had the changes of Alzheimer's disease. Studies of the clinical features of dementia, loss of adaptive behaviour skills, neuropsychological impairments, and neuropathological and neurochemical studies all indicate high rates of dementia amongst middle-aged people with Down syndrome. This association has previously been reviewed in detail (Oliver and Holland, 1986; Holland and Oliver, 1995).

Although initial neuropathological studies found that the vast majority of people with Down syndrome had evidence of significant plaques and tangles of the Alzheimer type in their brains if they had died after the age of 30 years, clinical studies have shown that not all people with Down syndrome develop the clinical features of Alzheimer's disease in later life. Lai and Williams (1989) found that prevalence rates in people over 50 years reached 75%. Holland *et al.* (1998), in a population-based prevalence study of 75 people with Down syndrome aged 30 years or older, reported prevalence rates increasing from approximately 1.0% at 30–39 years, to 10% at 40–49 years, and 40% at 50 years and over. Whilst studies differ in the exact rates reported, all agree that there is a proportion of people with Down syndrome who live into their 50s and 60s who do not have evidence of cognitive or functional decline suggestive of dementia.

The clinical diagnosis of dementia in people with Down syndrome is more problematic than for the general population because of the pre-existing ID. Thus, the absence of particular skills or the presence of a poor memory cannot by itself be taken as indicative of possible dementia. Rather, it is the development of such problems for the first time in adult life and evidence of progressive loss of function that is crucial to the diagnosis, together with the exclusion of other possible causation. In earlier studies the diagnosis of dementia in people with Down syndrome was made late in the course of the disease, as the early stages of dementia are hard to determine, despite detailed examination (Zigman *et al.*, 1987; Lai and Williams, 1989; Devenny *et al.*, 1992; Prasher, 1994). However, a more recent longitudinal study of older people with Down syndrome has reported that carers describe behavioural and personality changes in people with Down syndrome in their 30s and 40s. It has been proposed that these observed clinical changes may be precursors of what will become definite dementia in subsequent years (Holland *et al.*, 2000). The people with early behavioural changes have been found to have a greater degree of impairment on tests of executive function than an age-matched group with Down syndrome but without such behavioural changes, and to have an increased risk of subsequently developing dementia (Ball, 2005). On the basis of this evidence, whilst the later course of the dementia would appear similar to that of the general population, the early presentation in people with Down syndrome may be different and is primarily characterized by behavioural/personality changes. This observation, if confirmed, will be important as more effective treatments for dementia are developed.

The main hypothesis to account for the association between Down syndrome and Alzheimer's disease is the presence of the β amyloid precursor protein (*APP*) gene that is located on chromosome 21 (Tanzi *et al.*, 1987). Neuropathological studies of people with Down syndrome who have died at different ages, have found increased deposition of amyloid in early childhood prior to the later development of plaques and tangles (Mann, 1994; Rumble *et al.*, 1989). Whether excess amyloid deposition is sufficient to account for the subsequent development of Alzheimer's disease neuropathology is uncertain. As with the general population, other genetic factors, such as variants of the *ApoE* gene, have a modifying effect: the *ApoE 4* variant increases the risk for the subsequent development of Alzheimer's disease (Rubinzstein *et al.*, 1999). An alternative hypothesis relates to the role of superoxide dismutase (SOD) (the gene for which is also on chromosome 21). This enzyme is important in the disposal of free radicals that may have a damaging effect on cell membrane function. As yet, it is unknown whether the presence of the *SOD* gene in triplicate has a deleterious effect and whether that relates to the link with Alzheimer's disease.

Evidence of functional decline in an older person with Down syndrome requires full evaluation. Some studies have found that people with Down syndrome overlap in their symptoms of depression and dementia (Burt *et al.*, 1992; Prasher, 1995; Prasher and Filer, 1995). Similarly, hypothyroidism may superficially mimic dementia, and functional and behavioural symptoms respond to treatment of the thyroid disorder (Thase *et al.*, 1984). The differential diagnosis of decline in later life specifically in people with Down syndrome includes hypothyroidism, depression, and sensory impairments, in addition to Alzheimer's disease (see also the assessment section below).

Dementia in people with ID of any cause

Dementia has also been recognized for many years to occur in people with ID through causes other than Down syndrome (Bleuler, 1924; Heaton-Ward, 1967). Corbett (1979) suggested that there is a 'probable earlier appearance of dementia' in people with ID, but did not quote actual rates in his study. Studies of the prevalence of dementia have focused on different populations, and used differing methodologies, which makes comparisons difficult. Some studies have drawn their subjects from people resident in institutions (Reid and Aungle, 1974; Tait, 1983; Day, 1985; Day, 1987; Sansom et al., 1994), whereas others have studied epidemiological samples from the community and institutions (Lund, 1985), or whole populations living in a defined area (Moss and Patel, 1993; Cooper, 1997a). Some studies have relied on taking information/diagnoses from existing medical case notes (Day, 1985), whereas others included comprehensive psychiatric assessment and clearly defined diagnostic criteria (Sansom et al., 1994; Cooper, 1997a). The studies have examined different age groups; people aged 40 years and over (Day, 1985); aged 45 years and over (Reid and Aungle, 1974); aged 50 years and over (Moss and Patel, 1993); aged 60 years and over (Sansom et al., 1994); and aged 65 years and over (Day, 1987; Cooper, 1997a). All of these studies show the prevalence of dementia to be considerably higher in older people with ID, when compared with the age-matched general population. The three epidemiological studies provide similar prevalence findings. Lund (1985) reported 22.2% of people aged 65 years and over to have dementia; Cooper (1997a) reported 21.6% aged 65 years and over to have dementia. People with Down syndrome do not yet usually live beyond the age of 65 years, and so these two studies refer almost exclusively to people with ID of causes other than Down syndrome. In the study by Cooper (1997a), only five out of the 134 elderly people had Down syndrome: three out of the five people with Down syndrome had dementia, compared with 26 out of the 129 people with other underlying causes of their ID. Moss and Patel (1993) found 11.4% of people aged 50 years and over to have dementia. This included four out of the nine people in the study with Down syndrome, and eight out of the 96 people with ID of other causes. The study of Cooper (1997a) yielded a rate of dementia of 13.0% for people aged 50 years and over, which compares closely with the 11.4% reported by Moss and Patel (1993).

The prevalence of dementia increases with age. People with dementia have also been demonstrated more likely to be female, with more poorly controlled epilepsy, a larger number of additional physical disorders, and less likely to be smokers, compared with persons without dementia (Cooper, 1997a).

The reasons for these higher rates are unknown. Chromosome 21 is not known to be aetiological to ID of causes other than Down syndrome, and so related hypotheses are not generalizable to this group, and other hypotheses have not been tested. Perhaps other genetic factors are relevant. In the general population, a history of head injury increases the risk for dementia (Breteler *et al.*, 1992), an extreme example of this being dementia pugilistica (Roberts, 1969; Casson *et al.*, 1982; Casson *et al.*, 1984). Intellectual disabilities can be related to 'brain damage' caused by, for example, birth trauma, head injury, meningitis and other cerebral insults, and maybe these similar factors play a role in increasing rates of dementia. Another hypothesis relates to lack of 'reserve' in brain functioning. When functional and neuropsychological skills are already impaired (as in ID), perhaps even a very small brain insult can make a considerable difference, with the person being unable to compensate. High educational attainment has been demonstrated to be a protective factor against dementia (Katzman, 1993; Stern *et al.*, 1994), perhaps by increasing cortical density: maybe these theories can be extrapolated to people with ID.

Common cognitive symptoms of dementia include forgetfulness, impaired understanding, confusion, reduced self-care skills or increased need for prompting, forgetting names, geographical disorientation and temporal disorientation. Onset of incontinence, seizures, impaired mobility and weight loss are later manifestations.

In addition to memory changes and skill loss, non-cognitive symptoms have been reported to be commonly experienced by people with ID who have dementia. Cooper (1997c) found that 27.6% of 29 people with dementia experienced at least one type of psychotic symptom: persecutory delusions occurred in 20.7% and hallucinations in 20.7%. The commonest type of delusion was of money and other items being stolen from the subject (10.3%), whilst the commonest type of hallucination was of visual hallucinations of strangers in the person's house (13.8%). Non-psychotic symptoms were also common, including changed sleep pattern, loss of concentration, worry, change in appetite and onset of, or increase in, aggression. Similar findings have also been reported by Moss and Patel (1995).

Some of the psychopathology of dementia, such as aggression and sleep disturbance, can cause the person distress and present a significant management problem for carers, and may influence the viability of a person's place of residence (Reid and Aungle, 1974; Day, 1985; Cooper 1997c). As some of these non-cognitive symptoms may be responsive to pharmacological, psychological, social or developmental interventions or supports, it is essential that clinical assessments seek to detect such symptoms and also determine their likely causation and contributory factors.

From such assessments, appropriate management and care plans can be designed and agreed by professionals, carers, and the person with ID.

Mental ill-health other than dementia

The literature regarding mental ill-health amongst older people with ID is more limited than it is for dementia, and it is difficult to compare studies. Studies of people living in institutions include that of Day (1985) who reported the diagnoses documented in the case notes of 357 hospital residents aged 40 years and over, and found 109 (30%) to have a documented psychiatric diagnosis. Subsequently he interviewed staff to determine that one-fifth of the 99 hospital residents aged 65 years and over had a psychiatric disorder (diagnostic criteria were not defined) (Day, 1987). Sansom et al. (1994) examined 124 hospital residents with ID aged 60–94 years, and found 8.9% to meet DSM-III-R (American Psychiatric Association, 1987) criteria for affective disorders, and 6.5% to meet DSM-III-R criteria for schizophrenia (they did not study anxiety disorders or problem behaviours). It is unclear the extent to which these findings can be generalized to all older adults with ID, given the sampling bias.

Studies with representative samples (community as well as institution) include that of Corbett (1979), who employed ICD-8 criteria (World Health Organization, 1968) and interviewed the carers of subjects in a two-stage process. One hundred and ten subjects were aged 60 years or over, 62.9% of whom were free from mental ill-health (not including dementia). Schizophrenia was found in 5.4%, depression in 1.8%, manic depressive psychosis in 2.7%, childhood psychosis in 3.6% and personality disorder/problem behaviours in 22.7%. Patel et al. (1993) used a semi-structured interview to study the whole population of people with moderate to profound ID aged 50 years and over and living in Oldham, UK ($n = 105$). In total, 12 people were determined to have mental ill-health, meeting DSM-III-R criteria (excluding dementia). In addition, two other people were reported to have schizophrenia that could not be detected by the rating scale that was used, bringing the total to 14 out of 105. Surprisingly, no one was reported to have problem behaviours (it is unclear whether this is because of the diagnostic criteria which were employed). Of the 105 people, three were found to have agoraphobia, two had panic disorder, three had generalized anxiety disorder, five had major depression, one had dysthymia and one had hypomania. Cooper (1997b) studied the whole population of people with ID aged 65 years and over living in Leicestershire, UK, using a semi-structured psychiatric rating scale ($n = 134$). She used DCR (the operational criteria of ICD-10) (World Health Organization, 1993) to diagnose disorders, with some modifications. Mental ill-health (including dementia and euthymic participants with a past history of affective disorder) was found in 68.7%.

Schizophrenia/delusional disorder was present in 3.0%; a current diagnosis of depression was present in 6.0%; a past history of affective disorder in 15.7%; generalized anxiety disorder in 9.0%; agoraphobia in 3.7%; other phobias in 3.0%; behaviour disorder in 14.9%; and autism in 6.0%. This study also examined a younger cohort of adults with ID, and found the older cohort to have higher rates of dementia, depression and anxiety disorders, but equal rates of schizophrenia/delusional disorders, autism and problem behaviours in the two groups.

One would anticipate a higher prevalence of mental ill-health in older compared with younger adults with ID. Adults with ID have the same risk factors for mental ill-health that are present amongst the general population (e.g. genetic predisposition; associations with physical health; psychological predisposition; social factors and life events). Additionally, they have the risk factors for mental ill-health that are specific to ID (e.g. behavioural phenotypes; associations with epilepsy and physical disabilities; disadvantaged backgrounds leading to damaged psychological development; limited social networks, restricted social circumstances and stigma; developmental factors such as communication needs). Studies of people with genetic syndromes demonstrate how risks can be very specific to particular syndromes e.g. the association of Down syndrome and Alzheimer's disease, a genetic sub-type of Prader–Willi syndrome and affective psychotic illness in adult life (Boer *et al.*, 2002), velo-cardio-facial syndrome and schizophrenia (Murphy & Owen, 2001). Also, the current cohort of older people with ID are more likely to have grown up in an institution, rather than within families, with all the disadvantages that are acquired as a result of this.

Psychopathology

There are both similarities and differences in the psychopathology of mental ill-health in people with ID compared with the general population (Cooper *et al.*, 2003). Differences include the common occurrence of some symptoms in the presentation of mental ill-health in people with ID, which are unusual in the general population – e.g. increase in specific problem behaviours, or onset of problem behaviours (such as aggression), reduction in adaptive skills, reduction of speech, and increased reassurance-seeking behaviour. The intricacies of symptom dissection in people of average ability can often be determined with considerable sophistication, whereas this is less possible with someone with limited or no verbal communication skills; for example, delusions and hallucinations may be elicited in a person with ID, and sometimes auditory hallucinations can be determined to be occurring in either the second or third person; but it is extremely unlikely that passivity phenomena (the experience of replacement of will) could be distinguished from the belief of being controlled or influenced, or that thought interference could be distinguished from delusions of mind reading, or that delusional perception could be confidently determined. A person's developmental level may also preclude the development of certain types of psychopathology, which require quite complex analytic skills such as guilt, hopelessness, suicidal intent, worthlessness, distorted body image, and the awareness that phobic anxiety symptoms are out of keeping with the stimulus. Conversely, these symptoms are typical features of mental ill-health in people of average ability. The DC-LD (Royal College of Psychiatrists, 2001) manual was developed to provide diagnostic criteria for mental ill-health for adults with ID, to address this pathoplastic effect that increasing levels of ID has on the presentation of psychopathology within disorders. Further discussion is presented in the DC-LD manual itself, which is suitable for use with both older and younger adults with moderate to profound levels of ID (see also Chapter 1 by Sturmey.)

When measuring psychopathology, it is always essential to distinguish between trait and state findings, i.e. to demonstrate that a change has occurred. For example, if a person has, all their life, been socially withdrawn then this is a normal finding for them, and is not a symptom of mental ill-health. However, when social withdrawal occurs in a person who was previously sociable, then this indicates mental ill-health. If a person with lifelong social withdrawal becomes more socially withdrawn than is usual for them, then this too indicates mental ill-health. This is an important point, since many symptoms of mental ill-health can be present as lifelong traits in people with ID (as an integral part of the developmental disorder), whereas this is unusual in people of average ability. Some symptoms are always abnormal, e.g. delusions and hallucinations.

There are no comprehensive studies that report comparisons of psychopathology of different psychiatric disorders between older and younger adults with ID. This requires further research, as such differences have been reported to occur between older and younger adults of average ability. This is of clinical relevance, as an accurate understanding of clinical presentation is likely to lead to improved clinical practice and detection of mental ill-health.

Assessment and diagnosis

Comprehensive assessment is essential in order to detect mental ill-health and to understand its likely causation and contributory factors for that person, from which the most appropriate interventions and supports can be determined. The assessment must be thorough enough to include full details of the descriptive psychopathology and also to derive an aetiological formulation. The combination of having ID and increasing age is associated with excess physical morbidity, which may also present with change in behaviour, particularly in people with severe ID and limited language. Gastrointestinal problems, ear infections, eye disorders such as glaucoma, respiratory problems, or pain consequent upon age-related illness such as cancer are important to consider. This requires listening carefully and clarifying all of the information that is presented, but also then specifically asking about physical symptoms, psychopathology, present circumstances and background information, that might not have been volunteered. For example, if an older person with ID who has previously always been well, starts to become physically aggressive at home, then this is the likely problem that will be presented to the health care team. However, aggression can occur as a symptom of several types of mental ill-health or in response to physical illness. It would be inappropriate to assume that this was a problem behaviour, environmentally determined, without thorough enquiry including all other symptoms that are a feature of physical illness, dementia, schizophrenia, depression and anxiety disorders. As well as leading to a descriptive diagnosis, the assessment must include assessment of the likely aetiological factors for that person. For example a person may be experiencing a depressive episode, but the necessary management plan will differ between a person who has a long history of bipolar affective episodes, but no apparent psychological predisposition, social disadvantages or recent life events except discontinuation of their lithium, and a person who has recently been bereaved of their parent and moved into residential care and lost contact with their previous neighbourhood.

Assessments also require a full history to be taken from an informant who has known the person long enough to have knowledge of their usual premorbid personality and traits, as well as interviewing the person with ID her/himself. Information is collected regarding the descriptive psychopathology, the time scale and sequence of events and any associated factors including recent life events and changes in the care environment; past episodes of mental ill-health, their presentation, duration and successes/failures of treatments; past and current medical disorders and epilepsy history; details of current and past drugs that are taken for psychiatric and physical conditions (as some drugs can cause mental ill-health, and some drug side effects can mimic psychiatric disorders), the use of alcohol and recreational drugs; psychiatric disorders and ID that are present in family members; details of the individual's personal history, which indicates the way in which their personality has developed and their coping strategies; details of the person's social circumstances and social network; a developmental history, including the underlying cause of the person's ID and their current level of adaptive functioning; details of forensic history and past offences. A mental state examination should be conducted. A physical examination will be necessary in order to exclude any physical causes of the presentation, and similarly routine blood tests taken including full blood count, urea and electrolytes, liver function tests and thyroid function tests. Thyroid dysfunction, in particular, can mimic and/or precipitate all of the commoner types of psychiatric disorders. Any previous medical case notes the person has should be reviewed for additional relevant information. Additional investigations may well be required, but this is dependent upon the findings from the initial assessment.

The accurate diagnosis of dementia in people with ID has become increasingly important as specific treatments that at least temporarily may improve function have been developed (Prasher *et al.*, 2003; Prasher, 2004). Observer-rated scales such as the Dementia Questionnaire for Persons with Mental Retardation (DMR, Evenhuis 1992), the Dementia Scale for Down syndrome (Gedye, 1995), and more recently the CAMDEX-DS (Ball *et al.*, 2004) have been published. The last two of these scales emphasize the importance of functional change over time in arriving at a diagnosis of dementia, and a diagnosis of dementia made using the CAMDEX-DS has been shown to predict previous and subsequent cognitive decline. In contrast to the general population, the diagnosis relies more heavily on informant observation of change, as one-off findings on neuropsychological assessments such as the Mini Mental State Examination or the CAMCOG are of limited value. Diagnosis requires a comparison for each item of how the person performs now in comparison with their best performance in the past. As well as measuring all relevant psychopathology that can feature in dementia in this way, a comprehensive review of all psychopathology occurring in other possible psychiatric disorders and also symptoms/signs of physical disease is required. This is because dementia remains a diagnosis of exclusion.

If the individual's presentation is suggestive of dementia, more detailed physical investigations are required, in order to eliminate any reversible/treatable causes. This will necessitate additional blood tests to measure serum B12 and red cell folate, syphilis serology and the erythrocyte sedimentation rate. A urine sample should be checked for infection, and an electrocardiogram and chest X-ray taken. Cranial CT scan or MRI scan may be required to exclude other treatable causes of dementia, such as space occupying lesions, if the history indicates the need for these. These scans are not usually helpful in the diagnosis of dementia (other than to exclude other pathology), unless there has been a previous scan taken at some point in the past with which it can be compared (as scan findings are often abnormal in people with ID, regardless of the presence of dementia).

Once the diagnosis of dementia has been established, it may be important to measure its progress, in order to evaluate the effectiveness of any treatments that are used. Whereas the diagnosis of dementia requires a comparison of a person's symptoms and functioning now compared with the past, the progress of the disease can be assessed by comparing how the person performs on measures over time. This might include performance in cognitive tasks, such as measured by the Test for Severe Impairment (Albert and Cohen, 1992) together with adaptive behaviour skills, such as measured by the Vineland Scale (Sparrow *et al.*, 1984). Additionally, assessment of non-cognitive symptoms of dementia, such as anxiety, depression, or psychosis remains important whilst evaluating treatment outcomes, as often such non-cognitive symptoms can be ameliorated by effective management.

Professionals from a range of disciplines may contribute to the assessment, e.g. psychiatrists, psychologists, nurses and occupational therapists. Carers from the person's usual residential and day places will also contribute to this process, as will family members if there are any, together with the person with ID.

Conclusion

The life expectancy of people with ID is increasing, and many now live to middle and older age. Mental ill-health and physical ill-health are common amongst older people with ID, in view of having vulnerabilities associated with older age, in addition to those associated with ID, and also those that can affect the whole population. Dementia occurs commonly: for people with Down syndrome the risk for acquiring dementia is brought forward by about 30 years; for people with ID of other causes the risk is brought forward by about 15 years. Comprehensive assessment is essential in all cases when an older person with ID has changed in some way, in order to determine diagnosis and causation, from which the most appropriate interventions and supports can be devised and implemented. Services need to develop, within their local context, to ensure that they can meet the challenge of supporting the small but growing population of older persons with ID, whose needs do have some differences from the general population. Future research should be directed to understanding better the clinical and support needs of older persons with ID, and practices and policy to address needs.

Summary points

- The life expectancy of people with ID is increasing, and many now live to middle and older age.
- Mental ill-health is common amongst older people with ID: this is because they are at risk of the disorders that can affect the whole population, and also disorders associated with ID, and the disorders which are associated with older age.
- Dementia occurs commonly. This is particularly so for people with Down syndrome, whose risk for acquiring dementia is brought forward by about 30 years, but also for people with ID of other causes, whose risk is bought forward by about 15 years.
- Anxiety disorders and depression also occur commonly in older people; whereas schizophrenia/delusional disorders, problem behaviours and autism occur at a similar rate to that found in younger adults with ID.

- In addition to memory changes and skill-loss, non-cognitive symptoms are a common feature of dementia, including sleep disturbance, delusions and hallucinations, and aggression.
- Non-cognitive symptoms of dementia are important to determine, as many can be treated or modified; they are also a potential source of distress for the person with ID and stress for carers, and may affect the viability of a person continuing to live at their usual residence.
- Further research is required into differences in presentation of mental ill-health between older and younger adults with ID: a better understanding of this may lead to enhanced clinical practice with improved case detection, which in turn informs and directs the treatment/management/support plan.
- Comprehensive assessment is essential in all cases when the individual has changed in some way, in order to determine the diagnosis and aetiological formulation (and from there to plan treatment/management/supports).
- Services need to develop in order to meet the challenge of supporting this small but growing population of older persons with ID, whose needs do have some differences from the rest of the population.

REFERENCES

Albert, M. and Cohen, C. (1992). The Test for Severe Impairment: an instrument for assessment of people with severe cognitive dysfunction. *Journal of the American Geriatric Society*, **40**, 449–53.

American Psychiatric Association (1987). *Diagnostic and Statistical Manual of Psychiatric Disorders*, 3rd edn, revised. Washington, DC: American Psychiatric Association.

Balakrishnan, T. R. and Wolf, L. C. (1976). Life expectancy of mentally retarded persons in Canadian institutions. *American Journal on Mental Deficiency*, **80**, 650–62.

Ball, S. (2005). *The Course of Alzheimer's Disease in Adults with Down's Syndrome: Evidence for the Early Compromise of Frontal Lobe Function*. Thesis submitted to the University of Cambridge.

Ball, S. L., Holland, A. J., Huppert, F. A. *et al.* (2004). The modified CAMDEX informant interview is a valid and reliable tool for use in the diagnosis of dementia in adults with Down's Syndrome. *Journal of Intellectual Disability Research*, **48**, 611–20.

Bittles, A. H., Petterson, B. A., Sullivan, S. G. *et al.* (2002). The influence of intellectual disability on life expectancy. *Journal of Gerontology Series A – Biological Sciences and Medical Sciences*, **57**, 470–2.

Bleuler, E. (1916). Lehrbuch der Psychiatrie. Translated as *Textbook of Psychiatry* (1924) by Brill, A. A. New York: Dover Publications.

Boer, H., Holland, A. J., Whittington, J. *et al.* (2002). Psychotic illness in people with Prader–Willi syndrome due to chromosome 15 maternal uniparental disomy. *Lancet*, **359**, 135–6.

Böhmer, C. J., Klinkenberg-Knol, E. C., Niczen-de Boer, R. C. and Meuwissen, S. G. (1997). The age-related incidences of oesophageal carcinoma in intellectually disabled individuals in institutes in the Netherlands. *European Journal of Gastroenterology & Hepatology*, **9**, 589–92.

Breteler, M. M. B., Claus, J. J., van Duijn, C. M., Launer, L. T. and Hofman, A. (1992). Epidemiology of Alzheimer's disease. *Epidemiology Review*, **14**, 59–82.

Burt, D. B., Loveland, K. A. and Lewis, K. R. (1992). Depression and the onset of dementia in adults with mental retardation. *American Journal on Mental Retardation*, **96**, 502–11.

Casson, I. R., Sham, R., Campbell, E. A., Tarlau, M. and di Domenico, A. (1982). Neurological and CT evaluation of knocked-out boxers. *Journal of Neurology, Neurosurgery and Psychiatry*, **45**, 170–4.

Casson, I. R., Siegel, O., Sham, R. *et al.* (1984). Brain damage in modern boxers. *Journal of the American Medical Association*, **251**, 2663–7.

Center, J., Beange, H. and McElduff, A. (1998). People with mental retardation have an increased prevalence of osteoporosis: A population study. *American Journal on Mental Retardation*, **103**, 19–28.

Cooke, L. B. (1997). Cancer and learning disability. *Journal of Intellectual Disability Research*, **41**, 312–16.

Cooper, S.-A. (1997a). High prevalence of dementia amongst people with learning disabilities not attributed to Down's syndrome. *Psychological Medicine*, **27**, 609–16.

Cooper, S.-A. (1997b). Epidemiology of psychiatric disorders in elderly compared with younger people with learning disabilities. *British Journal of Psychiatry*, **170**, 375–80.

Cooper, S.-A. (1997c). Psychiatric symptoms of dementia amongst elderly people with learning disabilities. *International Journal of Geriatric Psychiatry*, **12**, 662–6.

Cooper, S.-A. (1998a). Clinical study of the effects of age on the physical health of adults with mental retardation. *American Journal on Mental Retardation*, **102**, 582–9.

Cooper, S.-A. (1998b). A population-based cross-sectional study of social networks and demography in older compared with younger adults with learning disabilities. *Journal of Learning Disabilities for Nursing, Health and Social Care*, **2**, 212–20.

Cooper, S.-A., Melville, C. A. and Einfeld, S. L. (2003). Psychiatric diagnosis, intellectual disabilities and Diagnostic Criteria for Psychiatric Disorders for Use with Adults with Learning Disabilities/Mental Retardation (DC-LD). *Journal of Intellectual Disability Research*, **47**, 3–15.

Corbett, J. A. (1979). Psychiatric morbidity and mental retardation. In James, F.-E. and Snaith, R. P. (eds.), *Psychiatric Illness and Mental Handicap*. London: Gaskell Press.

Day, K. (1985). Psychiatric disorder in the middle-aged and elderly mentally handicapped. *British Journal of Psychiatry*, **147**, 660–7.

Day, K. A. (1987). The elderly mentally handicapped in hospital: a clinical study. *Journal of Mental Deficiency Research*, **31**, 131–46.

Dayton, N. A., Doering, C. R., Hilferty, M. M., Maher, H. C. and Dolan, H. H. (1932). Mentality and life expectation in mental deficiency in Massachusetts: analysis of the fourteen-year period 1917–1930. *New England Journal of Medicine*, **206**, 550–70.

Devenny, D. A., Hill, A. L., Paxtot, O., Silverman, W. P. and Wisniewski, K. E. (1992). Ageing in higher functioning adults with Down's syndrome: an interim report in a longitudinal study. *Journal of Intellectual Disability Research*, **36**, 241–50.

Durvasula, S., Beange, H. and Baker, W. (2002). Mortality of people with intellectual disability in northern Sydney. *Journal of Intellectual and Developmental Disability*, **27**, 255–64.

Evenhuis, H. M. (1992). Evaluation of a screening instrument for dementia in ageing mentally retarded persons. *Journal of Intellectual Disability Research*, **36**, 337–47.

Evenhuis, H. M. (1995a). Medical aspects of ageing in a population with intellectual disability: I. Visual impairment. *Journal of Intellectual Disability Research*, **39**, 19–25.

Evenhuis, H. M. (1995b). Medical aspects of ageing in a population with intellectual disability: II. Hearing impairment. *Journal of Intellectual Disability Research*, **39**, 27–33.

Evenhuis, H. M. (1997). Medical aspects of ageing in a population with intellectual disability: II. Mobility, internal conditions and cancer. *Journal of Intellectual Disability Research*, **41**, 8–18.

Eyman, R. K., Grossman, H. J., Chaney, R. H. and Call, T. L. (1990). The life expectancy of profoundly handicapped people with mental retardation. *New England Journal of Medicine*, **323**, 584–9.

Fraser, J. and Mitchell, A. (1876). Kalmuc idiocy: report of a case with autopsy with notes on 62 cases. *Journal of Mental Science*, **22**, 169–79.

Gedye, A. (1995). *Dementia Scale for Down's Syndrome*. Vancouver, BC: Gedye Research and Consulting.

General Register Office for Scotland (2002). *Scotland's Population 2001*. General Register Office for Scotland: Edinburgh.

Hand, J. E. (1994). Report of a national survey of older people with lifelong intellectual handicap in New Zealand. *Journal of Intellectual Disability Research*, **38**, 275–87.

Heaton-Ward, W. A. (1967). *Mental Subnormality*, 3rd edn. Bristol: John Wright and Sons.

Hofman, A., Rocca, W. A., Brayne, C. *et al.* (1991). The prevalence of dementia in Europe: a collaborative study of 1980–1990 findings. *International Journal of Epidemiology*, **20**, 736–48.

Holland, A. J., Hon, J., Huppert, F. A., Stevens, F. and Watson, P. (1998). A population-based study of the prevalence and presentation of dementia in adults with Down's Syndrome. *British Journal of Psychiatry*, **172**, 493–8.

Holland, A. J., Hon, J., Huppert, F. A., Stevens, F. and Watson, P. (2000). Incidence and course of dementia in people with Down's Syndrome: findings from a population-based study. *Journal of Intellectual Disability Research*, **44**, 138–46.

Holland, A. J. and Oliver, C. (1995). Down's syndrome and the links with Alzheimer's disease. *Journal of Neurology, Neurosurgery and Psychiatry*, **59**, 111–15.

Hollins, S., Attard, M. T., von Fraunhofer, N., McGuigan, S. and Sedgwick, P. (1998). Mortality in people with learning disability: risks, causes, and death certification findings in London. *Developmental Medicine and Child Neurology*, **40**, 50–6.

Janicki, M. P., Dalton, A. J., Henderson, C. M. and Davidson, P. W. (1999). Mortality and morbidity among older adults with intellectual disability: health services considerations. *Disability & Rehabilitation*, **21**, 284–94.

Janicki, M. P., Davidson, P. W., Henderson, C. M. *et al.* (2002). Health characteristics and health services utilization in older adults with intellectual disability living in community residences. *Journal of Intellectual Disability Research*, **46**, 287–98.

Jervis, G. A. (1948). Early senile dementiath mongoloid idiocy. *American Journal of Psychiatry*, **105**, 102–6.

Kapell, D., Nightingale, B., Rodriguez, A. *et al.* (1998). Prevalence of chronic medical conditions in adults with mental retardation: comparison with the general population. *Mental Retardation*, **36**, 269–79.

Katzman, R. (1993). Education and the prevalence of dementia and Alzheimer disease. *Neurology*, **43**, 13–20.

Lai, F. and Williams, R. S. (1989). A prospective study of Alzheimer's disease in Down's syndrome. *Archives Neurology*, **46**, 849–53.

Lund, J. (1985). The prevalence of psychiatric morbidity in mentally retarded adults. *Acta Psychiatrica Scandinavica*, **72**, 563–70.

Mann, D. M. A. (1988). Alzheimer's disease and Down's syndrome. *Histopathology*, **13**, 125–37.

Mann, D. M. A. (1994). Association between Alzheimer Disease and Down's Syndrome: neuropathological observations. In Berg, J. M., Karlinsky, H., Holland, A. J. (eds.), *Alzheimer's Disease, Down Syndrome and their Relationship*. Oxford: Oxford Medical Publication, Oxford University Press, pp. 71–92.

McCurley, R., Mackay, D. N. and Scally, B. G. (1972). The life expectation of the mentally subnormal under community and hospital care. *Journal of Mental Deficiency Research*, **16**, 57–66.

McGrother, C., Thorp, C., Taub, N. and Machado, O. (2001). Prevalence, disability and need in adults with severe learning disability. *Tizard Learning Disability Review*, **6**, 4–13.

McGuigan, S. M., Hollins, S. and Attard, M. (1995). Age-specific standardized mortality rates in people with learning disability. *Journal of Intellectual Disability Research*, **39**, 527–31.

Miller, C. and Eyman, R. (1978). Hospital and community mortality rates among the retarded. *Journal of Mental Deficiency Research*, **22**, 137–45.

Moss, S. and Patel, P. (1993). The prevalence of mental illness in people with intellectual disability over 50 years of age, and the diagnostic importance of information from carers. *The Irish Journal of Psychology*, **14**, 110–29.

Moss, S. and Patel, P. (1995). Psychiatric symptoms associated with dementia in older people with learning disability. *British Journal of Psychiatry*, **167**, 663–7.

Murphy, K. C. and Owen, M. J. (2001). Velo-cardio-facial syndrome: a model for understanding the genetics and pathogenesis of schizophrenia. *British Journal of Psychiatry*, **179**, 397–402.

Oliver, C. and Holland, A. J. (1986). Down's syndrome and Alzheimer's disease: a review. *Psychological Medicine*, **16**, 307–22.

Patel, P., Goldberg, D. and Moss, S. (1993). Psychiatric morbidity in older people with moderate and severe learning disabilities II: The prevalence study. *British Journal of Psychiatry*, **163**, 481–91.

Patja, K. (2000). Life expectancy of people with intellectual disability: A 35-year follow-up study. *Journal of Intellectual Disability Research*, **44**, 590–9.

Patja, K., Eero, P. and Iivanainen, M. (2001b). Cancer incidence among people with intellectual disability. *Journal of Intellectual Disability Research*, **45**, 300–7.

Patja, K., Molsa, P. and Iivanainen, M. (2001a). Cause-specific mortality of people with intellectual disability in a population-based, 35-year follow-up. *Journal of Intellectual Disability Research*, **45**, 30–40.

Penrose, L. S. (1949). The incidence of mongolism in the general population. *Journal of Mental Science*, **9**, 10.

Prasher, V. P. (1994). Temporal association between clinical and neuropathological dementia in people with Down syndrome. *British Journal of Clinical and Social Psychiatry*, **9**, 24–5.

Prasher, V. P. (1995). Age specific prevalence, thyroid dysfunction and depressive symptomatology in adults with Down syndrome and dementia. *International Journal of Geriatric Psychiatry*, **10**, 25–31.

Prasher, V. P. (2004). Review of donepezil, rivastigmine, galantamine and memantine for the treatment of dementia in adults with Down Syndrome: implications for the intellectual disability population. *International Journal of Geriatric Psychiatry*, **19**, 509–15.

Prasher, V. P., Adams, C., Holder, R. and the Down Syndrome Research Group (2003). Long-term safety and efficacy of donepezil in the treatment of dementia in Alzheimer Disease in adults with Down's Syndrome: open label study. *International Journal of Geriatric Psychiatry*, **18**, 549–51.

Prasher, V. P. and Filer, A. (1995). Behavioural disturbance in people with Down's syndrome and dementia. *Journal of Intellectual Disability Research*, **39**, 432–6.

Puri, B. K., Lekh, S. K., Langa, A., Zamas, R. and Singh, I. (1995). Mortality in a hospitalised mentally handicapped population: a 10-year old survey. *Journal of Intellectual Disability Research*, **39**, 442–6.

Reid, A. H. and Aungle, P. G. (1974). Dementia in ageing mental defectives: a clinical psychiatric study. *Journal of Mental Deficiency Research*, **18**, 15–23.

Roberts, A. H. (1969). *Brain Damage in Boxers*. Pitman: London.

Royal College of Psychiatrists (2001). *[DC-LD] Diagnostic Criteria for Psychiatric Disorders for Use with Adults with Learning Disabilities/Mental Retardation*. London: Gaskell Press.

Rubinzstein, D., Hon, J., Stevens, F. *et al.* (1999). ApoE genotype and risk of dementia in Down's Syndrome. *Neuropsychiatric Genetics*, **88**, 344–7.

Rumble, B., Retallack, R., Hilbich, C. *et al.* (1989). Amyloid A4 protein and its precursor in Down's syndrome and Alzheimer's disease. *New England Journal of Medicine*, **320**, 1446–52.

Sansom, D. T., Singh, I., Jawed, S. H. and Mukherjee, T. (1994). Elderly people with learning disabilities in hospital: a psychiatric study. *Journal of Intellectual Disability Research*, **38**, 45–52.

Sparrow, S. S., Balla, D. A. and Cicchetti, D. V. (1984). *Vineland Adaptive Behaviour Scales. A Revision of the Vineland Social Maturity Scale by Edgar A. Doll*. Circle Pines, MN: American Guidance Service Inc.

Stern, Y., Gurland, B., Taternichi, T. K. *et al.* (1994). Influence of education and occupation on the incidence of Alzheimer's disease. *Journal of the American Medical Association*, **271**, 1004–10.

Strauss, D. and Eyman, R. K. (1996). Mortality of people with mental retardation in California with and without Down Syndrome, 1986–1991. *American Journal on Mental Retardation*, **100**, 643–53.

Strüwe, F. (1929). Histopathologische untersuchungen uber entstehung und wesen der senilen plaques. *Zeitshrift für die Gesamte Neurologie und Psychiatrie*, **122**, 291.

Tait, D. (1983). Mortality and dementia among ageing defectives. *Journal of Mental Deficiency Research*, **27**, 133–42.

Tanzi, R. E., Gusella, J. F., Watkins, P. C. *et al.* (1987). Amyloid β – protein gene: cDNA, mRNA distribution and genetic linkage near the Alzheimer locus. *Science*, **234**, 880–4.

Thase, M. E., Tigner, R., Smeltzer, D. J. and Liss, L. (1984). Age-related neuropsychological deficits in Down's Syndrome. *Biological Psychiatry*, **19**, 571–85.

van Schrojenstein Lantman-de Valk, H. M., van den Akker M., Maaskant, M. A. *et al.* (1997). Prevalence and incidence of health problems in people with intellectual disability. *Journal of Intellectual Disability Research*, **41**, 42–51.

Wolf, L. C. and Wright, R. E. (1987). Changes in life expectancy of mentally retarded persons in Canadian institutions: a 12-year comparison. *Journal of Mental Deficiency Research*, **31**, 41–59.

World Health Organization (1968). *Eighth Revision of the International Classification of Diseases: Glossary of Psychiatric Disorders*. Geneva: World Health Organization.

World Health Organization (1993). *The ICD-10 Classification of Mental and Behavioural Disorders: Diagnostic Criteria for Research*. Geneva: World Health Organisation.

Zigman, W. B., Schupf, N., Lubin, R. A. and Silverman, W. P. (1987). Premature regression of adults with Down's syndrome. *American Journal on Mental Deficiency*, **92**, 161–8.

11

People with intellectual disabilities who are at risk of offending

Glynis Murphy and Jonathan Mason

Introduction

In the past, particularly during the eugenics era, people with intellectual disabilities (ID) were often considered to be especially *likely* to break the law (Goddard, 1912; Clarke, 1894, quoted in Brown and Courtless, 1971). This belief probably led to a great many people with ID and/or mental health needs being incarcerated in hospitals and prisons for unjustifiably long periods (indeed some of the people detained probably should not have been there at all). At times, this became alarmingly clear, as in the well-known Baxstrom case, in which the US Supreme Court ruled in 1966 that 967 people (amongst whom there were disproportionate numbers of black southern migrants), detained in two hospitals for the 'criminally insane' in New York State, should be released, since all had been detained for longer than the maximum sentence for their original conviction (Steadman and Halfon, 1971). Following release to civil hospitals, most were later discharged to the community and extremely few re-offended, only 21 of the 967 people being returned to the secure hospitals in the first four years (Steadman and Halfon, 1971). Cases such as these, together with the advent of normalization (Emerson, 1992), the civil rights movement and the 'ordinary life' philosophy (Kings Fund, 1980; Department of Health 2001) have led to a changing attitude to people with ID and/or mental health needs who break the law. Here, the progress in the recognition of people with ID within the criminal justice system will be addressed, together with recent developments in the understanding of their needs.

Prevalence

Total population studies

Whether a larger proportion of people with ID commit crimes, than might be expected from the general population crime rates, can really only be investigated

Psychiatric and Behavioural Disorders in Intellectual and Developmental Disabilities, ed. Nick Bouras and Geraldine Holt. Published by Cambridge University Press. © Cambridge University Press 2007.

through total population studies. Several such studies exist and they throw some light on the issue of the prevalence of criminal offending in people with ID, though they are by no means conclusive. West and Farrington's long-term follow-up of working class boys, born in 1953 and living in London, is probably the most instructive, since it involved a total population of 411 boys and was prospective in nature (West and Farrington, 1973; Farrington, 1995). Over 30% of the participants were convicted of criminal offences in the period up to age 32 years and the peak age for offences was 17 years, rates decreasing thereafter. Those with convictions were more likely to have intellectual limitations (though it was unclear how many had IQs below 70) and to be achieving poor results at school, as well as being physically smaller, lighter, more hyperactive and impulsive at ten years. In addition, they were more likely to have come from larger, poorer families where parents had separated or were in constant conflict, had been convicted themselves and where harsh or erratic discipline was employed. By age 32, 6% of the sample had committed half of all the offences (Farrington and West, 1993) and these 'chronic offenders' could be remarkably well predicted from age 8–10 by 'troublesome' child behaviour, economic deprivation, lower cognitive ability, a convicted parent and poor child-rearing (Farrington, 1985).

A different research strategy was adopted by Hodgins (1992). She examined convictions for a Swedish birth cohort of 15 117 people born in Stockholm in 1953, who were followed up for 30 years. Evidence of ID was taken from registers of the children who were placed in special classes at school, as a result of ID (this included 1.5% of the men and 1.1% of the women). Hodgins reported that the likelihood of conviction for a man with ID was three times as high as for those without disabilities. For women with ID the likelihood was nearly four times as high as for women without disabilities. The odds ratios were even more extreme for violent offences (five times higher for men with ID and 25 times higher for women).

A further study by Hodgins et al. (1996) of a total population of over 300 000 people, in Denmark, born between 1944 and 1947, followed up at age 43 years, gave similar results: people with ID (excluding those with serious mental illness), who had had admissions to psychiatric wards, had an increased risk of committing offences of various kinds compared with people who had never been admitted (risk ratios were 5.5 and 6.9 for women and men respectively, for crimes entered onto the computerized criminal record system, which came into operation in 1978 in Denmark). There was no particular pattern to the crimes, according to the researchers.

Perhaps one of the more controversial works devoted to the analysis of the role of IQ in modern society is Herrnstein and Murray's (1994) book 'The Bell Curve'. Herrnstein and Murray attempt to analyse the effect of IQ on many of the most important areas of people's lives in contemporary American society, from schooling through to unemployment, welfare dependency, race, poverty and crime. It is their treatment of the mediating effects of IQ on crime that are of particular interest here. Using data based on a nationally representative sample of American youths aged between 14 and 22 in 1979 (originally totalling nearly 12 700 individuals), they postulated a direct negative correlation between IQ and crime, such that the more serious offenders tended to have a lower IQ than less serious offenders, who in turn had a lower IQ than non-offenders. Restricting their analysis to white males, Herrnstein and Murray note that those who fall into their category of 'very dull' (IQ 75 and below) are 12 times more likely to receive a custodial sentence than those whom they class as being 'very bright' (presumably with IQs of 125 or over). They also attempt to eliminate the commonly accepted argument that socio-economic status (SES) plays a significant mediating role. Seemingly, when IQ was controlled for, the men's SES had little or nothing to do with crime, such that higher SES was in fact associated with slightly higher self-reported crime. The real question, of course, is rather different: did the effect of IQ disappear when social deprivation was controlled for? Herrnstein and Murray do not comment on this.

Van Brunschot and Brannigan (1995) have criticized Herrnstein and Murray's hypothesized link between IQ and crime as being a 'mis-specified theory' and have noted that although there may be a link between IQ and delinquency, its root causes have been incorrectly evaluated. Within their discussion on the nature of the link between IQ and crime, Van Brunschot and Brannigan suggest that the effects of IQ on crime are mediated by gender and age in a fashion that is not 'readily explained by a reductionist perspective', and that the common notion of a causal relationship between IQ, school performance and crime is a spurious one. For example, they note that although there is a considerable amount of data to support at least the beginnings of a link between IQ and crime in men (i.e. that male offenders appear to have a lower IQ than male non-offenders), this is not the case for women offenders. Balthazar and Cook (1984) have found that not only is there no relationship between violent crime in females and IQ, but also that there is no relationship between imprisonment per se and IQ in women offenders. Van Brunschot and Brannigan state that either a different theory is required to explain female offending or that IQ does not hold the explanatory power attributed to it.

The extent to which all of these figures result from differences in arrest/conviction patterns rather than differences in criminal behaviour per se is uncertain; however, it may just be that people with disabilities are less good at evading the police (c.f. Robertson, 1988) and/or are more 'visible' or vulnerable to arrest (and even to wrongful conviction – see below). Moreover, retrospective surveys like Hodgins' are not able to distinguish cause from effect (this does not apply to the prospective West and Farrington study). It may be, for example, that having to attend a special school and/or being admitted to a psychiatric ward were more likely if the person showed challenging or anti-social behaviour and they were thus more likely to commit offences for reasons related to their challenging or anti-social behaviour, rather than their ID. Finally, the total population studies by both Hodgins, and Herrnstein and Murray, suffer from the difficulty of possible confounding variables, correlated with ID, which might raise the risk of offending. For example, poverty and social deprivation are associated with a raised prevalence of offending and are also known to be associated with ID. Interestingly, a recent study of self-report of offending in adolescents found that those with ID were no more likely to have offended than other adolescents, once poverty and social deprivation were taken into account (Dickson *et al.*, 2005).

In the UK, some total population studies have been undertaken focusing on people receiving ID services in particular geographical areas. Lyall *et al.* (1995b), in a small study in Cambridge, found that 2% of the 385 people, known to services for people with ID, had been in contact with the police as potential suspects over the previous year. McNulty *et al.* (1995), in another small study of two residential providers for people with ID (serving 180 residents), in London, found 9% of people had had contact with the police over the previous year, as suspects. In the Cambridge study, the contacts with police were for a range of offences (including assault and sexual offences) but none of the individuals was prosecuted and only one was formally cautioned, whereas in the London study, most were cautioned and about one-third were charged (however, the numbers in both studies were very small). The differences in figures between the Cambridge and London studies may partly have resulted from the fact that the London sample was entirely recruited from residential services. Arguably, people with challenging behaviour (including that of the offender type) were more likely to be in such services than living with families, probably resulting in a higher figure for the people living in residential services.

In a third and larger study, McBrien *et al.* (2003), based in a city with a general population of almost 200 000, examined the numbers of convictions and contacts (as suspects), with the Criminal Justice Service (CJS), of all 1326 adults known to ID services. It transpired that:
- A total of 0.8% of the 1326 were serving a current sentence.
- A total of 3% had a conviction of some kind (current or past).
- A further 7% had had contact with the CJS as a suspect but had no conviction.
- An additional 17% had challenging behaviour that was 'risky', in the sense that it could have been construed as offending.

This study suggests that about 10% of the people in touch with ID services will have had contact with the CJS at some time in their lives, as suspects. Vaughan *et al.* (2000), in a study of mentally disordered offenders and community teams in

Wessex (total population 1.8 million), found a slightly higher figure: 13% of the people known to ID teams fitted a definition of 'mentally disordered offender' (a larger percentage showed challenging behaviour).

In all probability, these kinds of studies over-estimate the proportion of all the people with ID at risk of offending, since many adults with mild disabilities lose touch with services when they leave school (Richardson and Koller, 1985) and the studies only count those in touch with services. In addition, the studies may miss a number of people with mild ID who are not known to disability services but who later become involved in the CJS.

Studies of people in the CJS

An alternative way of examining prevalence is to look at Criminal Justice Services and to ask how many people there have ID. A number of studies have examined the proportions of people with ID in the police station, in courts, in prisons and in hospitals following convictions for offences. Such figures can only be properly understood in the context of the filters that operate to keep people out of the CJS, e.g. it is known that where offending behaviour takes place in disability services, one of the filters operating is whether staff decide to report the person's behaviour to the police. Several studies have shown that staff may well be reluctant to report possible crimes, so that those reported to the police must be only a proportion of the total number committed (Lyall et al., 1995a; McBrien & Murphy, 2006).

Nevertheless, two UK studies have examined the numbers of people with ID appearing at police stations. For example, Gudjonsson et al. (1993) assessed the IQ of 156 people arrested for questioning at two London police stations, using a short form of the Wechsler Adult Intelligence Scale (WAIS-R). They found that 9% of the total sample had an IQ score below 70, and 34% had a score below 75 (representing the bottom 5% of the general population), suggesting that a significant proportion of those detained by the police had an intellectual impairment. Similar findings were reported by Lyall et al. (1995b), who screened 251 people appearing at a Cambridge police station for questioning. Participants were screened using a brief questionnaire (adapted from Clare and Gudjonsson, 1993), consisting of questions about the individual's reading and writing skills, whether they had received extra help at school and/or if they had attended a special needs school. They reported that 5% of the 251 people had attended a school for children with mild or severe ID and a further 10% had attended schools for children with emotional /behavioural difficulties or a learning support unit within a mainstream school. Again, the results suggested that substantial numbers of those appearing at police stations have ID.

In most jurisdictions, following questioning in the police station, if a person is charged with an offence, a court appearance will follow. Very few studies have been conducted which have assessed all those appearing before a court but, in two cohort studies in Australia, Hayes looked at the prevalence of people with ID appearing before magistrates' courts in New South Wales. In the first, she assessed 113 people appearing before four local (two urban and two rural) NSW magistrates' courts. A total of 14% of the suspects were found to score below IQ 70, and a further 9% scored between IQ 70 and 79 (Hayes, 1993). In the second study, Hayes (1996a) concentrated solely on two rural courts (thus incorporating a large aboriginal population) and demonstrated that 21% of those tested scored below IQ 70, and a further 36% scored between IQ 70 and IQ 79. In both studies, however, Hayes used the matrices section of the Kaufman Brief Intelligence Test (K-BIT) on the grounds that it was a culture-fair test (Hayes, 1996b), but many psychologists world argue that even the Matrices are not culture fair.

Following appearance in court, people with ID may be released unconvicted, or they may be convicted and subject to a variety of consequences, including imprisonment, hospitalization, probation or more minor consequences. Research that has examined the proportions of people in these parts of the CJS are discussed below.

Studies of people with ID in the prison system have a long history (Woodward, 1955, for example, quoted an analysis by Sutherland of over 300 studies conducted between 1910 and 1928 in the USA). The numerous investigations have led to divergent opinions as to the approximate number of people with ID in the prison system, some asserting that in the USA, for example, 10% is the correct prevalence figure (e.g. Brown and Courtless, 1971) while others argue that this simply reflects poor methodology (MacEachron, 1979). Figures from some of the recent studies are summarized in Table 11.1. Generally, it seems that studies from American prison populations produce higher prevalence rates than those from prisons in the UK. This may reflect the increased diversion from custody that takes place in the UK. It also seems that geographical differences exist within some countries, such that some states in the US record far higher prevalence rates than others (Noble and Conley, 1992). Variations in prevalence rates may also result from the use of different tests (for example, full individual IQ tests vs. quick screening tests), the administration of the tests by personnel with varying degrees of training, the time at which the tests are administered (for example, whether these are done at times when individuals may be highly stressed), the type of institution (it may be that some prisons are more prone to receive offenders with ID than others) and the methodology employed in the study (Noble and Conley, 1992).

Probably one of the least restrictive consequences following conviction is a sentence requiring the individual to report to a probation officer. The probation service, both in the UK and USA, provides for the supervision of offenders within the community. Little research has been done on the prevalence of mental disorder amongst those on probation but, where government policy emphasizes the least restrictive alternative and community-based treatment wherever possible (e.g. in

Table 11.1 Prevalence of offenders with developmental disabilities (DD) in prisons.

Author and year of study	Location of study	Number of participants	Test(s) used	% of prisoners with DD
Brown & Courtless, 1971	Inmates in US prisons	90 000 (80% of prison pop.)	Large variety	9.5%
MacEachron, 1979	Inmates in 2 US prisons	436 of the 3938 total pop.	Variety	1.5%–5.6% (depending on how measured)
Denkowski & Denkowski, 1985	20 prisons in USA*	19 1133	WAIS-R	0.2%–5.3% (state to state variations)
Coid, 1988	1 prison in England	Retrospective study, 10 000	None specified	0.34%
Gunn et al., 1991	UK, 16 prisons, 9 Young Offender Instns.)	404 youths 1365 men	None specified	0.4%
Murphy et al., 1995	1 London prison (remand)	157 men	WAIS-R	0% < IQ 70 5.7% < IQ 75
Birmingham et al., 1996	1 prison, northern UK (remand)	569 men	None specified	1%
Brooke et al., 1996	13 prisons and 3 YOIs in UK	750 youths and men	Quick test	1%
Singleton et al., 1998	1 in 34 of all UK male prisoners; 1 in 8 of all UK male remand prisoners; 1 in 3 UK women prisoners	3142 prisoners in total – i.e. 1437 remand and 1705 sentenced prisoners (2371 male and 771 female)	Quick test	—

* Denkowski and Denkowski also look at IQ scores on group tests in 16 other institutions. These have been omitted, YOI = Young Offender Institution.

the UK see Home Office, 1990, 1995a; Department of Health and Home Office, 1992; Department of Health, 1993; in the USA see the American Bar Association's Criminal Justice Mental Health Standards (1986) and Laski, 1992), the probation service may well provide supervision after conviction. Consequently, it may be the case that people with ID are increasingly appearing before the probation service, rather than being sent to hospital or prison and in the UK this has been confirmed by Mason and Murphy (2002a) who, in a preliminary study of 70 probationers in the south of England, found a prevalence rate of 6% with an IQ under 70 and a deficit in social functioning, with a further 11% scoring under IQ 75. Interestingly,

an earlier US study reported that a similar rate of 6% to 7% of people on probation and parole in Missouri had developmental disabilities (Wood, 1976, quoted in
Noble and Conley, 1992).

Characteristics of people with ID who offend

It is clear from the studies discussed above that, although the characteristics of
people with ID who offend are likely to vary with the setting in which the individuals
are studied, nevertheless, very few people with *severe* ID are to be found within any
part of the CJS. For example, only one of the Lyall *et al.*, 1995b, sample had severe
disabilities and most other studies seem to have identified very few people or no
one with severe disabilities (Noble and Conley, 1992; Lindsay *et al.*, 2002). Given
the estimates of the prevalence rates of some challenging behaviours which tend
to occur across the ability range, such as aggression (estimated to occur in 18%
of all those with ID in touch with services; Harris, 1993), this may be surprising.
However, it almost certainly results at least in part from the requirement in law, in
both the UK and USA, that the court must show not just *actus reus* but also *mens rea*
on the part of an individual before conviction. Moreover, in the UK and the US, for
state/federal prosecutions, decisions are made by the Crown Prosecution Service
(CPS) or the District Attorney (DA) about whether cases should go to court on a
number of criteria, including the likelihood of conviction and public interest. It is
probable that, where staff or carers do call the police when someone with severe
ID engages in potentially criminal behaviour, either the police themselves or the
CPS/DA judge it not to be in the public interest to proceed.

The vast majority of people with ID who are convicted of offences are young
and male, though no more so than might be expected when compared with other
offender populations without disabilities (Noble and Conley, 1992). Most studies,
however, have shown an over-representation of people from ethnic minorities with
ID in courts/prisons, more than would be predicted from other suspects or offenders
without disabilities (Hayes, 1993, 1996a; Noble and Conley, 1992). Quite why this
occurs is unclear but it may reflect poorer access to defence lawyers by people from
ethnic minorities.

The kinds of crimes which people with ID commit has been a matter of dispute
for years. Early assertions, drawn from Walker and McCabe's (1973) data on people
detained under the Mental Health Act 1959 in England, in a particular year, claimed
that sexual offences and arson were particularly common amongst people with ID
(Prins, 1980, p. 92; Robertson, 1981). In fact, this did not follow from Walker and
McCabe's data (even though researchers such as Lindsay *et al.*, 2002, continue to
assert that people with ID are particularly likely to be sexual offenders). All that
the Walker and McCabe figures showed was that a disproportionate number of

the sexual and arson offences *of their sample* were committed by the proportion of people detained under the Mental Health Act on the grounds of 'mental subnormality' and 'severe mental subnormality' (as they were then termed). However, this should not be interpreted as having any implications for the proportion of *all* sexual and arson offences committed since, first, not all such crimes are reported to the police (especially in the case of sexual offences) and second, it is known that only a small minority of such offenders are diverted into hospitals under the Mental Health Act in England (so that a hospitalized group is a biased sample of all such offenders with mental health needs or ID). Similar arguments have been put by Noble and Conley (1992) in relation to data from various studies in the USA. Assertions of the same kind, drawn from assessments of people referred for forensic evaluations (Rasanen *et al.*, 1995; Hawk *et al.*, 1993) can be subject to the same criticism.

The only way to derive a true picture of the types of crimes committed by people with ID would be through the offence records for a total population sample (and even then, only *documented* offences would be counted). In fact, this is a difficult task: following school-leaving age, the numbers of people with mild degrees of ID, in touch with services, drops by three-quarters to two-thirds, as people 'blend' into the 'ordinary' community, apparently needing no further services (Richardson and Koller, 1985). In the absence of a total population sample, the most that can be said is that, where the types of offences of people with ID have been analysed, the range seems similar to those of other offenders (Hodgins *et al.*, 1996; Glaser and Deane, 1999; Barron *et al.*, 2004). It is possible that, amongst sexual offenders, those with ID commit somewhat fewer penetrative offences (Murray *et al.*, 1992) and somewhat more often involve victims who are younger and male children (Blanchard *et al.*, 1999).

However, MacEachron (1979) compared offenders with ID with those with borderline abilities in two US prisons and found no significant differences in the severity of the most recent offence, the length of current sentence, the degree of recidivism, participation in rehabilitation programmes, recommendations for parole, degree to which parole had ever been revoked and the use of probation as a juvenile. The only significant distinction found in types of crime was that those with disabilities had fewer violent incidents in prison, than the comparison group.

Little further information can be considered to provide a reliable guide to offences committed by people with ID. Studies conducted in police stations, courts and prisons, examining all suspects and/or offenders, have obtained only small samples of people with ID on the whole, so very little can be deduced from them about the kinds of crimes committed by people with ID. Likewise, reports from treatment facilities for people with ID usually describe only small numbers of people (usually around 20–40) and these are usually a highly selected sample, considered in need of psychological and/or psychiatric treatment in secure settings, so that they tend to include disproportionately serious offenders (for example, 40% of Day's (1988) sample had been convicted of sex offences and 10% had been convicted of arson but these were a highly selected group).

Some characteristics have been confirmed in almost all studies, however. It appears that the social background of people with ID who have offended is very often characterized by social deprivation. Most of the investigations referred to above reported a high incidence of social deprivation and family breakdown/disorder in childhood (e.g. Day, 1988; Winter *et al.*, 1997; Barron *et al.*, 2004), long histories of anti-social or 'challenging behaviour' (e.g. Day, 1988; Winter *et al.*, 1997), high rates of adult unemployment (Murphy *et al.*, 1995; Barron *et al.*, 2004) and a raised incidence of abuse in their own histories (Lindsay *et al.*, 2001; Barron *et al.*, 2004; Lindsay *et al.*, 2004). Nevertheless, relatively few of the studies have included comparison groups of non-disabled offenders, so that any findings on social background are difficult to interpret. MacEachron (1979), in her study of people in prison in Maine and Massachusetts, found that, compared with people in the borderline range for IQ, those with ID were on average slightly older (in their thirties), less well educated, less likely to be abusing drugs, and were from larger families (the average number of children was seven). Otherwise, the groups were very similar (for example, both groups were highly likely to be unemployed, equally likely to have other disabilities, and equally unlikely to be married). Moreover, in attempts to predict offence severity and length of sentence from intellectual, social and legal variables, MacEachron found few differences between the disabled and non-disabled groups and she concluded that the intellectual differences between the two groups were fairly immaterial, with the social and legal variables 'more germane to the problem of being an offender than . . . intelligence'.

It seems likely that there is a high prevalence of mental health needs amongst people with ID who have committed offences (Noble and Conley, 1992; McGee and Menolascino, 1992). Studies from specialist treatment units and from prisons in the UK and the USA have reported very high rates of mental health problems in those with ID (Day, 1988; Murphy *et al.*, 1991; Steiner, 1984; White and Wood, 1988; Lindsay *et al.*, 2002; O'Brien, 2002; Lindsay *et al.*, 2004). While this may not be surprising in health service facilities and prisons, it remains to be seen whether the same holds true for people who are questioned at the police station but who are living in the community (recent studies, such as Winter *et al.*, 1997, have included samples too small to determine this accurately).

Vulnerabilities of people with ID in the CJS

In a number of countries, the disadvantages which people with ID suffer in the Criminal Justice System are beginning to be documented. Some of these are reflected in the legal process: for instance, Brown and Courtless (1971) found 8% of defendants with ID were not represented by a lawyer. Some disadvantages are more subtle, however, and relate to the suspects' understanding of their rights in detention and their understanding of the legal process.

In the UK, on arrest, the police are required to 'caution' individuals. The exact words of the caution change from time to time and in England they were altered in 1994, when the right to silence was modified. The newer caution (current words) are as follows:

You do not have to say anything. But it may harm your defence if you do not mention when questioned something which you later rely on in court. Anything you do say may be given in evidence.

Studies in England have demonstrated that many people with ID did not fully understand the older (simpler) caution (Clare and Gudjonsson, 1991). It is very unlikely therefore that they will understand the new caution and several studies have demonstrated that even the general population (Clare *et al.*, 1998) and non-disabled suspects frequently struggle to understand the new caution (Fenner *et al.*, 2002). Indeed the middle sentence of the current English caution is so complex that some of the police were unable to give a full account of its meaning (Clare *et al.*, 1998).

In addition, in England, when suspects arrive at the police station, they are given a written 'Notice to Detained Persons', which reiterates the caution and also tells them that they have a right to have someone informed of their arrest, to have a legal representative and to consult the Codes of Practice (Home Office, 1995b; for revised Codes, see Home Office, 2006). However, analysis of the written 'Notice' has shown that it requires a reading age which people with ID are very unlikely to attain (Gudjonsson, 1991) and it contains such complex wording that many people with ID cannot understand it, even if they have it read to them, which the police are not obliged to do. As a result, Clare and Gudjonsson (1992) developed an experimental version of the 'Notice', with simplified wording and demonstrated that it was far easier to understand than the version in use in police stations (the Home Office declined to adopt the new version, however).

Similarly, in the USA, since the Miranda vs. Arizona case of 1966, suspects have to be warned before interrogation that they have a right to remain silent, that what they do say may be used in court and that they have a right to a lawyer (the so-called 'Miranda rights'). Suspects are allowed to waive these rights if the waiver is made 'voluntarily, knowingly and intelligently' (Fulero and Everington, 1995). Much as in the case of the English 'Notice to Detained Persons', the written form of the Miranda warning is too complex in wording and reading level for people with ID to be able to comprehend it (Fulero and Everington, 1995). Moreover, when tested on the Grisso (1981) scales designed to assess understanding of the Miranda rights,

Fulero and Everington (1995) found that even people with mild ID obtained very poor scores, compared with both juvenile and adult samples. They concluded that most people with ID would not have been competent to waive their rights.

Turning to people's possible vulnerabilities on questioning, people with ID may be able to accurately recount an event that has occurred (Perlman et al., 1994; Kebbel and Hatton, 1999) but they tend to be more suggestible and acquiescent, on average, than people without such disabilities, under questioning (Heal and Sigelman, 1995; Finlay and Lyons 2001). Beail (2002) has argued that the usual tests employed to assess acquiescence and suggestibility need to be interpreted with care but, nevertheless, in the police station, such vulnerabilities would make it more likely that people would acquiesce to suggestions made to them by the police and be led by leading questions into self-incrimination (Clare and Gudjonsson, 1993; Cardone and Dent, 1996; Everington and Fulero, 1999). This in turn makes it more probable that people with ID would be vulnerable to making false confessions, as indeed appears to be the case (Gudjonsson, 1992; Perske, 1991). This tendency to false confessions may be exacerbated by the fact that many people with ID misunderstand legal terms which are basic to the legal process: Smith (1993), for example, found that about 20% of the people referred for pre-trial competency assessments in South Carolina did not understand the terms 'guilty' and 'not guilty', such that some actually had the meanings of the words reversed. Some people with ID may also misunderstand the likely events in the criminal justice process, thinking for example that if they make a false confession, even to a serious crime, in the police station, they will be allowed to go home and will be able to correct it later in court (Clare and Gudjonsson, 1995).

In England and Wales, in recognition of some of these vulnerabilities of people with ID, special provisions were brought in, under the *Police and Criminal Evidence Act 1984*, in particular the audio-taping of police interviews (so that the manner of police questioning could be analysed) and the provision of an 'Appropriate Adult' (AA) for 'vulnerable' suspects (including those with developmental disabilities). Somewhat similar provisions were also made in Australia (Baroff et al., 2004).

In England and Wales, the Appropriate Adult's (AA) role in the police station is to protect vulnerable suspects from their tendency to 'provide information which is unreliable, misleading or self-incriminating' (Home Office, 1995b; 2006). However, there appear to have been two main problems with the Appropriate Adult scheme:

- Firstly, it was difficult for the police to evaluate when someone had a developmental disability (see below) so that many people were not provided with an Appropriate Adult, even though they were entitled to one (Bean and Nemitz, 1994; Medford et al., 2000).

- Secondly, Appropriate Adults, who may be parents, carers, or social workers who have never met the individual in question, often did not speak during the police interview and seemed unclear about their role (Pearse and Gudjonsson, 1996). Many areas have since brought in Appropriate Adult training schemes, in order to improve the effectiveness of this important provision.

Diversion out of the CJS

In most countries, diversion out of the Criminal Justice System can occur at a number of points. For example, the police may decide not to proceed with a case involving a person with ID or, following an appearance in court, the person might be referred to community-based services for people with ID or sent to hospital, either on remand or once convicted (Denkowski *et al.*, 1983; Laski, 1992; James, 1996).

In England and Wales, courts can only divert people to hospital if it has been established in court that the individual is unfit to plead or if she/he falls within the broad category of 'mental disorder' (for admission for assessment) or the specific categories of 'mental illness', 'psychopathic disorder', 'mental impairment' or 'severe mental impairment' of the Mental Health Act (MHA) 1983. Usually, those with ID would be admitted under 'mental impairment', or 'severe mental impairment', which requires the presence of ID and 'abnormally aggressive or seriously irresponsible conduct'. People diverted from courts into hospitals who are classified under 'mental illness' far outnumber those classified under 'mental impairment' or 'severe mental impairment'. While the numbers of those with mental illness diverted from courts and detained under the MHA are increasing, the numbers with mental impairment and severe mental impairment are decreasing: on a census day at the end of March 2004, out of a total of 14 000 people detained under the MHA 1983, only 1092 were detained under mental impairment/severe mental impairment.

In the UK, Canada, the USA, Australia and elsewhere, people with ID can be found 'unfit to plead' (UK) or 'not competent to stand trial' (USA) and can be diverted out of the CJS (Rasch, 1990; Bonnie, 1992; Murphy and Clare, 2003; Baroff *et al.*, 2004). In England and Wales, this procedure was based on criteria set out in *R* v. *Pritchard 1836*, where it was established that the crucial issues were whether the accused could understand the proceedings so as to make a defence, challenge a juror, and comprehend the evidence (Mackay, 1990). Nowadays fitness to plead is usually said to be based on five criteria: ability to plead; ability to understand the evidence; ability to understand the court proceedings; ability to instruct a lawyer; and knowing that a juror can be challenged (Grubin, 1991a; Mackay and Kearns, 2000). The criteria in the USA and Australia are very similar (Baroff *et al.*, 2004).

From 1964, under the *Criminal Procedure (Insanity) Act 1964*, in England and Wales, people who were found unfit to plead were detained in hospital (often in high-security hospitals) and were supposed to return to court once they became fit to plead. In fact, this happened relatively rarely for people with ID. Grubin (1991a), in a survey of the 286 people found unfit to plead between 1976 and 1988, reported that 21% had ID (the remainder had serious mental health needs). A disproportionate number of those with ID remained in hospital without ever returning to court for a trial (40% of those people who still remained in hospital without a trial by 1989 had ID – Grubin, 1991b). This of course had major civil rights implications, particularly since the evidence that the person had committed a crime was often unclear. There was subsequently a change in the law in England and Wales, such that the facts of the case had to be tried, according to the *Criminal Procedure (Insanity and Fitness to Plead) Act 1991*, and only then could someone be detained if they were deemed unfit to plead. The same Act also allowed community treatment as well as hospital treatment; nevertheless, relatively few people have been found unfit to plead, perhaps because diversion from the CJS, through use of the *Mental Health Act 1983*, often allowed more flexibility. Mackay and Kearns (2000) found that the number of people found unfit to plead rose from an average of 12 per year across England and Wales, to 33 per year, after the changes to the legislation, only a quarter of these being people with ID (the remainder had mental health problems).

In the USA and Canada, in contrast, 'competence' hearings were very much more common than in England and Wales, so that they were estimated to arise in between 2 and 8% of felony cases in the USA for example (Hoge *et al.*, 1992), meaning that there were thousands of competency hearings per year (Steadman *et al.*, 1982). Trial judges were required to order competence evaluations whenever significant doubts were raised as to the defendant's mental competence, and failure of defence lawyers to consider such an evaluation could invalidate subsequent conviction, if competence was later established as an issue (Bonnie, 1992). Commonly, competence was judged on the 'Dusky' criterion: 'whether the defendant has sufficient present ability to consult with his lawyer with a reasonable degree of rational understanding and whether he has a rational as well as factual understanding of the proceedings against him' (*Dusky* v. *United States, 1960*). More recently the criteria have been considered to be three-fold: understanding the nature and seriousness of the charge, understanding the nature and purpose of the court proceedings, and being able to assist one's lawyer in providing a defence (Baroff *et al.*, 2004).

In the early years of competence hearings, difficulties arose in the USA that mirrored some of those in the UK: for example, one study found that 50% of those found 'incompetent' and sent to hospital in Michigan were never released (Hess and Thomas, 1963), and McGarry (1971) reported that, after being found 'incompetent', more people left hospital, in Massachusetts, by dying than by any other route. Subsequently, following the case of *Jackson* v. *Indiana*, in 1972, the US Supreme Court ruled that those held in hospital following an incompetency hearing could not be kept there for an unreasonable length of time. Thereafter, the average length of time in hospital following incompetency hearings fell to around six months to a year and people with mental health needs were frequently treated in hospital and returned to court rapidly, as had been the original intention (Steadman *et al.*, 1982). Where someone's competence to stand trail was considered 'untreatable', as presumably it might be for people with intellectual disabilities, the state was required to proceed with a civil commitment or drop the charges.

Some studies have shown that as few as 2% of defendants with ID have pre-trial evaluations of competence to stand trial (Brown and Courtless, 1971), though recent figures suggested this had increased somewhat (Smith and Broughton, 1994). In practice, competence to stand trial has often been assessed by informal interview, although a number of formal test protocols have been developed for the purpose (Grisso, 1986), including at least one which is highly sophisticated, the McArthur Adjudicative Competency Assessment or McCAT-CA (Hoge *et al.*, 1997). Only two measures have been designed specifically for people with ID, however, one being a brief screening test (Smith and Hudson, 1995) and the other a more thorough assessment, the Competence Assessment for Standing Trial for Defendants with Mental Retardation (CAST-MR) (Everington and Luckasson, 1987; Everington, 1990).

When competence is assessed in people with ID referred for evaluation, it appears that about 35% are judged not competent to stand trial (Petrella, 1992; Smith and Broughton, 1994). For example, in an analysis of a five-year cohort of the 160 people thought to have ID, who were evaluated for competence in South Carolina, it was found that they were typically male (93%), black (66%) and young (mean age 28 years) and had frequently spent many months in detention before evaluation and/or court appearances (Smith and Broughton, 1994). Approximately two-thirds were judged competent and one-third not competent to stand trial (this latter group had a lower mean IQ of 58, compared to those judged competent, who had a mean IQ of 64). Those judged not competent were far less often sent to jail (0%, as opposed to 55% of those judged competent), less often put on probation (13%, compared with 31%) and mostly were dismissed back home (47%, compared with 7%) or referred to the department of 'Mental Retardation' (40%, as compared with 7%).

In addition to 'competence' in the USA, 'culpability' or criminal responsibility may be assessed. Essentially, the former refers to whether the defendant understands the charges and court proceedings and can instruct his/her lawyer, while the latter refers to whether the defendant knew right from wrong at the time of the offence (Smith and Broughton, 1994). Criminal responsibility is usually judged by the

McNaughten rule, the so-called right-wrong test (which states that a person is not legally responsible if she/he was 'labouring under such a defect of reason from disease of the mind, as not to know the nature and quality of the act he was doing; or, if he did know it, that he did not know what he was doing was wrong' (Grisso, 1986). Mental health professionals have often been accused of confusing competence to stand trial and culpability (Johnson *et al.*, 1990) and a number of investigations have addressed the extent to which the two characteristics co-occur in particular individuals (Johnson *et al.*, 1990; Petrella, 1992; Smith and Broughton, 1994). In general, for people with ID, it appears that it is rarer to be judged not criminally responsible than to be judged not competent to stand trial and, amongst those judged not responsible, most will have also been judged not competent (though these relationships are different for people with mental health problems – see Johnson *et al.*, 1990).

Improvements in practice

At present, people with ID who break the law generally enter the CJS much as other people would, though perhaps with more confusion and less appreciation of their circumstances than most. Essentially, their treatment within the CJS depends on the extent to which their disability is recognized by those coming into contact with them, as it is this factor which will often determine their course through the system. Most research, though, has demonstrated that the identification of people with ID in the CJS is poor in the pre-trial phase: according to Brown and Courtless (1971) in the USA only 2% of such defendants had a pre-trial psychological assessment, while Denkowski and Denkowski (1985) reported that 38% of US States did not attempt to identify defendants with ID. Similarly, in England where some special provisions (such as an *Appropriate Adult*) exist for people with ID and/or mental health needs in the police station, Gudjonsson *et al.* (1993) found that only about one-fifth of the people who needed this special help were identified and others have suggested even lower rates of identification nationally (Bean and Nemitz, 1994). Likewise, reports from court diversion schemes in the UK (James, 1996) have shown that very few people assessed in these projects have ID, implying that many cases may simply be missed: Cooke (1991), for example, in Scotland, reported that in a consecutive series of 150 offenders referred for psychological/psychiatric treatment before prosecution (so called 'primary diversion') none appeared to have ID and Joseph and Potter (1993) in a London diversion scheme, operating at two magistrates' courts, found only four people (2%) had ID (formal assessment was not employed). Moreover, *after* conviction, McAfee and Gural (1988), in their survey of the States' Attorneys General, concluded that protections for people with ID were also very poor, with many states providing little in the way of treatment or training (see also Denkowski *et al.*, 1983), and they were forced to conclude that the CJS 'appears to have adopted an informal, inconsistent and inequitable response' to the problems of individuals with ID who are accused of a crime.

Nevertheless, special protections before and during trials do exist and there is some evidence that they are being increasingly recognized and more often used, though not yet to anything like their full extent. Thus, for example, in some police stations in the UK, people brought in for questioning are screened by the custody sergeant in order to try to ensure that the protections available at the police station are made available (Clare, 2003). Likewise, a brief screening test for the presence of ID has been developed in Australia (Hayes, 2002) and in the UK (Mason and Murphy, 2002b), and a brief screening test to assess competence to stand trial has been developed in the USA (Smith and Hudson, 1995), in order to allow rapid screening of all those who will appear in court and may need a full competency assessment. In addition, there is beginning to be an increase in the willingness of agencies in the CJS and health services to work together, to provide support for those proceeding through the CJS (for example, Hollins *et al.*, 1996a and 1996b) and to ensure treatment for those people with ID who may otherwise be likely to remain at risk of offending (Churchill *et al.*, 1997; Clare and Murphy, 1998).

Assessment, treatment and risk management

Early attempts to provide assessment and treatment for people with ID who were at risk of offending concentrated on behavioural and medical methods, with limited success (Murphy *et al.*, 1983; Clarke, 1989; Scotti *et al.*, 1991; Cooper, 1995; Murphy, 1997). Increasingly, however, specific measures have been developed for the psychological assessment of people at risk of aggression (Benson & Ivins 1992; Walker and Cheseldine, 1997; Taylor, 2002); people who set fires (Murphy and Clare, 1995); and men who engage in sexually abusive behaviour (Lindsay *et al.*, 2004). Recently, cognitive-behavioural treatment (CBT) has been seen as the method of choice (Clare and Murphy, 1998) and a number of studies have now demonstrated that such techniques as anger management training are effective in reducing self-rated anger (Benson *et al.*, 1986; Rose *et al.*, 2000; Whitaker, 2001; Taylor *et al.*, 2002; Taylor *et al.*, 2004), and that cognitive-behavioural treatment for sexual offenders can reduce recidivism (Lindsay and Smith, 1998) and cognitive distortions (Lindsay *et al.*, 1998a, b, c; Rose *et al.*, 2002; see Lindsay, 2004, for a review). Nevertheless, very few of the studies investigating the effectiveness of CBT in reducing offending-type behaviour have involved control or comparison groups of any kind (Benson *et al.*, 1986; Lindsay and Smith, 1998; Rose *et al.*, 2000; Taylor *et al.*, 2002). Even fewer have involved a randomized control trial (RCT), as noted by Barron *et al.* (2002), Lindsay (2002) and Taylor (2002), although one small RCT has appeared that examined the effectiveness of anger management training (Willner *et al.*, 2002).

Whether or not treatment can be provided for people with ID at risk of offending, services frequently employ risk assessment and risk management methods, so as to ensure public safety and to reduce the risk of re-offending. As Halstead (1997) and Johnston (2002) have commented, many services for people with ID simply employ structured clinical judgments of risk for this purpose and, while this method of risk assessment may have some face validity, there have been criticisms that such methods are not as good as actuarial methods in predicting risk, at least in the non-disabled population (Grove, 2000; Monahan, 2002).

For non-disabled offenders, risk is predicted using measures that combine actuarial historical variables (such as age, gender, numbers of previous offences), with clinical variables (such as diagnoses, PCL-R scores). The result is that a variety of measures abound, such as the Violence Risk Appraisal Guide (VRAG) (Quinsey *et al.*, 1998) and the Sex Offender Risk Appraisal Guide (SORAG) (Quinsey *et al.*, 1995), the Historical Clinical Risk-20 (HCR-20) (Webster *et al.*, 1995), the Sexual Violence Risk-20 (SVR-20) (Boer *et al.*, 1997), the SONAR, the Static-99 (Hanson & Thornton, 1999) and the Rapid Risk Assessment of Sexual offence Recidivism (RRASOR) (Hanson, 1997). A number of large-scale studies have found that these instruments do predict risk well and that the instruments are often equally good in their predictive ability for non-disabled offenders (Barbaree *et al.*, 2001; Sjostedt and Langstrom, 2002; Harris *et al.*, 2003). Nevertheless, research into the use of these instruments is only just beginning in relation to people with ID at risk of offending (Lindsay & Beail, 2004): for example, Harris and Tough (2004) have found that the RRASOR did predict sexual offending amongst men with ID and sexually abusive behaviour, while Quinsey *et al.* (2004) reported that the VRAG was a good predictor of violent and sexual behaviours in people with ID transferred from institutions to community settings. However, McMillan *et al.* (2004) noted that clinical prediction was as good as actuarial prediction of violent incidents within a forensic institution.

Increasingly, there have been attempts to improve prediction of re-offending by non-disabled offenders, by including dynamic factors (such as mood) in the risk measure, to supplement the normally static actuarial and clinical factors. Attempts to do this for people with ID are just beginning (Boer *et al.*, 2004) and some measures have shown some initial success: Lindsay *et al.* (2004), for example, have developed a measure called Dynamic Risk Assessment and Management System (DRAMS) which is showing promise as a predictor of aggressive incidents in residential settings.

Conclusion

It seems clear that people with ID are liable to break the law from time to time but are less likely to do so than used to be supposed in the early 1900s. The precise prevalence of people with ID in the various parts of the Criminal Justice System varies with the laws, social policy and the presence of alternative rehabilitative systems in place in the area studied. In the UK, USA and Australia, it seems to be beginning to be accepted that people with ID should not be in prison, at least partly because of their increased risk of victimization there. Moreover, it is increasingly recognized that people with ID are especially vulnerable in the police station and the courts and that they need special provisions there. In a number of jurisdictions, protections for people with ID have been set up but it seems that everywhere the identification and operation of the protective features of the system currently fall well short of the ideal. Meanwhile, assessment and treatment for people with ID at risk of offending is a growing area of research, with cognitive-behavioural methods showing considerable promise. It has to be acknowledged, however, that some areas of research, such as that on risk assessment, are really only just beginning for people with ID. There is a long way to go therefore, but some improvements in practice can be seen which suggest that there is a growing awareness of the difficulties of people with ID who are at risk of offending, whether they are in the Criminal Justice System or in mental health services.

Summary points

- It is unclear whether people with ID are more or less likely to offend than people without disabilities.
- Risk factors, such as poverty, social deprivation, being young and being male, for offending in the non-disabled population are also risk factors in people with ID.
- People with ID who offend may not have their offence brought to the attention of the Criminal Justice System (CJS).
- Of those who do come to the attention of the CJS, only a proportion will proceed to court.
- People with severe ID are unlikely to have contact with the CJS.
- In the absence of total population studies, it appears that the range of offences committed by people with ID is similar to that of other offenders.
- The evidence suggests that there is a high prevalence of mental health needs amongst people with ID who offend, although community studies are awaited.
- People with ID are disadvantaged in the CJS and are vulnerable in prison.
- In most countries, diversion out of the CJS can occur at a number of points.
- Identification of people with ID in the CJS tends to be poor in the pre-trial phase.

- Increasingly, cognitive-behaviour therapy is being used to reduce the risk of offending by people with ID.
- Research into the use of risk assessment instruments is at an early stage.

REFERENCES

American Bar Association (1986). *Criminal Justice Mental Health Standards*. Washington, DC: American Bar Association.

Balthazar, M. R. & Cook, R. J. (1984). An analysis of the factors related to the extent of violent crimes committed by incarcerated females. *Journal of Offender Counselling, Services and Rehabilitation*, **9**(1–2), 103–18.

Barbaree, H. E., Seto, M. C., Langton, C. M. & Peacock, E. J. (2001). Evaluating the predictive accuracy of six risk assessment instruments for adult sexual offenders. *Criminal Justice and Behaviour*, **28**, 490–521.

Baroff, G., Gunn, M. & Hayes, S. (2004). Legal issues. In W. R. Lindsay, J. L. Taylor & P. Sturmey (eds.), *Offenders With Developmental Disabilities*. Chichester: John Wiley & Sons, pp. 37–65.

Barron, P., Hassiotis, A. & Banes, J. (2002). Offenders with intellectual disability: the size of the problem and therapeutic outcomes. *Journal of Intellectual Disability Research*, **46**, 454–63.

Barron, P., Hassiotis, A. & Banes, J. (2004). Offenders with intellectual disability: a prospective comparative study. *Journal of Intellectual Disability Research*, **48**, 69–76.

Beail, N. (2002). Interrogative suggestibility, memory and intellectual disability. *Journal of Applied Research in Intellectual Disabilities*, **15**, 129–37.

Bean, P. & Nemitz, T. (1994). *Out of Depth and Out of Sight*. London: Mencap.

Benson, B. A. & Ivins, J. (1992). Anger, depression and self-concept in adults with mental retardation. *Journal of Intellectual Disability Research*, **36**, 169–75.

Benson, B. A., Johnson Rice, C. & Miranti, S. V. (1986). Effects of anger management training with mentally retarded adults in group treatment. *Journal of Consulting & Clinical Psychology*, **54**, 728–9.

Birmingham, L., Mason, D. & Grubin, D. (1996). Prevalence of mental disorder in remand prisoners: consecutive case study. *British Medical Journal*, **313**: 1521–4.

Blanchard, R., Watson, M., Choy, A. *et al.* (1999). Paedophiles: mental retardation, maternal age and sexual orientation. *Archives of Sexual Behaviour*, **28**, 111–27.

Boer, D. P., Hart, S. D., Kropp, P. R. & Webster, C. D. (1997). *Manual for the Sexual Violence Risk-20: Professional Guidelines for Assessing Risk of Sexual Violence*. Vancouver, BC: British Columbia Institute on Family Violence & Mental Health Law & Policy Institute, Simon Fraser University.

Boer, D. P., Tough, S. & Haaven, J. (2004). Assessment of risk manageability of intellectually disabled sex offenders. *Journal of Applied Research in Intellectual Disabilities*, **17**, 275–84.

Bonnie, R. J. (1992). The competence of criminal defendants: a theoretical reformulation. *Behavioural Sciences and the Law*, **10**, 291–316.

Brooke, D., Taylor, C., Gunn, J. & Maden, A. (1996). Point prevalence of mental disorder in unconvicted male prisoners in England and Wales. *British Medical Journal*, **313**, 1524–7.

Brown, B. S. & Courtless, T. F. (1971). *The Mentally Retarded Offender*. Washington, DC: US Government Printing Office, Dept of Health Education and Welfare Publication, No. 72–90–39.

Cardone, D. & Dent, H. (1996). Memory and interrogative suggestibility: The effects of modality of information presentation and retrieval conditions upon the suggestibility scores of people with learning disabilities. *Legal and Criminological Psychology*, 1, 34–42.

Churchill, J., Brown, H., Craft, A. & Horrocks, C. (1997). *There Are No Easy Answers: The Provision of Continuing Care and Treatment to Adults with Learning Disabilities who Sexually Abuse Others*. Chesterfield: ARC/NAPSAC.

Clare, I. C. H. (2003). Psychological vulnerabilities of adults with mild learning disabilities: implications for suspects during police detention and interviewing. Unpublished Ph.D. thesis, University of London.

Clare, I. C. H. & Gudjonsson, G. H. (1991). Recall and understanding of the caution and rights in police detention among persons of average intellectual ability and persons with a mental handicap. *Proceedings of the First DCLP Annual Conference*, 1, 34–42. Leicester: British Psychological Society (Issues in Criminological and Legal Psychology Series, No. 17).

Clare, I. C. H. & Gudjonsson, G. H. (1992). *Devising and Piloting an Experimental Version of the 'Notice to Detained Persons'*. The Royal Commission on Criminal Justice, Research Study No. 7. London: HMSO.

Clare, I. C. H. & Gudjonsson, G. H. (1993). Interrogative suggestibility, confabulation, and acquiescence in people with mild learning disabilities (mental handicap): Implications for reliability during police interview. *British Journal of Clinical Psychology*, 32, 295–301.

Clare, I. C. H. & Gudjonsson, G. H. (1995). The vulnerability of suspects with intellectual disabilities during police interviews: a review and experimental study of decision-making. *Mental Handicap Research*, 8, 110–28.

Clare, I. C. H., Gudjonsson, G. H. & Harari, P. M. (1998). Understanding of the current police caution (England and Wales). *Journal of Community and Applied Social Psychology*, 8, 323–9.

Clare, I. C. H. & Murphy, G. (1998). Working with offenders or alleged offenders with intellectual disabilities. In E. Emerson, A. Caine, J. Bromley & C. Hatton (eds.), *Clinical Psychology and People with Intellectual Disabilities*. Chichester: John Wiley and Sons, pp. 154–76.

Clarke, D. J. (1989). Anti-libidinal drugs and mental retardation: a review. *Medicine, Science and Law*, 29, 136–48.

Coid, J. (1988). Mentally abnormal prisoners on remand – rejected or accepted by the NHS? *British Medical Journal*, 296, 1779–82.

Cooke, D. J. (1991). Treatment as an alternative to prosecution: offenders diverted for treatment. *British Journal of Psychiatry*, 158, 785–91.

Cooper, A. J. (1995). Review of the role of two anti-libidinal drugs in the treatment of sex offenders with mental retardation. *Mental Retardation*, 33, 42–8.

Day, K. (1988). A hospital-based treatment programme for male mentally handicapped offenders. *British Journal of Psychiatry*, 153, 636–44.

Denkowski, G. C. & Denkowski, K. M. (1985). The mentally retarded offender in the state prison system: Identification, prevalence, adjustment and rehabilitation. *Criminal Justice and Behaviour*, 12, 55–70.

Denkowski, G.C., Denkowski, K.M. & Mabli, J. (1983). A 50-state survey of the current status of residential programmes for mentally retarded offenders. *Mental Retardation,* **21**, 197–203.

Department of Health (1993). *Services for People with Learning Disabilities and Challenging Behaviour or Mental Health Needs* (Chairman: Professor Jim Mansell). London: HMSO.

Department of Health (2001). *Valuing People: A New Strategy for Learning Disability for the 21st Century.* London: HMSO.

Department of Health and Home Office (1992). *Review of Health and Social Services for Mentally Disordered Offenders and Others Requiring Similar Services* (Chairman Dr. J. Reed). London: HMSO.

Dickson, K., Emerson, E. & Hatton, C. (2005). Self-reported anti-social behaviour: prevalence and risk factors amongst adolescents with and without intellectual disability. *Journal of Intellectual Disability Research,* **49**, 820–6.

Emerson, E. (1992). What is normalization? In H. Brown and H. Smith (eds.), *Normalisation: A Reader for the Nineties.* London: Routledge, pp. 1–18.

Everington, C. T. (1990). The competence assessment for standing trial for defendants with mental retardation (CAST-MR). *Criminal Justice and Behaviour,* **17**, 147–68.

Everington, C. T. & Fulero, S. M. (1999). Competence to confess: Measuring understanding and suggestibility of defendants with mental retardation. *Mental Retardation,* **37**, 212–20.

Everington, C. & Luckasson, R. (1987). *Competence Assessment for Standing Trial for Defendants with Mental Retardation: CAST-MR.* Oxford, OH: Miami University, Dept. of Educational Psychology.

Farrington, D. P. (1985). Predicting self-reported and official delinquency. In D. P. Farrington and R. Tarling (eds.), *Prediction in Criminology.* Albany, NY: State University of New York Press, pp. 150–73.

Farrington, D.P. (1995). The development of offending and anti-social behaviour from childhood: key findings from the Cambridge study in delinquent development. *Journal of Child Psychology and Psychiatry,* **360**, 929–64.

Farrington, D. P. & West, D. J. (1993). Criminal, penal and life histories of chronic offenders: risk and protective factors and early identification. *Criminal Behaviour and Mental Health,* **3**, 492–523.

Fenner, S., Gudjonsson, G. H. & Clare, I. C. H. (2002). Understanding of the current police caution (England and Wales) among suspects in police detention. *Journal of Community and Applied Social Psychology,* **12**, 83–93.

Finlay, W. M. L. & Lyons, E. (2002). Acquiescence in interviews with people who have mental retardation. *Mental Retardation,* **40**, 14–29.

Fulero, S. M. & Everington, C. (1995). Assessing competence to waive Miranda rights in defendants with mental retardation. *Law and Human Behaviour,* **19**, 533–43.

Glaser, W. & Deane, K. (1999). Normalisation in an abnormal world: a study of prisoners with an intellectual disability. *International Journal of Offender Therapy and Comparative Criminology,* **43**, 338–56.

Goddard, H. H. (1912). How shall we educate mental defectives? *The Training School Bulletin,* **9**, 43.

Grisso, T. (1981). *Juveniles' Waiver of Rights: Legal and Psychological Competence.* New York, NY: Plenum Press.

Grisso, T. (1986). *Evaluating Competencies: Forensic Assessments and Instruments.* New York, NY: Plenum Press.

Grove, W. M. (2000). Clinical versus mechanical prediction: a meta-analysis. *Psychological Assessment,* **12**, 19–30.

Grubin, D. H. (1991a). Unfit to plead in England and Wales 1976–1988, a survey. *British Journal of Psychiatry*, **158**, 540–8.

Grubin, D. H. (1991b). Unfit to plead, unfit for discharge: Patients found unfit to plead who are still in hospital. *Criminal Behaviour and Mental Health*, **1**, 282–94.

Gudjonsson, G. H. (1991). The 'Notice to Detained Persons', PACE Codes and reading ease. *Applied Cognitive Psychology*, **5**, 89–95.

Gudjonsson, G. H. (1992). *The Psychology of Interrogations, Confessions and Testimony.* Chichester: John Wiley & Sons.

Gudjonsson, G., Clare, I. C. H., Rutter, S. & Pearse, J. (1993). *Persons at Risk during Interviews in Police Custody: The Identification of Vulnerabilities.* The Royal Commission of Criminal Justice, Research Study no. 12. London: HMSO

Gunn, J., Maden, A. & Swinton, M. (1991). Treatment needs of prisoners with psychiatric disorders. *British Medical Journal*, **303**, 338–41.

Halstead, S. (1997). Risk assessment and management in psychiatric practice: inferring predictors of risk. A view from learning disability. *International Review of Psychiatry*, **9**, 217–24.

Hanson, R. K. (1997). *The Development of a Brief Actuarial Risk Scale for Sexual Offence Recidivism.* Ottawa, ON: Dept. of the Solicitor General of Canada.

Hanson, R. K. & Thornton, D. (1999). *Static-99: Improving Actuarial Risk Assessment for Sex Offenders.* Ottawa, ON: Dept. of the Solicitor General of Canada.

Harris, G. T., Rice, M. E., Quinsey, V. L. *et al.* (2003). A multi-site comparison of actuarial risk instruments for sex offenders. *Psychological Assessment,* **15**, 413–25.

Harris, G. T. & Tough, S. (2004). Should actuarial risk assessments be used with sex offenders who are intellectually disabled? *Journal of Applied Research in Intellectual Disabilities*, **17**, 235–41.

Harris, P. (1993). The nature and extent of aggressive behaviour amongst people with learning difficulties (mental handicap) in a single health district. *Journal of Intellectual Disability Research*, **37**, 221–42.

Hawk, G. L., Rosenfield, B. D. & Warren, J. I. (1993). Prevalence of sexual offences among mentally retarded criminal defendants. *Hospital and Community Psychiatry*, **44**, 784–6.

Hayes, S. (1993). *People with an Intellectual Disability and the Criminal Justice System: Appearances Before the Local Courts* (Research Report 4). Sydney: New South Wales Reform Commission Report.

Hayes, S. C. (1996a). *People with an Intellectual Disability and the Criminal Justice System: Two Rural Courts.* Research Report Number 5. Sydney: NSW Law Reform Commission.

Hayes, S. C. (1996b). Recent research on offenders with learning disabilities. *Tizard Learning Disability Review*, **1**, 7–15.

Hayes, S. C. (2002). Early intervention or early incarceration? Using a screening test for intellectual disability in the Criminal Justice System. *Journal of Applied Research in Intellectual Disabilities*, **15**, 120–8.

Heal, L. W. & Sigelman, C. K. (1995). Response biases in interviews of individuals with limited mental ability. *Journal of Intellectual Disability Research*, **39**, 331–40.

Herrnstein, R. J. & Murray, C. (1994). *The Bell Curve: Intelligence and Class Structure in American Life*. New York, NY: Free Press.

Hess, J. H. & Thomas, H. E. (1963). Incompetency to stand trial. Procedures, results and problems. *American Journal of Psychiatry*, **119**, 713–20.

Hodgins, S. (1992). Mental disorder, intellectual deficiency and crime: evidence from a birth cohort. *Archives of General Psychiatry*, **49**, 476–83.

Hodgins, S., Mednick, S. A., Brennan, P. A., Schulsinger, F. & Engberg, M. (1996). Mental disorder and crime. *Archives of General Psychiatry*, **53**, 489–96.

Hoge, S. K., Bonnie, R. J., Poythress, N. & Monahan, J. (1992). Attorney-client decision-making in criminal cases: Client competence and participation as perceived by their attorneys. *Behavioural Sciences and the Law*, **10**, 385–94.

Hoge, S. K., Bonnie, R. J., Poythress, N. *et al.* (1997). The MacArthur adjudicative competency study: Development and validation of a research instrument. *Law and Human Behaviour*, **21**, 141–79

Hollins, S., Clare, I. C. H., Murphy, G. & Webb, B. (1996a). *You're Under Arrest*. London: Gaskell Press.

Hollins, S., Murphy, G., Clare, I. C. H. & Webb, B. (1996b). *You're On Trial*. London: Gaskell Press.

Home Office (1990). *Provisions for Mentally Disordered Offenders (Circular 66/90)*. London: Home Office.

Home Office (1995a). *Mentally Disordered Offenders: Inter-Agency Working (Circular 12/95)*. London: Home Office.

Home Office (1995b). *Police and Criminal Evidence Act 1984. Codes of Practice*. Revised Edition. London: HMSO.

Home Office (2006). *Police and Criminal Evidence Act 1984: Codes of Practice*. Revised edn. London: The Stationery Office.

James, A. (1996). *Life on the Edge: Diversion and the Mentally Disordered Offender*. London: Mental Health Foundation.

Johnson, W. G., Nicholson, R. A. & Service, N. M. (1990). The relationship of competency to stand trial and criminal responsibility. *Criminal Justice and Behaviour*, **17**, 169–85.

Johnston, S. J. (2002). Risk assessment in offenders with intellectual disability: the evidence base. *Journal of Intellectual Disability Research*, **46**, 47–56.

Joseph, P. L. A. & Potter, M. (1993). Diversion from custody. I: Psychiatric assessment at the magistrates' court. *British Journal of Psychiatry*, **162**, 325–30.

Kebbell, M. R. & Hatton, C. (1999). People with mental retardation as witnesses in court: a review. *Mental Retardation*, **37**, 179–87.

King's Fund Centre (1980). *An Ordinary Life: Comprehensive Locally-Based Residential Services for Mentally Handicapped People*. London: King's Fund Centre.

Laski, F. J. (1992). Sentencing the offender with mental retardation: Honouring the imperative for intermediate punishments and probation. In R. W. Conley, R. Luckasson & G. N. Bouthilet (eds.), *The Criminal Justice System and Mental Retardation.* Baltimore, MD: Paul H. Brookes, pp. 137–52.

Lindsay, W. L. (2004). Sex offenders: conceptualisation of the issues, services, treatment and management. In W. R. Lindsay, J. L. Taylor & P. Sturmey (eds.), *Offenders with Developmental Disabilities.* Chichester: John Wiley & Sons, pp. 163–85.

Lindsay, W. R. (2002). Research and literature on sex offenders with intellectual and developmental disabilities. *Journal of Intellectual Disability Research,* **46**, 74–85.

Lindsay, W. R. & Beail, N. (2004). Risk assessment: actuarial prediction and clinical judgement of offending incidents and behaviour for intellectual disability services. *Journal of Applied Research in Intellectual Disabilities,* **17**, 229–34.

Lindsay, W. R., Law, J., Quinn, K., Smart, N. & Smith, A. H. W. (2001). A comparison of physical and sexual abuse histories: sexual and non-sexual offenders with intellectual disability. *Child Abuse and Neglect,* **25**, 989–95.

Lindsay, W. R., Marshall, I., Neilson, C. Q., Quinn, K. & Smith, A. H. W. (1998b). The treatment of men with a learning disability convicted of exhibitionism. *Research in Developmental Disabilities,* **19**, 295–316.

Lindsay, W. R., Murphy, L., Smith, G. *et al.* (2004). The dynamic risk assessment and management system: an assessment of immediate risk of violence for individuals with offending and challenging behaviour. *Journal of Applied Research in Intellectual Disabilities,* **17**, 267–74.

Lindsay, W. R., Neilson, C. Q., Morrison, F. & Smith, A. H. W. (1998a). The treatment of six men with a learning disability convicted of sexual offences with children. *British Journal of Clinical Psychology,* **37**, 83–98.

Lindsay, W. R., Olley, S., Jack, C., Morrison, F. & Smith, A. H. W. (1998c). The treatment of two stalkers with intellectual disabilities using a cognitive approach. *Journal of Applied Research in Intellectual Disabilities,* **11**, 333–44.

Lindsay, W. R. & Smith, A. (1998). Responses to treatment for sex offenders with intellectual disability: a comparison of men with 1- and 2-year probation sentences. *Journal of Intellectual Disability Research,* **42**, 346–53.

Lindsay, W. R., Smith, A. H. W., Law, J. *et al.* (2002). A treatment service for sex offenders and abusers with intellectual disability: characteristics of referrals and evaluation. *Journal of Applied Research in Intellectual Disability,* **15**, 166–74.

Lyall, I., Holland, A. J. & Collins, S. (1995a). Offending by adults with learning disabilities: identifying need in one health district. *Mental Handicap Research,* **8**, 99–109.

Lyall, I., Holland, A. J., Collins, S. & Styles, P. (1995b). Incidence of persons with a learning disability detained in police custody: A needs assessment for service development. *Medicine, Science and the Law,* **35**, 61–71.

MacEachron, A. E. (1979). Mentally retarded offenders: prevalence and characteristics. *American Journal of Mental Deficiency,* **84**, 165–76.

MacKay, R. D. (1990). Insanity and fitness to stand trial in Canada and England: a comparative study. *Journal of Forensic Psychiatry,* **1**, 277–303.

MacKay, R. D. & Kearns, G. (2000). An upturn in fitness to plead? Disability in relation to the trial under the 1991 Act. *Criminal Law Review,* July, 532–46.

Mason, J. & Murphy, G. H. (2002a). People with intellectual disabilities on probation: an initial study. *Journal of Community & Applied Social Psychology,* **12**, 44–55.

Mason, J. & Murphy, G. H. (2002b). People with an intellectual disability in the criminal justice system: developing an assessment tool for measuring prevalence. *British Journal of Clinical Psychology,* **41**, 315–20.

McAfee, J. K. & Gural, M. (1988). Individuals with mental retardation and the Criminal Justice System: The View from States' Attorneys General. *Mental Retardation,* **26**, 5–12.

McBrien, J., Hodgetts, A. & Gregory, J. (2003). Offending and risky behaviour in community services for people with intellectual disabilities in one Local Authority. *Journal of Forensic Psychiatry,* **14**, 280–97.

McBrien, J. & Murphy, G. (2006). Police and carers' views on reporting of alleged offences by people with intellectual disabilities. *Psychology, Crime and Law,* **12**, 127–44.

McGarry, A. L. (1971). The fate of psychotic offenders returned for trial. *American Journal of Psychiatry,* **127**, 1181–4.

McGee, J. J. & Menolascino, F. J. (1992). The evaluation of defendants with mental retardation in the Criminal Justice System. In R. W. Conley, R. Luckasson & G. N. Bouthilet (eds.), *The Criminal Justice System and Mental Retardation.* Baltimore, MD: Paul H. Brookes, pp. 55–77.

McMillan, D., Hastings, R. & Coldwell, J. (2004). Clinical and actuarial prediction of physical violence in a forensic intellectual disability hospital: a longitudinal study. *Journal of Applied Research in Intellectual Disabilities,* **17**, 255–65.

McNulty, C., Kissi-Deborah, R. & Newsom-Davies, I. (1995). Police Involvement with Clients having Intellectual Disabilities: A Pilot Study in South London. *Mental Handicap Research,* **8**, 129–36.

Medford, S., Gudjonsson, G. & Pearse, J. (2000). *The Identification of Persons at Risk in Police Custody: The Use of Appropriate Adults by the Metropolitan Police.* London: Published by the Metropolitan Police.

Monahan, J. (2002). The McArthur studies of violence risk. *Criminal Behaviour and Mental Health,* **12**, 67–72.

Murphy, G. (1997). Treatment and risk management. In J. Churchill, A. Craft and H. Brown (eds.), *There Are No Easy Answers.* ARC and NAPSAC, New York: Dorset Press, pp. 108–29.

Murphy, G. & Clare, I. C. H. (1995). Analysis of motivation in people with mild learning disabilities (mental handicap) who set fires. *Psychology, Crime and the Law,* **2**, 153–64

Murphy, G. & Clare, I. C. H. (2003). Adults' capacity to make legal decisions. In R. Bull and D. Carson (eds.), *Handbook of Psychology in Legal Contexts,* 2nd edn. Chichester: John Wiley & Sons, pp. 31–66.

Murphy, W. D., Coleman, E. M. & Haynes, M. R. (1983). Treatment and evaluation issues with the mentally retarded sex offender. In J. D. Greer & I. R. Stuart (eds.), *The Sexual Aggressor: Current Perspectives on Treatment.* New York: Nostrand-Rheinhold, pp. 21–41.

Murphy, G., Harnett, H. & Holland, A. J. (1995). A survey of intellectual disabilities amongst men on remand in prison. *Mental Handicap Research,* **8**, 81–98.

Murphy, G., Holland, A., Fowler, P. & Reep, J. (1991). MIETS: A service option for people with mild mental handicaps and challenging behaviour or psychiatric problems. 1. Philosophy, service and service users. *Mental Handicap Research*, **4**, 41–66.

Murray, G. J., Briggs, D. & David, C. (1992). Psychopathic disorders, mentally ill and mentally handicapped sex offenders: a comparative study. *Medicine, Science and Law*, **32**, 331.

Noble, J. H. & Conley, R. W. (1992). Toward an epidemiology of relevant attributes. In R. W. Conley, R. Luckasson & G. N. Bouthilet (eds.), *The Criminal Justice System and Mental Retardation*. Baltimore, MD: Paul H. Brookes, pp. 17–53.

O'Brien, G. (2002). Dual diagnosis in offenders with intellectual disability: setting research priorities – a review of research findings concerning psychiatric disorder (excluding personality disorder) among offenders with intellectual disability. *Journal of Intellectual Disability Research*, **46**, 21–30.

Pearse, J. & Gudjonsson, G. H. (1996). How appropriate are Appropriate Adults? *Journal of Forensic Psychiatry*, **7**, 570–80.

Perlman, N. B., Ericson, K. I., Esses, V. M. & Isaacs, B. J. (1994). The developmentally handicapped witness. *Law and Human Behaviour*, **18**, 171–87.

Perske, R. (1991). *Unequal Justice?* Nashville, TN: Abingdon Press.

Petrella, R. C. (1992). Defendants with mental retardation in the forensic services system. In R. W. Conley, R. Luckasson and G. N. Bouthilet (eds.), *The Criminal Justice System and Mental Retardation*. Baltimore, MD: Paul H. Brookes, pp. 79–96.

Prins, H. (1980). *Offenders, Deviants or Patients? An Introduction to the Study of Socio-Forensic Problems*. London: Tavistock Publications.

Quinsey, V. L., Book, A. & Skilling, T. A. (2004). A follow-up of deinstitutionalised men with intellectual disabilities and histories of anti-social behaviour. *Journal of Applied Research in Intellectual Disabilities*, **17**, 243–53.

Quinsey, V. L., Harris, G. T., Rice, M. E. & Cromier, C. A. (1998). *Violent Offenders: Appraising and Managing Risk*. Washington, DC: American Psychological Association.

Quinsey, V. L., Rice, M. E. & Harris, G. T. (1995). Actuarial prediction of sexual recidivism. *Journal of Interpersonal Violence*, **10**, 85–105.

Rasanen, P., Hakko, H. & Vaisanen, E. (1995). The mental state of arsonists as determined by forensic psychiatric examinations. *Bulletin of the American Academy of Psychiatry and Law*, **23**, 547–53.

Rasch, W. (1990). Criminal responsibility in Europe. In R. Bluglass and P. Bowden (eds.), *Principles and Practice in Forensic Psychiatry*. London: Churchill-Livingstone, pp. 299–305.

Richardson, S. A. & Koller, H. (1985). Epidemiology. In A. M. Clarke, A. D. B. Clarke & J. M. Berg (eds.), *Mental Deficiency: The Changing Outlook*. London: Methuen.

Robertson, G. (1981). The extent and pattern of crime amongst mentally handicapped offenders. *Apex: Journal of the British Institute of Mental Handicap*, **9**, 100–3.

Robertson, G. (1988). Arrest patterns among mentally disordered offenders. *British Journal of Psychiatry*, **153**, 313–16.

Rose, J., Jenkins, R., O'Connor, C., Jones, C. & Felce, D. (2002). A group treatment for men with intellectual disabilities who sexually offend or abuse. *Journal of Applied Research in Intellectual Disabilities*, **15**, 138–50.

Rose, J., West, C. & Clifford, D. (2000). Group interventions for anger in people with intellectual disabilities. *Research in Developmental Disabilities*, **21**, 171–81.

Scotti, J. R., Evans, I. M., Meyer, L. H. & Walker, P. (1991), A meta-analysis of intervention research with problem behaviour: treatment validity and standards of practice. *American Journal on Mental Retardation*, **29**, 136–48.

Singleton, N., Meltzer, H., Gatward, R., Coid, J. & Deasy, D. (1998). *Psychiatric Morbidity Among Prisoners*. London: The Stationery Office.

Sjostedt, G. & Langstrom, N. (2002). Assessment of risk for criminal recidivism among rapists: a comparison of four different measures. *Psychology, Crime & Law*, **8**, 25–40.

Smith, S. A. (1993). Confusing the terms "guilty" and "not guilty": Implications for alleged offenders with mental retardation. *Psychological Reports*, **73**, 675–8.

Smith, S. A. & Broughton, S. F. (1994). Competency to stand trial and criminal responsibility: an analysis in South Carolina. *Mental Retardation*, **32**, 281–7.

Smith, S. A. & Hudson, R. L. (1995). A quick screening test of competency to stand trial for defendants with mental retardation. *Psychological Reports*, **76**, 91–7.

Steadman, H. J. & Halfon, A. (1971). The Baxstrom patients: Backgrounds and outcomes. *Seminars in Psychiatry*, **3**, 376–85.

Steadman, H. J., Monahan, J. & Hartson, E. (1982). Mentally disordered offenders: a national survey of patients and facilities. *Law and Human Behaviour*, **6**, 31–8.

Steiner, J. (1984). Group counselling with retarded offenders. *Social Work*, **29**, 181–2.

Taylor, J. (2002). A review of the assessment and treatment of anger and aggression in offenders with intellectual disability. *Journal of Intellectual Disability Research*, **46**, 57–73.

Taylor, J. L., Novaco, R. W., Gillmer, B. & Robertson, A. (2004). Treatment of anger and aggression. In W. R. Lindsay, J. L. Taylor & P. Sturmey (eds.), *Offenders with Developmental Disabilities*. Chichester: John Wiley & Sons, pp. 201–20.

Taylor, J. L., Novaco, R. W., Gillmer, B. & Thorne, I. (2002). Cognitive-behavioural treatment of anger intensity among offenders with intellectual disabilities. *Journal of Applied Research in Intellectual Disabilities*, **15**, 151–65.

Van Brunschot, E. G. & Brannigan, A. (1995). IQ and crime: Dull behaviour and/or misspecified theory. *The Alberta Journal of Educational Research*, **61** (3), 316–21.

Vaughan, P. J., Pullen, N. & Kelly, M. (2000). Services for mentally disordered offenders in community psychiatry teams. *Journal of Forensic Psychiatry*, **11**, 571–86.

Walker, T. & Cheseldine, S. (1997). Towards outcome measurements monitoring effectiveness of anger management and assertiveness training in a group setting. *British Journal of Learning Disabilities*, **25**, 134–7.

Walker, N. & McCabe, S. (1973). *Crime and Insanity in England*, Vol. 2. Edinburgh: Edinburgh University Press.

Webster, C. D., Eaves, D., Douglas, K. S. & Wintrup, A. (1995). *The HCR-20: The Assessment of Dangerousness and Risk*. Vancouver: Simon Fraser University & British Columbia Forensic Psychiatric Services Commission.

West, D. J. & Farrington, D. P. (1973). *Who Becomes Delinquent?* London: Heinemann.

Whitaker, S. (2001). Anger control for people with learning disabilities: a critical review. *Behavioural and Cognitive Psychotherapy*, **29**, 277–93.

White, D. L. & Wood, H. (1988). Lancaster County MRO programme. In J. A. Stark, F. J. Menolascino, M. H. Albarelli & V. C. Gray (eds.), *Mental Retardation/Mental Health: Classification, Diagnosis, Treatment, Services*. New York, NY: Springer Verlag.

Willner, P., Jones, J., Tams, R. & Green, G. (2002). A randomised controlled trial of the efficacy of a cognitive-behavioural anger management group for clients with learning disabilities. *Journal of Applied Research in Intellectual Disabilities*, **15**, 224–35.

Winter, N., Holland, A. J. & Collins, S. (1997). Factors predisposing to suspected offending by adults with self-reported learning disabilities. *Psychological Medicine*, **27**, 595–607.

Woodward, M. (1955). The role of low intelligence in delinquency. *British Journal of Delinquency*, **5**, 281–303.

12

Behavioural phenotypes: growing understandings of psychiatric disorders in individuals with intellectual disabilities

Robert M. Hodapp and Elisabeth M. Dykens

Introduction

In writing about behavioural phenotypes, we can see just how far the field has come in only a few short years. In the first edition of this volume, published in 1999, we began our chapter with the paradox that geneticists had discovered over 750 different genetic disorders associated with intellectual disabilities (ID), but that behavioural work lagged far behind. We lamented the so-called 'two cultures' of behavioural work in ID (Hodapp & Dykens, 1994), noting how researchers who were more biomedically oriented versus more behaviourally oriented rarely intersected one with another.

But much has changed over the past five to ten years. Consider the sheer number of research articles on behaviours of the most prominent genetic disorders of ID. Using computer searches comparing the 1980s to the 1990s, one sees remarkable, almost exponential, increases. From the 1980s to the 1990s, the numbers of behavioural research articles on Williams syndrome increased from ten to 81; on Prader–Willi syndrome from 24 to 86; on fragile X syndrome from 60 to 149. Even in Down syndrome, the sole aetiology featuring a longstanding tradition of behavioural research, the amount of behavioural research almost doubled – from 607 to 1140 articles – over these two decades. The years since 2000 have shown even more pronounced increases, particularly with regards to Williams and Prader–Willi syndromes.

Granted, such progress is uneven, with many more studies performed on Down syndrome than on almost all other syndromes combined. In addition, the field knows a fair amount about behaviour in persons with Williams syndrome, Prader–Willi syndrome, and fragile X syndrome, but far less about 5p−, velocardiofacial, Rubenstein–Taybi, Smith–Magenis, and Angelman syndromes (Dykens, Hodapp, & Finucane, 2000 for a review). Furthermore, we do not possess even a single

Psychiatric and Behavioural Disorders in Intellectual and Developmental Disabilities, ed. Nick Bouras and Geraldine Holt. Published by Cambridge University Press. © Cambridge University Press 2007.

behavioural study for most of the remaining genetic aetiologies of ID. Still, in spite of such gaps, progress has been rapid in aetiology-based behavioural research, a trend that could not have been predicted even as recently as the 1980s.

Given the rapid developments in aetiology-based behavioural research, this chapter begins by defining the concept of a behavioural phenotype and illustrating how that concept can be profitably used when considering psychiatric and behavioural problems in people with ID. As we hope to show, behavioural phenotypes provide a critical starting point for the description, understanding, and treatment of psychopathology in individuals with ID.

Behavioural phenotypes

To understand the ways in which genetic syndromes relate to maladaptive behaviour (or behaviour in general), we need to discuss the issue of 'behavioural phenotypes'. Although researchers differ in their definitions of the term, we provide the following working definition. For our purposes, a behavioural phenotype 'may best be described as the heightened *probability* or *likelihood* that people with a given syndrome will exhibit certain behavioural or developmental sequelae relative to those without the syndrome' (Dykens, 1995, p. 523). This definition leads to several additional issues.

(1) Within-syndrome variability

Given that behavioural phenotypes involve probability statements, not every individual with a given syndrome will exhibit that syndrome's characteristic behaviour. Consider language abilities in Down syndrome. For many years, studies have found that persons with Down syndrome (both children and adults) show specific deficits in grammar, expressive language, and articulation, but such deficits are not found in every person with this syndrome. For example, Rondal (1995) provided an in-depth examination of the language of Françoise, a 32-year old woman whose IQ is 64. Although Françoise has trisomy 21, she nevertheless utters sentences such as (translated), 'And that does not surprise me because dogs are always too warm when they go outside' ('Et ça m'étonne pas parce que les chiens ont toujours trop chaud quand ils vont à la porte'; Rondal, 1995, p. 117). Such complicated sentences, though common in Françoise's speech, rarely occur in the speech of most adults with Down syndrome. Similarly in the realm of maladaptive behaviour-psychopathology, most – but rarely all – individuals with the genetic syndrome show that syndrome's 'characteristic' behaviours. Within-syndrome variability is the rule, not the exception.

Table 12.1 Genetic aetiologies with possibly unique maladaptive behaviour-psychopathology.

Aetiology	Behaviour(s) possibly unique to a particular syndrome	References-reviews
Prader–Willi syndrome	hyperphagia, food ideation,	Dykens, 1999
Lesch–Nyhan syndrome	extreme self-mutilation,	Anderson & Ernst, 1994
Smith–Magenis syndrome	putting objects into bodily orifices, self-hugging	Dykens et al., 1997 Finucane et al., 1994
Velocardiofacial (VCF) syndrome	schizophrenia or schizoaffective disorder,	Murphy, 2002; 2004
Rett syndrome	stereotypic hand movements (described as 'hand-washing' or 'hand-wringing')	Kerr & Ravine, 2003; Wales et al., 2004; Van Acker (1991)
Angelman syndrome	'puppet-like' gait, attraction to water,	Clayton-Smith & Laan, 2003
5p– (cri du chat) syndrome	inappropriate laughter, 'cat-cry' during infancy	Carlin, 1990; Gersh et al., 1995

Additional information from Barnard et al., 2002; Hodapp, 1997; Udwin & Dennis, 1995.

(2) Total vs. partial specificity from one syndrome to another

In most studies of behavioural phenotypes, researchers examine a particular aetiology to discover its unique behaviours. Recently, however, we have come to appreciate that different genetic disorders vary in their effects. Sometimes a one-to-one correspondence is evident, such that a particular behaviour is unique to one and only one genetic aetiology. Table 12.1 gives examples of this first, totally specific sense of behavioural phenotypes. The hyperphagia found in Prader–Willi syndrome; the extreme self-mutilation in Lesch–Nyhan syndrome; the high rates of schizophrenia in adults with velocardiofacial syndrome; the insertion of foreign objects into bodily orifices (along with the 'self-hugging') of Smith–Magenis syndrome: all appear unique to only one aetiology.

At other times, a few separate aetiologies will share a propensity for a particular behaviour. This situation, called 'partial specificity', occurs when two or more different aetiologies share a predisposition to a particular outcome (Hodapp, 1997). Although, as Table 12.1 illustrates, totally specific behavioural phenotypes do indeed exist, genetic disorders probably more often show partial specificity in their effects. Such thinking follows the developmental psychopathology principle of 'equifinality', the idea that, when considering psychiatric disorders, many roads lead to a single outcome (Cicchetti, 1990; Loeber, 1991). Or, as the clinical geneticist John

Opitz (1985) noted, 'The causes are many, but the final common developmental pathways are few' (p. 9).

This situation shows itself often in examining maladaptive behaviour in different genetic aetiologies. In many cases, a particular aetiological group more often shows a particular behaviour or psychiatric diagnosis compared with mixed or non-specific groups, but the behaviour or diagnosis also occurs in more than one single syndrome. For example, hyperactivity seems common in individuals with fragile X syndrome (Munir & Wilding 2000) and with Williams syndrome (Einfeld *et al.*, 2001), even as hyperactivity is less often seen in mixed groups or in other genetic disorders (e.g. Prader–Willi syndrome; Dykens *et al.*, 1992). Although compared with mixed groups a specific behavioural outcome may more commonly occur in a particular genetic aetiology, that outcome may also be associated with other genetic aetiologies.

(3) Diversity of behavioural domains

Just as there may be total and partial specificity, so too do behavioural phenotypes relate to a variety of domains. Like much aetiology-based research, this chapter is concerned with maladaptive behaviour and psychiatric disorders. But other behaviours are also affected by aetiology.

Several examples serve to illustrate the interesting, at times surprising, predispositions of certain syndromes and specific areas of functioning. Consider the case of Prader–Willi syndrome. Best known for its hyperphagia and obesity (Dykens, 1999), Prader–Willi syndrome also predisposes affected individuals to obsessions and compulsions that are similar in number and severity to those shown by non-intellectually impaired subjects with obsessive-compulsive disorder (OCD; Dykens *et al.*, 1996). But other areas of functioning are also affected. Specifically, many individuals with Prader–Willi syndrome show high-level skills in putting together jigsaw puzzles (Dykens, 2002). Such skills generally exceed mental age levels, and oftentimes are even in advance of typical children of equal chronological ages (CA-matches). To complicate matters further, it seems the case that such high-level skills are mostly shown by individuals with the paternal deletion (not the maternal disomy) form of Prader–Willi syndrome (Dykens, 2002).

Other aetiologies may show less pronounced but still interesting cognitive or linguistic profiles. Children with Down syndrome generally have relative weaknesses in expressive versus receptive language abilities (Miller, 1999), and in grammar versus other aspects of language (Chapman & Hesketh, 2000). Although exact behavioural profiles remain unresolved for Down syndrome and for most other disorders, suffice to say that maladaptive behaviour-psychopathology is but one of many direct effects of genetic disorders of ID.

(4) Indirect behavioural effects

In addition to their direct effects, genetic disorders also show indirect effects. These indirect effects relate to a variety of people in the individual's surrounding environment, including parents, siblings, teachers, and peers. The important point is that, if individuals with a certain aetiology are more prone to exhibit specific behaviours, then surrounding persons may be more likely to respond in certain ways (Hodapp, 1999). If, for example, children with Prader–Willi syndrome are likely to show hyperphagia, food ideation, temper tantrums, and a variety of obsessions and compulsions (Dykens et al., 1996; Dykens & Kasari, 1997), then might not these children elicit specific reactions from their parents and families?

Although a review of family work is beyond the scope of this chapter, certain child characteristics do seem associated with increased family stress. In the few studies performed so far, the main child characteristic relating to familial stress is the child's degree of maladaptive behaviour. Thus, families of children with Prader–Willi syndrome (Hodapp et al., 1997) and with 5p– syndrome (Hodapp et al., 1997) both displayed greater stress levels when their children showed more maladaptive behaviours.

Conversely, children with Down syndrome seem to elicit more favourable reactions from their parents (Hodapp et al., 2001). Granted, such reactions may partially relate to 'other-than-behavioural' characteristics of Down syndrome. Down syndrome is a prevalent condition, occurs more often in older and more experienced mothers, and has a greater number of more active parent groups. This syndrome is also more of a 'known' syndrome to professionals and lay people alike.

Still, at least part of what has been called a 'Down syndrome advantage' (Seltzer & Ryff, 1994) seems to relate to the personalities of most children with this disorder. Particularly prior to the adolescent years, most parents spontaneously describe their child with Down syndrome as 'cheerful', 'sociable', 'loveable', 'nice', and 'gets on well with people' (Carr, 1995; Hornby, 1995). In addition, most studies find that, compared with children with other types of ID or to non-specific groups, children with Down syndrome show lesser levels of maladaptive behaviour-psychopathology (Dykens & Kasari, 1997; Meyers & Pueschel, 1991). Partly as a result, compared with parents of children with other disabilities, parents generally consider their children with Down syndrome as more rewarding and as less stressful to parents (Hodapp et al., 2001). Genetic syndromes indirectly affect parents, teachers, siblings, and others in the child's everyday environment.

(5) Effects of developmental, contextual, or other influences

Developmental, contextual, and 'other genetic' factors must all be considered when one ponders why a particular phenotypic behaviour occurs. Different behaviours will become more apparent at some ages than at others, and certain contexts and practices may alter the prevalence or intensity of particular behaviours.

Consider two recently discovered examples, both involving Prader–Willi syndrome. Dimitropoulos *et al.* (2001) found that the obsessions and compulsions common in Prader–Willi syndrome only began during the preschool period (2–5 years) and that by 4–5 years, children with Prader–Willi syndrome showed significantly more compulsive behaviours than both the Down syndrome and the typically developing comparison groups. At the other end of the age spectrum, Dykens (2004) noted a mellowing of many maladaptive behaviours as adults with Prader–Willi syndrome got older. Compared with both teens (10–20 years) and younger adults (20–30 years), adults aged 30 and older showed lower scores on the Yale-Brown Obsessive-Compulsive Scales, on skin-picking, and on several domains of Achenbach's (1991) Child Behaviour Checklist (CBCL). Although age-related changes have only begun to be studied in many different genetic syndromes, their effects serve to qualify any conclusions about genetic disorder effects on maladaptive (and other) behaviours.

In a similar way, one needs to remember that any particular genetic disorder involves an anomaly on only one small portion of the entire genome. Thus, the deletion in Williams syndrome, Prader–Willi syndrome, or other deletion syndromes occurs only on a single chromosome; the trisomy that is Down syndrome involves only the 21st pair, which is but one of the individual's 23 pairs of chromosomes. The remainder of that person's genome has been left unchanged (and presumably also affects the child's behaviour). Yet such attention to 'background genetics' has to date remained mostly unexamined in behavioural phenotype studies, even as behaviour geneticists have examined the background genetics of many complex human traits in non-disabled groups.

Implications

Given these five issues concerning behavioural phenotypes, we end this chapter with examples of research that will likely constitute the future of behavioural phenotypic work in the field of psychiatric and behavioural disorders in people with ID.

Differentiating among the maladaptive behaviours of different syndromes

In investigating the total versus partial specificity of different genetic disorders of ID, researchers are increasingly comparing maladaptive behaviours across different aetiological groups. In one study, for example, Dykens and Kasari (1997) examined the CBCL scores of three groups of children with Prader–Willi syndrome, Down syndrome, and a non-specific group. Two findings were of interest. First, children with Prader–Willi syndrome showed much higher rates of maladaptive behaviour than either the non-specific group or the group with Down syndrome. Second, using a small set of behaviours, the three groups could be reliably differentiated, with correct classification occurring in 91% of children with Prader–Willi syndrome, 80% for the Down syndrome group, and 70% for the non-specific group. If the field is ever to ascertain which behaviours are totally specific and which are partially specific, more studies are necessary that compare the maladaptive behaviour of various aetiological groups.

In considering studies that compare across different groups, we have also been struck by the complexity of the entire issue of control and contrast groups. Reviewing existing behavioural studies of genetic syndromes, Hodapp and Dykens (2001) found a wide variety of practices in published research. Some studies featured no control groups (using the person with the genetic disorder as their own control), whereas others examined performance compared with mental age or to chronological age-matched typical controls. Most often, perhaps, studies compared a group with a specific genetic disorder to a group with ID from either mixed or unknown causes. Other studies compared those with a specific genetic syndrome with those with Down syndrome, a practice that we feel often underestimates the degree to which Down syndrome shows its own, aetiology-related behavioural phenotype. Finally, an occasional study examined groups with a genetic syndrome to groups without ID, but who are special or unusual in a specific way (e.g. individuals with OCD, or with special skills in specific areas). Granted, multiple approaches can be used to discover information, and different designs differ in the questions that they can best address. Even so, more thought seems needed concerning the entire control or contrast group issue in aetiology-based behavioural research.

Differences within specific aetiological groups

Some of the most exciting phenotypic studies currently examine individuals with the same aetiology, but who differ in one or more aspects of behaviour. To date, two factors most likely explain within-syndrome behavioural differences. The first involves slight genetic variations (Einfeld, 2004). In 5p– syndrome, the exact location of the deletion seems to determine whether or not infants will have the syndrome's characteristic 'cat-cry' (Gersh *et al.*, 1995). Also in 5p– syndrome, it appears that those children who have the translocation form of the disorder may be more prone to social withdrawal (Dykens & Clarke, 1997).

In Prader–Willi syndrome, a distinction exists between individuals who have a deletion on the chromosome 15 contributed from the father (i.e. paternal deletion), and those who have two chromosome 15s from the mother (i.e. uniparental maternal disomy (UPD)). Individuals with UPD more often suffer from psychotic disorders that first appear in early adulthood (Clarke *et al.*, 1998; Vogels *et al.*, 2004).

Such psychotic symptoms occur more often in UPD versus deleted cases, and the nature, causes, and course of such psychotic disorders are currently being investigated (Verhoeven et al., 2003).

In addition, behaviour in Prader–Willi may also be affected differently by different types of deletion. Butler et al. (2004) noted that individuals with the syndrome have one of two distinct types of deletions. In the first type (TI, or Type I deletion), individuals have a larger deletion than in TII (Type II) deletions. Behaviourally, individuals with Type I deletions showed lower adaptive behaviour scores and several specific obsessive-compulsive behaviours. Although preliminary, such within-syndrome genetic differences appear to be an important avenue of research in coming years in Prader–Willi syndrome and in other genetic syndromes of intellectual disabilities.

The second within-syndrome factor concerns other, non-genetic characteristics that may operate differently in a particular syndrome. In Prader–Willi syndrome, an individual's weight may relate to psychopathology, but differently than expected. It now appears that those individuals who are less obese show higher maladaptive behaviour scores (Dykens & Cassidy, 1995). These thinner (as compared with heavier) subjects showed more problems in confused and distorted thinking, anxiety, sadness, fearfulness, and crying. Why such differences occur is less clear: thinner individuals may be upset that their syndrome has not 'gone away' once they have controlled their weight; increased tensions and distress may accompany the continual need to avoid eating, or other explanations may relate to specific neuropeptides. Clearly, though, within-syndrome work will increasingly characterize studies of maladaptive behaviour-psychopathology in the years to come.

Using total and partial specificity to understand mechanisms

As advances in identifying and describing genetic aetiologies continue, researchers from a variety of professions can search for the mechanisms associated with maladaptive behaviour. These mechanisms can be described on a number of levels, all the way from the production of proteins to the development and functioning of brain structures. Both totally and partially specific effects will be of interest in these searches. By identifying totally specific effects, researchers will be able to home in on a single pathway; for example, how the disomy or either of the two deletion types associated with chromosome 15 leads to hyperphagia. Conversely, evidence that two or more aetiologies lead to a certain behaviour may indicate that researchers need to examine commonalities: what protein has not been produced, or what other mechanism disrupted, that leads to a single outcome? Although such thoughts remain speculative, both total and partial specificity should eventually aid in the search for the mechanisms leading to psychopathology on any number of levels.

Therapeutic advances

If the search for mechanisms seems a far-off affair, behavioural knowledge may be helpful right now in intervening with individuals with different aetiologies. Recent years have seen a move in this direction, with suggestions for both educational and therapeutic interventions that are partially based on the person's genetic aetiology.

The intervention proposals arise from specific strengths and weaknesses shown by children with different syndromes. Consider Down syndrome. In addition to weaknesses in grammar, expressive language, and articulation, these children show relative strengths in visual short-term memory (Hodapp *et al.*, 1999; Pueschel *et al.*, 1986). Such visual strengths have led Buckley (1999) and others to advocate for reading instruction in this group. In essence, if children with Down syndrome possess relative strengths in certain visual skills, it would seem plausible that reading – a visual system of language – might prove particularly beneficial to them. Although children with Down syndrome do have problems in certain aspects of reading (Hodapp & Freeman, 2003), it remains unclear as to which is the best way to teach reading in this group, or whether the effects of the child's being able to read might spill over into other areas of language development. Moreover, while several aetiology-based educational interventions have been proposed, no rigorous evaluations have yet been performed (Hodapp & Fidler, 1999).

In psychotherapy, too, different aetiological groups will be prone to different types of maladaptive behaviour and may benefit from different treatment approaches. Compare, for example, individuals with Williams syndrome with those with fragile X syndrome (Dykens & Hodapp, 1997). Persons with Williams syndrome often show generalized anxiety and worry about anticipated or future events (Dykens, 2003), but are also very social and have relatively intact verbal skills. As a result, successful interventions may need to focus on team or 'buddy' systems at work and school, on expressing thoughts and feelings within therapy, and in both individual and group sessions. Conversely, in fragile X syndrome, social anxiety and lack of eye contact may impede team or buddy approaches, and make much less successful a therapeutic focus on either feelings or group work. Aetiology-related propensities to different types of psychopathology, as well as to different cognitive-linguistic interests and strengths, will lead to markedly different therapeutic approaches.

Conclusion

Even compared with five to ten years ago, behavioural work has exploded concerning genetic syndromes of ID. In many ways, we have moved beyond the 'cultural divide' that earlier characterized behavioural work, when biomedically oriented workers and behaviourally oriented workers worked in relative isolation from one another.

Instead, recent years have witnessed increased inter-disciplinary collaboration, with different researchers joining together to better understand gene-brain-behaviour relations as they develop over time.

Looking ahead, such inter-disciplinary collaborations will result in many benefits. These advances will encompass descriptions of newly discovered disorders (as has recently occurred in Smith–Magenis syndrome), understandings of the various biological 'pathways' to psychopathology (as may be occurring in velocardiofacial syndrome; Murphy, 2004), and new intervention and treatment considerations (as has occurred across a variety of aetiologies). In short, although we have a long way to go, we are heartened by the significant advances that have occurred in recent years. As the past decade has shown, examining behavioural phenotypes constitutes one excellent way to achieve new understandings of psychiatric disorders in persons with ID.

Summary points

- Genetic disorders have increasingly been linked to specific types of maladaptive behaviour-psychopathology.
- Both across- and within-syndrome findings are of interest and lead to better specification of both how psychopathology arises and how it can be treated.

REFERENCES

Achenbach, T. M. (1991). *Manual for the Child Behavior Checklist 4–18–and 1991 Profiles.* Burlington, VT: University of Vermont Press.

Anderson, L. T. & Ernst, M. (1994). Self-injury in Lesch–Nyhan disease. *Journal of Autism and Developmental Disorders,* **24**, 67–81.

Barnard, L., Pearson, J., Ripon, L. & O'Brien, G. (2002). Behavioural phenotypes of genetic syndromes: Summaries, including notes on management and therapy. In G. O'Brien (ed.), *Behavioural Phenotypes in Clinical Practice* (pp. 169–227). London: MacKeith Press.

Buckley, S. (1999). Promoting the cognitive development of children with Down syndrome: The practical implications of recent psychological research. In J. A. Rondal, J. Perera & L. Nadel (eds.), *Down's Syndrome: A Review of Current Knowledge* (pp. 99–110). London: Whurr Publishers Ltd.

Butler, M. G., Bittel, D. C., Kibiryeva, N., Talebizadeh, Z. & Thompson, T. (2004). Behavioral differences among subjects with Prader–Willi syndrome and type I or type II deletion and maternal disomy. *Pediatrics,* **113**, 565–73.

Carlin, M. E. (1990). The improved prognosis in cri-du-chat (5p−) syndrome. In W. I. Fraser (ed.), *Proceedings of the 8th Congress of the International Association of the Scientific Study of Mental Deficiency* (pp. 64–73). Edinburgh: Blackwell.

Carr, J. (1995). *Down's Syndrome: Children Growing Up*. Cambridge: Cambridge University Press.

Chapman, R. S. & Hesketh, L. J. (2000). Behavioral phenotype of individuals with Down syndrome. *Mental Retardation and Developmental Disabilities Research Reviews*, **6**, 84–95.

Cicchetti, D. (1990). A historical perspective on the discipline of developmental psychopathology. In J. Rolf, A. S. Masten, D. Cicchetti, K. H. Neuchterlein & S. Weintraub (eds.), *Risk and Protective Factors in the Development of Psychopathology* (pp. 2–28). Cambridge: Cambridge University Press.

Clarke, D. J., Boer, H., Webb, T. *et al.* (1998). Prader–Willi syndrome and psychotic symptoms: I. Case descriptions and genetic studies. *Journal of Intellectual Disability Research*, **42**, 440–50.

Clayton-Smith, J. & Laan, L. (2003). Angelman syndrome: A review of the clinical and genetic aspects. *Journal of Medical Genetics*, **40**, 87–95.

Dimitropoulos, A., Feurer, I. D., Butler, M. G. & Thompson, T. (2001). Emergence of compulsive behavior and tantrums in children with Prader–Willi syndrome. *American Journal on Mental Retardation*, **106**, 39–51.

Dykens, E. M. (1995). Measuring behavioral phenotypes: Provocations from the 'New Genetics.' *American Journal on Mental Retardation*, **99**, 522–32.

Dykens, E. M. (1999). Prader–Willi syndrome. In H. Tager-Flusberg (ed.), *Neurdevelopmental Disorders* (pp. 137–54). Cambridge, MA: MIT Press.

Dykens, E. M. (2002). Are jigsaw puzzles 'spared' in persons with Prader–Willi syndrome? *Journal of Child Psychology and Psychiatry*, **43**, 343–52.

Dykens, E. M. (2003). Anxiety, fears, and phobias in persons with Williams syndrome. *Developmental Neuropsychology*, **23**, 291–316.

Dykens, E. M. (2004). Maladaptive and compulsive behavior in Prader–Willi syndrome: New insights from older adults. *American Journal on Mental Retardation*, **109**, 142–53.

Dykens, E. M. & Cassidy, S. B. (1995). Correlates of maladaptive behavior in children and adults with Prader–Willi syndrome. *American Journal of Medical Genetics*, **60**, 546–9.

Dykens, E. M. & Clarke, D. (1997). Correlates of maladaptive behavior in individuals with 5p– (cri du chat) syndrome. *Developmental Medicine and Child Neurology*, **39**, 752–6.

Dykens, E. M., Finucane, B. & Gayley, C. (1997). Cognitive and behavioral profiles in persons with Smith–Magenis Syndrome. *Journal of Autism and Developmental Disorders*, **27**, 203–11.

Dykens, E. M. & Hodapp, R. M. (1997). Treatment issues in genetic mental retardation syndromes. *Professional Psychology: Research and Practice*, **28**, 263–70.

Dykens, E. M., Hodapp, R. M. & Finucane, B. (2000). *Genetics and Mental Retardation Syndromes: A New Look at Behavior and Interventions*. Baltimore, MD: Paul H. Brookes Publishing Company.

Dykens, E. M., Hodapp, R. M., Walsh, K. K. & Nash, L. (1992). Adaptive and maladaptive behavior in Prader–Willi Syndrome. *Journal of the American Academy of Child and Adolescent Psychiatry*, **31**, 1131–6.

Dykens, E. M. & Kasari, C. (1997). Maladaptive behavior in children with Prader–Willi syndrome, Down syndrome, and non-specific mental retardation. *American Journal on Mental Retardation*, **102**, 228–37.

Dykens, E. M., Leckman, J. F. & Cassidy, S. (1996). Obsessions and compulsions in persons with Prader–Willi syndrome: A case-controlled study. *Journal of Child Psychology and Psychiatry,* **37**, 995–1002.

Einfeld, S. L. (2004). Behaviour phenotypes of genetic disorders. *Current Opinion in Psychiatry,* **17**, 343–9.

Einfeld, S. L., Tonge, B. J. & Rees, V. W. (2001). Longitudinal course of behavioral and emotional problems in Williams syndrome. *American Journal on Mental Retardation,* **106**, 73–81.

Finucane, B. M., Konar, D., Haas-Givler, BV., Kurtz, M. & Scott, C. I. (1994). The spasmodic upper body squeeze: A characteristic behavior of Smith–Magenis syndrome. *Developmental Medicine and Child Neurology,* **36**, 78–83.

Gersh, M., Goodart, S. A., Pasztor, L. M. *et al.* (1995). Evidence for a distinctive region causing a cat-like cry in patients with 5p deletions. *American Journal of Human Genetics,* **56**, 1404–10.

Hodapp, R. M. (1997). Direct and indirect behavioral effects of different genetic disorders of mental retardation. *American Journal on Mental Retardation,* **102**, 67–79.

Hodapp, R. M. (1999). Indirect effects of genetic mental retardation disorders: theoretical and methodological issues. *International Review of Research in Mental Retardation,* **22**, 27–50.

Hodapp, R. M. & Dykens, E. M. (1994). Mental retardation's two cultures of behavioral research. *American Journal on Mental Retardation,* **98**, 675–87.

Hodapp, R. M. & Dykens, E. M. (2001). Strengthening behavioral research on genetic mental retardation disorders. *American Journal on Mental Retardation,* **106**, 4–15.

Hodapp, R. M., Dykens, E. M. & Masino, L. L. (1997). Families of children with Prader–Willi syndrome: Stress-support and relations to child characteristics. *Journal of Autism and Developmental Disorders,* **27**, 11–24.

Hodapp, R. M., Evans, D. W. & Gray, F. L. (1999). Intellectual development in children with Down syndrome. In J. Rondal, J. Perera & L. Nadel (eds.), *Down Syndrome: A Review of Current Knowledge* (pp. 124–32). London: Whurr.

Hodapp, R. M. & Fidler, D. J. (1999). Special education and genetics: Connections for the 21st century. *The Journal of Special Education,* **33**, 130–7.

Hodapp, R. M. & Freeman, S. F. N. (2003). Advances in educational strategies for children with Down syndrome. *Current Opinion in Psychiatry,* **16**, 511–16.

Hodapp, R. M., Ly, T. M., Fidler, D. J. & Ricci, L. A. (2001). Less stress, more rewarding: Parenting children with Down syndrome. *Parenting: Science and Practice,* **1**, 317–37.

Hodapp, R. M., Wijma, C. A. & Masino, L. L. (1997). Families of children with 5p– (cri du chat) syndrome: Familial stress and sibling reactions. *Developmental Medicine and Child Neurology,* **39**, 757–61.

Hornby, G. (1995). Fathers' views of the effects on their families of children with Down syndrome. *Journal of Child and Family Studies,* **4**, 103–17.

Kerr, A. M. & Ravine, D. (2003). Breaking new ground with Rett syndrome. *Journal of Intellectual Disability Research,* **47**, 580–7.

Loeber, R. (1991). Questions and advances in the study of developmental pathways. In D. Cicchetti & S. Toth (eds.), *Models and Integrations. Rochester Symposia on Developmental Psychopathology,* Vol. 3 (pp. 97–117). Rochester, NY: University of Rochester Press.

Meyers, B. A. & Pueschel, S. M. (1991). Psychiatric disorders in persons with Down syndrome. *Journal of Nervous and Mental Disease,* **179,** 609–13.

Miller, J. (1999). Profiles of language development in children with Down syndrome. In J. F. Miller, M. Leddy & L. A. Leavitt (eds.), *Improving the Communication of People with Down syndrome* (pp. 11–39). Baltimore, MD: Paul H. Brookes Publishing Company.

Munir, F. & Wilding, J. (2000). A neuropsychological profile of attention deficits in young males with fragile X syndrome. *Neuropsychologia,* **38,** 1261–70.

Murphy, K. C. (2002). Schizophrenia and velo-cardio-facial syndrome. *Lancet,* **359,** 193–8.

Murphy, K. C. (2004). The behavioural phenotype in velo-cardio-facial syndrome. *Journal of Intellectual Disability Research,* **48,** 524–30.

Opitz, J. M. (1985). Editorial comment: The developmental field concept. *American Journal of Medical Genetics,* **21,** 1–11.

Pueschel, S. R., Gallagher, P. L., Zartler, A. S. & Pezzullo, J. C. (1986). Cognitive and learning processes in children with Down syndrome. *Research in Developmental Disabilities,* **8,** 21–37.

Rondal, J. (1995). *Exceptional Language Development in Down Syndrome.* Cambridge: Cambridge University Press.

Seltzer, M. M. & Ryff, C. D. (1994). Parenting across the lifespan: The normative and non-normative cases. *Life-span Development and Behavior,* **12,** 1–40.

Udwin, O. & Dennis, J. (1995). Psychological and behavioural phenotypes in genetically determined syndromes: A review of research findings. In G. O'Brien & W. Yule (eds.), *Behavioural Phenotypes* (pp. 90–208). London: MacKeith Press.

Van Acker, R. (1991). Rett Syndrome: A review of current knowledge. *Journal of Autism and Developmental Disorders,* **21,** 381–406.

Vogels, A., De Hert, M., Descheemaeker, M. J. *et al.* (2004). Psychotic disorders in Prader–Willi syndrome. *American Journal of Medical Genetics, Part A,* **127A,** 238–43.

Verhoeven, W. M. A., Tuinier, S. & Curfs, L. (2003). Prader–Willi syndrome: Cycloid psychosis in a genetic subtype? *Acta Neuropsychiatrica,* **15,** 32–7.

Wales, L., Charman, T. & Mount, R. H. (2004). An analogue assessment of repetitive hand behaviours in girls and young women with Rett syndrome. *Journal of Intellectual Disability Research,* **48,** 672–8.

13

Mental health problems in people with autism and related disorders

Celine Saulnier and Fred Volkmar

Introduction

The issue of psychiatric co-morbidity in adolescents with autism and related disorders is a complex one (Volkmar and Klin, 2005). On the one hand it does appear that, as with other developmental disorders, a process of diagnostic overshadowing has tended to occur, i.e. a tendency to overlook co-morbid conditions given the significance of the individual's other developmental problems (Dykens, 2000).

On the other hand it is also quite clear that, of itself, a condition like autism will be associated with a range of additional symptoms which may not, necessarily, rise to the level of 'disorder'. For example, problems with attention are frequently seen in autism and Asperger's syndrome, but it remains unclear whether such difficulties are sufficient to achieve an additional diagnosis of attention deficit hyperactivity disorder (ADHD). Nevertheless some researchers have proposed that such a combination may prove to be a robust subtype (Landgren et al., 1996). This problem is further compounded when the issue is co-morbid diagnosis of conditions, like anxiety or depression, in lower-functioning adolescents, i.e. in individuals with little or no expressive language. Additionally much of the data on psychiatric co-morbidity in adolescence rests largely on case reports. As noted elsewhere (Volkmar & Woolston, 1997; Kent et al., 1999; Slone et al., 1999) this literature is difficult to interpret given the bias for positive associations to be published; the critical issue is whether rates of a given disorder in larger (ideally epidemiologically representative) samples can demonstrate significant elevations in the rates of co-morbid conditions (Fombonne, 2003). A final problem relates to some basic differences in approaches to co-morbidity, e.g. DSM-IV (American Psychiatric Association, 2000) tends, on balance, to encourage multiple diagnoses whereas the ICD-10 system (World Health Organization, 1993), conversely, discourages this practice (Volkmar et al., 2002).

Psychiatric and Behavioural Disorders in Intellectual and Developmental Disabilities, ed. Nick Bouras and Geraldine Holt. Published by Cambridge University Press. © Cambridge University Press 2007.

Interest in the problem of psychiatric co-morbidity has centred particularly on Asperger's syndrome – both for historical and practical reasons. Early interest focused on Asperger's as a possible 'transitional' condition between autism and schizophrenia (Klin & Volkmar, 2003). The verbal accessibility of individuals with Asperger's syndrome also made it much easier to apply usual diagnostic models and criteria to them. To date the strongest available data suggest that adolescents with Asperger's syndrome are at increased risk for mood disorders – particularly depression (Ghaziuddin *et al.*, 1998; Volkmar *et al.*, 1998; Kim *et al.*, 2000). This observation is also consistent with the observation of Rourke and Tsatsanis (2000) that adolescents with the Non-verbal Learning Disability profile (commonly associated with Asperger's) are at high risk for depression and suicide ideation. Some case reports have also suggested that adolescents with Asperger's may be at higher risk for bipolar disorder (Frazier *et al.*, 2002; Duggal, 2003). Despite early interest in the possible co-occurrence of Asperger's and psychotic conditions, the available evidence is quite limited and consists largely of case reports (Taiminen, 1994; Ghaziuddin *et al.*, 1995) and the issue remains to be clarified using epidemiologically based samples.

For adolescents with autism, particularly for those more cognitively able, an increased risk for depression has also been noted (Kim *et al.*, 2000). Despite the impression that autism might represent a form of schizophrenia, it appears that rates of schizophrenia in adolescents with autism are not increased as compared with the general population (Volkmar & Cohen, 1991).

Attention deficit hyperactivity disorder

Symptoms of hyperactivity, impulsivity, and inattention are often observed in individuals with autism. However, the exclusionary criteria listed in the Diagnostic and Statistical Manual for Mental Disorders, 4th edition, Text Revision (DSM-IV-TR, APA, 2000) continues to rule out ADHD as a co-morbid diagnosis with any of the pervasive developmental disorders (PDDs). As a result, there has been a great deal of controversy over whether ADHD can, in fact, co-occur with the PDDs. Studies comparing groups of individuals with ADHD-like symptoms with and without PDD have suggested that individuals with PDD who present with symptoms of inattention, hyperactivity, and impulsivity do actually meet criteria for ADHD above and beyond the typical symptoms associated with PDD (Goldstein & Schwebach, 2004). Frazier *et al.* (2001) found that the individuals with PDD and ADHD presented with more severe impairments that required additional medical and psychological care than individuals with PDD alone, thus emphasizing the need for the co-morbid diagnosis so as to develop the most appropriate and effective treatments.

Differentiating between ADHD and pervasive developmental disorder, not otherwise specified (PDD-NOS) becomes more complicated than between ADHD and autism. The diagnostic term PDD-NOS captures a heterogeneous group of individuals that are more or less defined by negative, rather than positive, symptoms (e.g. not meeting criteria for autism). Thus, with the heterogeneity of symptoms comes an overlap with similar disorders, including ADHD. Just as individuals with PDD-NOS are likely to present with symptoms of inattention, hyperactivity, and impulsivity, individuals with ADHD are likely to experience social vulnerabilities. For this reason, it is often difficult to diagnostically distinguish the two disorders and researchers are divided on how to conceptualize the overlap in symptoms.

In an attempt to better differentiate PDD-NOS from ADHD, Luteijn *et al.* (2000) compared a group of individuals with PDD-NOS (without intellectual disabilities) with four age- and gender-matched clinical samples. The comparison groups included individuals with high-functioning autism, ADHD, ADHD and PDD-NOS (combined), and a clinical control group. Results indicated that both the PDD-NOS and the combined groups had significantly more impairments in socialization, communication, and stereotyped behaviours than the ADHD group. There were no differences in social interaction between the PDD-NOS group and the combined group, with both being socially impaired. There were also no significant differences in attention problems between the ADHD and the PDD-NOS groups, but the combined group had significantly more inattention symptoms than those with only ADHD. These results highlight the unique impairments in individuals who suffer from both ADHD and PDD-NOS, suggesting the benefit of allowing a dual diagnosis for treatment purposes.

With the extreme variability in PDD-NOS also comes the overlap with individuals who have multiple impairments that involve social vulnerabilities. For instance, there is a sub-group of children who suffer from a combination of social, cognitive, and affective impairments who have been conceptualized as having Multiplex Developmental Disorder (MDD) (Cohen *et al.*, 1994). The social impairments in these individuals are not necessarily the core symptoms as seen in autism, but rather are a by-product of the early developmental delays in other areas. Nonetheless, individuals with MDD and PDD-NOS can be difficult to distinguish and since there is currently insufficient empirical research on MDD as a diagnostic classification, those individuals with MDD are often classified as a sub-group of PDD-NOS.

Learning disabilities

Although language impairments are part of the diagnostic criteria for autism, they are neither specific nor central to the disorder. As a result, the boundaries between specific language disorders and autism can be blurred, most notably between pragmatic language impairment (PLI) and high-functioning autism (HFA) or Asperger's syndrome.

Whether PLI is distinct from or synonymous with autism, particularly in higher functioning individuals, has been an ongoing clinical debate (Bishop & Norbury, 2002). When comparing children with PLI with children with HFA, Bishop and Norbury (2002) found several of the PLI children to also meet criteria for autism based on their socialization impairments. However, some of the PLI children did not have autism suggesting that, despite the overlap, the two disorders are distinct. It is also important to consider pragmatic language impairments in Asperger's syndrome, as these deficits tend to be just as severe as those observed in HFA despite the common conceptualization of Asperger's syndrome being the milder of the two disorders (Ramberg *et al.*, 1996).

Just as individuals with classic autism suffer from language impairments, higher functioning individuals, particularly those with Asperger's syndrome, can suffer from non-verbal processing impairments or non-verbal learning disability (NLD). In fact, research has shown that the neuropsychological profiles of individuals with Asperger's syndrome are distinct from those with high-functioning autism in that the former have specific deficits that tend to be consistent with NLD (Klin *et al.*, 1995). These deficits include poor visual–perceptual–organizational skills, impaired holistic processing skills, and impaired arithmetic and psychomotor skills in conjunction with significantly higher verbal abilities, often in the average to above average range. Although NLD profiles are often observed in Asperger's syndrome, they are not exclusive to the disorder. Furthermore, individuals with NLD can exhibit social impairments, making diagnostic distinctions problematic.

There is general agreement that intellectual disabilities (ID) are the most frequently associated learning difficulty observed in autism – affecting perhaps 70% of cases (Volkmar & Klin, 2005). Interestingly although a broader spectrum of disabilities – including social, communication, and learning problems – seems to be inherited, it appears that intellectual disabilities per se are not (Rutter, 2005).

Depression and anxiety

Affective impairments in autism have been described as early as Kanner's (1943) initial report. However, impairments in the ability to interpret and even express emotions certainly do not make individuals with autism immune from experiencing affective disorders such as anxiety and depression (Ghaziuddin *et al.*, 2002). In fact, of the psychiatric disorders, depression appears to be the most common co-morbid disability for adolescents and adults with autism spectrum disorders, with rates of

2% or more noted in the literature (Ghaziuddin *et al.*, 1992; Lainhart & Folstein, 1994). Why the rate of depression is higher in autism than would be expected in the general population remains unclear. Biological, genetic, and social influences are all likely contributing factors. For instance, the risk of developing depression in autism may be confounded by existing medical conditions. It is well documented in the literature that 25–30% of individuals with autism will suffer from seizures and that the majority of individuals on the spectrum will have some form of ID (Volkmar & Klin, 2005), with both disorders commonly associated with depression in the general population (Ghaziuddin *et al.*, 2002). Depression also tends to be prevalent in parents of children with autism spectrum disorders, suggesting a genetic link. The onset of depressive episodes, particularly in mothers, has been found to begin prior to the child's birth, ruling out parental stress as the only accountable factor (Micali *et al.*, 2004; Ghaziuddin *et al.*, 2002).

Co-morbidity rates between Asperger's syndrome and depression appear to be much higher than those found in more classic autism. In a preliminary report, Ghaziuddin *et al.* (1998) reported that 37% of cases met criteria for depression. Again, various factors could be associated with this high percentage. As in autism, psychogenetic theories come into question with many parents of children with Asperger's syndrome suffering from depressive disorders. Social factors, however, certainly play a role as well. Adolescents and adults with Asperger's syndrome, although socially disabled, often have some awareness of their vulnerabilities and an intent to interact with others. Yet, these individuals are often ostracized, bullied, and teased by their peers, which can foster both depression and anxiety when their attempts to interact repeatedly fail (Volkmar *et al.*, 2000).

Diagnosing depression in lower-functioning autism can be more complicated, especially for individuals with limited language abilities. In these cases, it is important to look for the more vegetative symptoms of depression, such as changes in appetite, weight, irritability and behaviour (Ghaziuddin *et al.*, 2002). It is also important to consider family history and to ensure that individuals who are genetically vulnerable to depression are observed closely for symptoms.

Many individuals with autistic spectrum disorders are also prone to anxiety. As with ADHD and language disorders, there is conflicting research as to whether symptoms such as heightened fear responses, obsessions and compulsions, and specific phobias are simply concomitant features of autism (Rumsey *et al.*, 1985) or co-morbid anxiety disorders (Muris *et al.*, 1998).

Kim *et al.* (2000) reported on the prevalence and correlates of anxiety and mood problems in groups of more able children and adolescents with PDD. Compared with a large community the children with autism and Asperger's syndrome demonstrated greater rates of both anxiety and depression.

The number of psychiatric difficulties was related, to some extent, to early developmental discrepancies; the results suggested increased risk of mood problems of various types. Similar findings have been reported by others both in terms of an increased risk for anxiety problems in general and in terms of specific difficulties, e.g. obsessive-compulsive disorder, in particular (Fontenelle *et al.*, 2004; Gillott *et al.*, 2001; McDougle *et al.*, 1990). A major point of differentiation of more typical obsessive phenomena from those observed in Asperger's syndrome (e.g. in the form of all-encompassing special interests) has related to the general observation that, in contrast to children without major social disability, the obsessive symptoms are 'ego dystonic', i.e. disliked by the individual whereas this is not true in Asperger's. On the other hand, it is the case that at least some aspects of these difficulties (including both anxiety and obsessive features) may respond to some of the same pharmacological interventions useful in more typical obsessive-compulsive disorder (McDougle *et al.*, 1990).

Other conditions

Vocal and motor tics can be present in autism and related disorders. Tourette syndrome has been found to co-occur in over 6% of autism cases, which is greater than would be expected by chance (Baron-Cohen *et al.*, 1999). Genetic factors again come into question, with first-degree relatives of individuals with autism presenting with anxiety, tics, obsessions, and compulsions (Micali *et al.*, 2004; Bolton *et al.*, 1998).

Schizophrenia

The debate over the relationship between autism and schizophrenia dates back to when autism was first documented. Over the years, the two disorders have been described as being related, distinct, or variations in between (Kanner, 1943; Volkmar and Cohen, 1991; Konstantareas & Hewitt, 2001). Certainly the question re-emerges with the broadening of the autism spectrum to include more high functioning individuals who present with atypical thought processing and affective behaviours typically indicative of schizophrenia. Volkmar and Cohen (1991) reviewed the cases of 163 adolescents and adults with autism and found only one individual to also qualify for a diagnosis of schizophrenia. This percentage was consistent with the rate of schizophrenia in the general population, thus ruling out co-morbidity as a common occurrence. More recently, Konstantareas and Hewitt (2001) compared groups of individuals with autism and schizophrenia and found half of the autism group to have affective symptoms diagnostic of schizophrenia. Yet, one must consider whether these symptoms are manifestations of higher-functioning autism or distinct enough to merit a co-morbid diagnosis.

Conclusion

In summary, the relationship between autistic spectrum disorders and other psychiatric disorders is a complex one, both in terms of the equivocal research studies investigating the prevalence of co-morbid disorders, as well as the extreme heterogeneity observed across the autism spectrum. For more prototypical or classic autism, intellectual disabilities and, thus, subsequent medical complications (e.g. seizures) appear to be the most prevalent. Attentional problems and language impairments can be observed in classic autism, but these difficulties are also widely manifested in the broader spectrum disorders (i.e. PDD-NOS and Asperger's syndrome). In fact, some individuals with PDD-NOS often exhibit attentional and behavioural impairments to the degree of meriting an additional diagnosis of ADHD. Probably the most research, as well as the most consistent findings, has focused on co-morbid conditions with Asperger's syndrome. Individuals with Asperger's syndrome tend to present with symptoms of anxiety and depression, particularly in adolescence and young adulthood, often to the degree of requiring medication and/or psychotherapeutic treatment for these specific symptoms. Therefore, it is important to be aware of and better understand the nature and prevalence of co-morbid conditions in the autistic spectrum disorders, for the sake of enhancing treatment and prognosis for the disorder.

Summary points

- There is a strong relationship between autism and ID but it appears that the associated ID arises as a result of autism.
- Most of the work on co-morbidity in autism and related conditions has focused on Asperger's syndrome.
- In Asperger's there is reasonably clear evidence of higher rates of attentional problems (particularly in school-age children) and depression (particularly in adolescents and young adults).
- Historically one of the interests in Asperger's related to the notion that it might be a 'bridge' between autism and schizophrenia, but the suggestion of increased risk for schizophrenia in this condition rests largely on case reports. Controlled studies have not clearly demonstrated this association.
- Individuals with autism do not appear to be at increased risk for schizophrenia.

- Individuals with difficulties that fall into the 'broader spectrum' of social disability (PDD-NOS/atypical autism) exhibit a range of problems, including higher rates of attention and affective disorders.

REFERENCES

American Psychiatric Association (2000). *Diagnostic and Statistical Manual of Mental Disorders* (4th edn., Text Rev.). Washington, DC: author, pp. 69–84.

Baron-Cohen, S., Scahill, V. L., Izaguirre, J., Hornsey, H. & Robertson, M. M. (1999). The prevalence of Gilles de la Tourette syndrome in children and adolescents with autism: A large-scale study. *Psychological Medicine*, **29**, 1151–9.

Bishop, D. V. & Norbury, C. F. (2002). Exploring the borderlands of autistic disorder and specific language impairment: a study using standardised diagnostic instruments. *Journal of Child Psychology & Psychiatry & Allied Disciplines*, **43**(7), 917–29.

Bolton, P. F., Pickles, A., Murphy, M. & Rutter, M. (1998). Autism, affective and other psychiatric disorders: Patterns of familial aggregation. *Psychological Medicine*, **28**(2), 385–95.

Cohen, D., Towbin, K., Mayes, L. & Volkmar, F. R. (1994). Developmental Psychopathology of multiplex developmental disorder. In *Developmental Follow-up: Concepts, Genres, Domains, and Methods*. S. L. Friedman & H. C. Haywood. (eds). New York: Academic Press, pp. 155–79, 1995.

Duggal, H. S. (2003). Bipolar disorder with Asperger's disorder [comment]. *American Journal of Psychiatry*, **160**(1), 184–5.

Dykens, E. M. (2000). Psychopathology in children with intellectual disability. *Journal of Child Psychology & Psychiatry & Allied Disciplines*, **41**(4), 407–17.

Fombonne, E. (2003). Epidemiological surveys of autism and other pervasive developmental disorders: An update. *Journal of Autism and Developmental Disorders*, **33**(4), 365–82.

Fontenelle, L. F., Mendlowicz, M. V., de Menezes, G. B., dos Santos Martins, R. R. & Versiani, M. (2004). Asperger Syndrome, Obsessive-Compulsive Disorder, and Major Depression in a Patient with 45,X/46,XY Mosaicism. *Psychopathology*, **37**(3), 105–9.

Frazier, J. A., Biederman, J., Bellordre, C. A. *et al.* (2001). Should the diagnosis of attention-deficit/hyperactivity disorder be considered in children with pervasive developmental disorder? *Journal of Attention Disorders*, **4**(4), 203–11.

Frazier, J. A., Doyle, R., Chiu, S. & Coyle, J. T. (2002). Treating a child with Asperger's disorder and comorbid bipolar disorder[comment]. *American Journal of Psychiatry*, **159**(1), 13–21.

Ghaziuddin, M., Ghaziuddin, N. & Greden, J. (2002). Depression in persons with autism: implications for research and clinical care. *Journal of Autism & Developmental Disorders*, **32**(4), 299–306.

Ghaziuddin, M., Leininger, L. & Tsai, L. (1995). Brief report: thought disorder in Asperger syndrome: comparison with high-functioning autism. *Journal of Autism & Developmental Disorders*, **25**(3), 311–17.

Ghaziuddin, M., Tsai, L. & Ghaziuddin, N. (1992). Comorbidity of autistic disorder in children and adolescents. *European Child & Adolescent Psychiatry,* **1**(4), 209–13.

Ghaziuddin, M., Weidmer-Mikhail, E. & Ghaziuddin, N. (1998). Comorbidity of Asperger's syndrome: A preliminary report. *Journal of Intellectual Disability Research,* **42**(4), 279–83.

Gillott, A., Furniss, F. & Walter, A. (2001). Anxiety in high-functioning children with autism. *Autism,* **5**(3), 277–86.

Goldstein, S. & Schwebach, A. J. (2004). The comorbidity of pervasive developmental disorder and attention deficit hyperactivity disorder: Results of a retrospective chart review. *Journal of Autism and Developmental Disorders,* **34**(3), 329–39.

Kanner, L. (1943). Autistic disturbances of affective contact. *Nervous Child,* **2**, 217–50.

Kent, L., Evans, J., Paul, M. & Sharp, M. (1999). Comorbidity of autistic spectrum disorders in children with Down syndrome. *Developmental Medicine & Child Neurology,* **41**(3), 153–8.

Kim, J. A., Szatmari, P., Bryson, S. E., Streiner, D. L. & Wilson, F. J. (2000). The prevalence of anxiety and mood problems among children with autism and Asperger's syndrome. *Autism,* **4**(2), 117–32.

Klin, A. & Volkmar, F. R. (2003). Asperger syndrome: Diagnosis and external validity. *Child and Adolescent Psychiatric Clinics of North America,* **12**(1), 1–13.

Klin, A., Volkmar, F. R., Sparrow, S. S., Cicchetti, D. V. & Rourke, B. P. (1995). Validity and neuropsychological characteristics of Asperger syndrome: Convergence with nonverbal learning disabilities syndrome. *Journal of Child Psychology and Psychiatry,* **36**(7), 1127–40.

Konstantareas, M. M. & Hewitt, T. (2001). Autistic disorder and schizophrenia: Diagnostic overlaps. *Journal of Autism and Developmental Disorders,* **31**(1), 19–28.

Lainhart, J. E. & Folstein, S. E. (1994). Affective disorders in people with autism: a review of published cases. *Journal of Autism and Developmental Disorders,* **24**(5), 587–601.

Landgren, M., Pettersson, R., Kjellman, B. & Gillberg, C. (1996). ADHD, DAMP and other neurodevelopmental/psychiatric disorders in 6-year-old children: epidemiology and comorbidity. *Developmental Medicine & Child Neurology,* **38**(10), 891–906.

Luteijn, E., Serra, M., Jackson, S. *et al.* (2000). How unspecified are disorders of children with a pervasive developmental disorder not otherwise specified? A study of social problems in children with PDD-NOS and ADHD. *European Child & Adolescent Psychiatry,* **9**(3), 168–79.

McDougle, C. J., Price, L. H. & Goodman, W. K. (1990). Fluvoxamine treatment of coincident Autistic Disorder and Obsessive Compulsive Disorder: A case report. *Journal of Autism and Developmental Disorders,* **20**, 537–43.

Micali, N., Chakrabarti, S. & Fombonne, E. (2004). The broad autism phenotype: Findings from an epidemiological survey. *Autism* **8**(1), 21–37.

Muris, P., Steerneman, P., Merckelbach, H., Holdrinet, I. & Meesters, C. (1998). Comorbid anxiety symptoms in children with pervasive developmental disorders. *Journal of Anxiety Disorders,* **12**(4), 387–93.

Ramberg, C., Ehlers, S., Nyden, A., Johansson, M. & Gillberg, C. (1996). Language and pragmatic functions in school-age children on the autism spectrum. *European Journal of Disorders of Communication,* **31**(4), 387–413.

Rourke, B. P. & Tsatsanis, K. D. (2000). Nonverbal learning disabilities and Asperger's syndrome. In A. Klin & F. R. Volkmar (eds.), *Asperger Syndrome* (pp. 231–53). New York, NY: The Guilford Press.

Rumsey, J. M., Rapoport, J. L. & Sceery, W. R. (1985). Autistic children as adults: psychiatric, social, and behavioral outcomes. *Journal of the American Academy of Child and Adolescent Psychiatry,* **24**(4), 465–73.

Rutter, M. (2005). Genetic factors in autism. In *Handbook of Autism and Pervasive Developmental Disorders*, 3rd edn, ed. F. Volkmar, A. Klin, R. Paul & D. Cohen. New York, NY: Wiley.

Slone, M., Durrheim, K., Kaminer, D. & Lachman, P. (1999). Issues in the identification of comorbidity of mental retardation and psychopathology in a multicultural context. *Social Psychiatry and Psychiatric Epidemiology,* **34**(4), 190–4.

Taiminen, T. (1994). Asperger's syndrome or schizophrenia: Is differential diagnosis necessary for adult patients? *Nordic Journal of Psychiatry,* **48**(5), 325–8.

Volkmar, F. R. & Cohen, D. J. (1991). Comorbid association of autism and schizophrenia. *American Journal of Psychiatry,* **148**, 1705–7.

Volkmar, F. R. & Klin, A. (2005). Issues in the classification of autism and related conditions. In *Handbook of Autism and Pervasive Developmental Disorders*, 3rd edn, ed. F. Volkmar, A. Klin, R. Paul & D. Cohen New York, NY: Wiley.

Volkmar, F. R., Klin, A. & Pauls, D. (1998). Nosological and genetic aspects of Asperger Syndrome. *Journal of Autism and Developmental Disorders,* **28**(5), 457–63.

Volkmar, F. R., Klin, A., Schultz, R. T., Rubin, E. & Bronen, R. (2000). Clinical case conference: Asperger's disorder. *American Journal of Psychiatry,* **157**(2), 262–7.

Volkmar, F. R., Scwab-Stone, M. & First, M. (2002). Classification in child psychiatry: Principles and issues. In M. Lewis (ed.), *Child and Adolescent Psychiatry: A Comprehensive Textbook*, 3rd edn (pp. 499–506). Baltimore, MD: Williams & Wilkins.

Volkmar, F. R. & Woolston, J. L. (1997). Comorbidity of psychiatric disorders in children and adolescents. In S. Wetzler & W. C. Sanderson (eds.), *Treatment Strategies for Patients with Psychiatric Comorbidity* (pp. 307–22). New York, NY: John Wiley & Sons, Inc.

World Health Organization (1993). In Mental and behavioral disorders (including disorders of psychological development). *International Classification of Diseases: Tenth Revision.* Chapter V. Geneva: Author, pp. 147–54.

14

Self-injurious behaviour

John Hillery and Philip Dodd

Introduction

People who self-injure present a major challenge to services and carers. The behaviour can cause negative emotions in observers. Even experienced clinicians can find themselves conflicted.

Tsiouris *et al.* (2003) have reservations that the behaviour as manifested by people with intellectual disabilities (ID) can be considered an Axis I psychiatric diagnosis in the context of DSM IV (American Psychiatric Association, 1994). Favazza and Rosenthal (1993) classified self-mutilation in general into three basic types: major, superficial and stereotypic. They claim that the stereotypic type is most commonly seen in institutionalized people with ID, although the authors admit that not all self injury in people with ID is of this type.

Indeed, we know that people with ID can show myriad forms of self injury. It can be resistant to treatment. Kahng *et al.* (2002) in reviewing the literature on behavioural intervention stated that, though there is much research 'the disorder persists'. Self-injurious behaviour can be responsible for much medical, psychological and social morbidity.

Definition

Variations in the definition make comparison between epidemiological studies difficult. The definitions used generally include the requirement that the actions cause tissue damage. Oliver *et al.* (1987) reported that the 'tissue damage' criterion proved robust when judging the ability of different informants to agree on caseness.

Definitions also vary according to the frequency and severity of the self-injury (e.g. Borthwick-Duffy, 1994 vs. O'Brien, 2003).

Psychiatric and Behavioural Disorders in Intellectual and Developmental Disabilities, ed. Nick Bouras and Geraldine Holt. Published by Cambridge University Press. © Cambridge University Press 2007.

Rojahn (1994) makes a strong case for his assertion that the term self-injurious behaviour stands for a heterogeneous group of behaviours with little in common.

The Diagnostic Criteria for Psychiatric Disorders for Use with Adults with Learning Disabilities/Mental Retardation [DC-LD] (Royal College of Psychiatrists, 2001) includes diagnostic criteria for problem behaviour, of which self-injury is one. One of the unique features of the DC-LD classification is to include self-injury as a diagnosis. This is appropriate given the strict hierarchical system that is used, based on a set of operationalized diagnostic criteria (see also Chapter 1 by Sturmey).

Epidemiology

As well as the problems with definition, differences in the methodology of the studies and the populations studied results in widely varying prevalence rates in available epidemiological studies.

Prevalence rates as low as 1.7 per cent (Rojahn, 1986) and as high as 41 per cent (Saloviita, 1988) have been reported. Rojahn (1994) points out that studies based on service system databases are biased in favour of those who proclaim an urgent need for service and against those who do not take up services, for whatever reason. Even with the effort to correct for bias by using geographically based populations (e.g. Hillery & Mulcahy, 1997, 14 per cent; Deb *et al.*, 2001, 24 per cent), there is still a wide variation in prevalence.

It seems apparent from the results given above that for future epidemiological studies to be useful, consensus must occur on parameters for choosing populations for study and on the definition of what constitutes a case.

Widespread adoption of the diagnostic criteria for self-injury as set down in the DC-LD (Royal College of Psychiatrists, 2001) should help to standardize future studies.

Consequences of self-injurious behaviour

Exhibiting self-injurious behaviour may bring short-term positive results for the individual, but in the long term the outcomes are usually negative. Physical morbidity can be a direct result of the behaviour. Other authors have pointed out that this behaviour disorder is a cause of increased stress to relatives (Quine & Pahl, 1985) and puts people displaying it at increased risk of abuse from carers (Maurice & Trudel, 1982). The displaying of self-injurious behaviour puts people at increased risk of institutionalization (Lakin *et al.*, 1983).

People who display self-injurious behaviour have also been shown more likely to be given psychotropic medication (Deb *et al.*, 2001) and are more likely to be kept on medication (Chadsey-Rusch & Sprague, 1989). Griffen *et al.* (1986)

expressed concern about the high number of people in their survey of self-injurious behaviour who were in physical restraint. However, more recently, the observation that self-restraint or the preference for imposed restraint being associated with self-injury has been made, and warrants further investigation (Foreman *et al.*, 2001).

It has been shown that individuals who self-injure are more likely to experience unsuccessful community relocation following de-institutionalization (Sutter *et al.*, 1980; Hemming, 1982). Self-injurious behaviour is a common reason for people with ID being excluded from community-based educational services and vocational training (Shlalock *et al.*, 1985, Oliver *et al.*, 1987). The conclusion from available research is that exhibiting self-injurious behaviour considerably decreases a person's quality of life.

Issues related to self-injurious behaviour

Studies of self-injurious behaviour have generally found an inverse relationship between IQ and the likelihood of a person displaying such behaviour. Studies suggest a relationship between self-injurious behaviour and age. In a review of studies, Rojahn (1994) reported a curvilinear relationship with a higher prevalence in adolescents and adults than in young children and the elderly. Rojahn suggested that this may be because of under-reporting of self-injurious behaviour in the very young, owing either to the behaviours not being fully developed (the 'cocoon' stage) or to a reluctance by informants to label childhood behaviours as self-injurious behaviour even when the topography is the same as that of behaviours which would be labelled as such if they occurred in an adult. Indeed, a more recent study, using videotaped data collection, has shown that 4.6 per cent of children with a developmental disability, under the age of forty months, exhibited self-injurious behaviour (Berkson *et al.* 2001).

Though most studies have not shown a connection between self-injurious behaviour and gender, more recently, Deb *et al.* (2001) found a significant association with female gender.

Though environmentalists such as Wolfensberger (1972) have strongly championed the benefits of de-institutionalization, with the implication that institutional environments are responsible for behavioural disorders such as self-injurious behaviour, these ideas have not been supported by research. Hillery and Mulcahy (1997) reported that the occurrence of self-injurious behaviour was not related to environment but that its severity was greater in those living in residential centres. These findings endorse the opinion of Emerson (1992) that little direct evidence exists to support the view that non-normative or institutional environments are a major cause of self-injurious behaviour but that self-injurious behaviour leads to people being placed in more restrictive environments.

Though the evidence is limited (Murphy, 1994), efforts to link the occurrence of the behaviour to specific medical diagnoses or known neurobiological disturbances continue. Symons *et al.* (2000), in reporting an association between self-injurious behaviour and sleep disturbance, relate this to possible neurochemical dysregulation. In another paper, Symons and co-workers (2003) describe a finding of high levels of cortisol, corelated to severity of self-injury and hypothesize a relationship of the behaviour to stress-related analgesia. It has been reported the behaviour has a greater prevalence in those with an ID (Emerson, 1990).

Self-injurious behaviour has also been associated with certain genetically transmitted conditions including Lesch–Nyhan syndrome (Lesch & Nyhan, 1964) and fragile X syndrome (Turk, 1992), as well as Cornelia de Lange syndrome (Bryson *et al.*, 1971), Prader–Willi syndrome (Clarke, Waters & Corbett, 1989; Bhargava *et al.*, 1996), Rett syndrome (Oliver *et al.*, 1987), Smith–Magenis syndrome (McNaught & Turk, 1993) and phenylketonuria (Fitzgerald *et al.*, 2000).

Theories on the causation of self-injurious behaviour

Hypotheses on the aetiology of self-injurious behaviour remain mostly theoretical and contradictory. This illustrates the impracticality of attempting to generate one aetiologic theory for a heterogeneous concept whose presentation is a sign of a range of different symptoms (Rojahn, 1994). Several authors have suggested ways in which available theoretical information can be related to practical experience in order to generate working hypotheses useful for treatment. The conflict between behavioural theories and those relating self-injurious behaviour to underlying mental illness, neurochemical imbalance and/or biologically transmitted conditions is changing to an understanding of their inter-relatedness. Halliday and Mackrell (1998) set out a systems model based on the work of Bronfenbrenner (1979).

The list of theories as to aetiology is long and diverse and includes self-injurious behaviour as a learned behaviour, a form of communication, a result of neurochemical imbalance, a symptom of organic illness (e.g. Carr & Smith, 1995), a symptom of intermittent physical discomfort (e.g. Taylor *et al.*, 1993), a symptom of mental illness (e.g. Tsiouris *et al.* 2003; Ross & Oliver, 2001), a consequence of stereotypies (Wieseler *et al.*, 1985), a compulsive behaviour (King, 1993), a symptom of grief or post-traumatic stress (Hollins & Esterhuyzen, 1997; Bonell-Pascual *et al.*, 1999), or caused by over-sensitivity to sensory input (Reisman, 1993). Though it is acknowledged that an institutional environment is probably not a cause for self-injury, ecology (the interaction of people with their environment) is an important factor in its initiation and maintenance (Murphy, 1994). The main theories are addressed in greater detail below.

Behavioural theories

Behavioural theories are generally based on operant conditioning (Oliver, 1993). A behaviour occurs and may be positively reinforced with a reward (e.g. attention) or by the removal of an unwanted demand. The initial behaviour may be displayed by accident (e.g. as part of a tantrum) or on purpose, but for a reason unrelated to the eventual reinforcer (e.g. as a response to the pain of otitis media). A relationship between people exhibiting self-injury and their carers and the environment, involving operant conditioning on both sides, has been hypothesized. Thus subtle interactions between the person exhibiting the behaviour and their carers or other aspects of the environment (e.g. noise) may promote the behaviour, while not being obvious on superficial observation. Oliver (1993) proposed that some people have factors that make them vulnerable to developing such behaviour, including sensory and physical disability, having a syndrome known to be associated with self-injurious behaviour and/or having an increased degree of ID. Other factors are also involved in the development and maintenance of the behaviour. These include factors such as expressive communication problems, operant vulnerability and operant susceptibility and pre-existing neurotransmitter disturbance. Expressive communication problems are the extent to which a person can influence the behaviour of others through verbal or other forms of communication. Deficits in this may lead to aberrant behaviour being used as a communicative tool. Operant vulnerability is an increased likelihood that a person will be exposed to a situation or circumstance that will cause them to display the behaviour in the first place. Operant susceptibility refers to the enhanced potency of certain issues outside the person to act as reinforcers and maintain self-injurious behaviour in susceptible people.

A related alternative view is summarized by Halliday and Mackrell (1998) who posit that self-injury is the 'person's best attempt to deal with abusive, neglecting or traumatic behaviour' and is 'essentially communicative and functionally adaptive'.

Neurochemical theories

Neurochemical theories concern three separate types of neurotransmitters: dopamine, opiates and serotonin. The dopamine theory postulates that self-injurious behaviour is the result of dopamine receptor over-sensitivity (Schroeder, 1996). The D1 receptors are thought to be the principal dopamine receptors involved in the genesis and maintenance of self-injurious behaviour. This has important implications for pharmacotherapy as most neuroleptics have little effect at these receptors. The neuroleptic, clozapine, is more active at these receptors and has been successfully used to treat self-injurious behaviour (Symons *et al.*, 2001; Schroeder *et al.*, 1995; see also Chapter 19 by King).

Studies showing raised plasma beta-endorphin in people displaying self-injurious behaviour (Sandman *et al.*, 1990), or a therapeutic behaviour-attenuating response to the administration of opiate-blocking agents (Sandman *et al.*, 1990; Roth *et al.*, 1996), support hypotheses of raised endogenous opiates as a cause or contributor to individuals with ID displaying self-injurious behaviour. Two theories have been put forward. One suggests that a high level of circulating endogenous opiates allows the person to display self-injurious behaviour without suffering painful consequences, thus the behaviour can be used by the person to influence his or her environment. The other is that when people self-injure, they induce a release of endogenous opiates and this serves as a pleasurable positive reinforcer for the behaviour. The initial behaviour may occur for a variety of reasons, but its repetition is encouraged by the opiate feedback. The latter theory is supported by the work of Sandman and Hetrick (1995) who reported that plasma levels of beta-endorphin were raised in individuals directly after they self-injured.

Though the proposal that self-injurious behaviour is secondary to serotonin imbalance is somewhat tenuous (Murphy, 1994) there is supporting evidence. People who have syndromes associated with self-injurious behaviour such as Cornelia de Lange syndrome (Gillberg & Coleman, 1992) have been shown to have hyposerotoninaemia. There are also case reports of a treatment response to serotonin-raising medication such as clomiprimine (Lewis *et al.*, 1996).

It has been generally accepted that one aetiologic theory cannot determine assessment and treatment in individual cases. Many people with ID are exposed to events that could initiate a response of self-injurious behaviour or have factors that are associated with it, without ever displaying it. Neurotransmitter abnormalities may affect the way that people respond to their environment.

Implications of theory and research for assessment and therapy

Murphy (1994), in reviewing non-pharmaceutical treatment approaches, concluded that effective treatment programmes using up-to-date techniques (functional analysis, constructional approaches and functional communication training) were feasible but that success was not guaranteed. Iwata *et al.* (1994) stated that the only treatments that have been consistently effective in treating self-injury have been those based on punishment in the form of aversive stimulation, but that concerns exist about the appropriateness and safety of their use. Though they caution that omission of failed treatment interventions may skew the data,

Kahng *et al.* (2002) report their review of the behavioural literature as showing that most such treatments have been effective to a certain degree. They also point out that increased use of functional assessment approaches coincides with an increase in the use of reinforcement-based interventions and the decrease in the use of punishment-based interventions. The aim of behavioural assessment is to formulate and test hypotheses as regards the function of the behaviour. The hypotheses are developed by carrying out an in-depth review of the behaviour called a functional analysis. The aim is to produce a treatment plan that will facilitate the individual in developing more productive ways of achieving the same end. The positive reinforcement strategies developed by behaviourists such as Carr and Durand (1985) and La Vigna and Donnellan (1986) are examples of this approach.

Aman (1993), in reviewing the efficacy of psychotropic drugs for self-injurious behaviour, concluded that the available research showed tenuous success for such treatment. Other authors have questioned the appropriateness of intervention with psychotropic medication (Emerson *et al.*, 1994) in view of the fact that much of the behaviour involved does not have a proven neurochemical and/or psychopathological basis, although more recent work is providing a stronger evidence base for continued medication use (Aman & Madrid, 1999). It is probable that a combination of approaches aimed at the individual is most likely to succeed. Unless an obvious remediable cause explains the behaviour, assessment should take account of all the aetiologic factors already outlined. Thus assessment approaches should be multifactorial and multidisciplinary. Tsiouris *et al.* (2003), in championing the benefits of diagnosis and treatment of psychiatric disorders in people exhibiting self-injurious behaviour, caution against the use of psychotropics in treatment of self-injurious behaviour unless an identifiable psychiatric disorder is present.

Several authors have proposed practical approaches that integrate behavioural and neurochemical theory. Mace and Mauk (1995) outlined a schedule for what they called bio-behavioural diagnosis and treatment. This involved a range of assessments: psychological, paediatric, psychiatric and neurochemical. Patients were placed in a diagnostic category subtype on the basis of the results and were then treated according to the diagnostic category with behavioural therapy or psychotropic medication or a combination of each, depending on the subtype. In claiming an improved success rate for treatment, the authors emphasized the need for transdisciplinary work in dealing with the complex problem of self-injurious behaviour. Gardner and Sovner (1994) outlined a 'multimodal functional approach'. They emphasized the importance of data keeping and review in the context of the possible known aetiologic factors. Thompson *et al.* (1994) summarized the evidence supporting the use of psychotropic medications in self-injurious behaviour treatment regimes. These authors stress that if treatment takes account of the effects of psychotropics on learning, and the neurochemical theories on aetiology, then interventions are more likely to succeed, and inappropriate use of psychotropic agents can be avoided.

Aman (1993) recommended that, in view of the possible serious side-effects of these drugs, a behavioural programme should always be tried before introduction of medication. A behaviour monitoring programme should remain in place during treatment with psychotropic medication and should combine systematic direct observations and the use of a suitable rating tool. Different approaches were recommended depending on whether the cause of the patient's ID is known or if a physical or mental illness is suggested by assessment.

Despite the evidence of a significant prevalance of self-injurious behaviour in young children (Berkson et al., 2001), little has been done to develop targeted early intervention treatments.

Conclusion

Self-injurious behaviour causes physical and mental morbidity for the people who display it, stress for their carers and uses valuable resources. Dispite the wide-ranging research literature there is a lack of clarity and consensus to aid clinicians in assessment and intervention. This should encourage multidisciplinary co-operation but also carries a risk of antagonistic unifactorial approaches, especially where available clinical inputs have a narrow base of training and experience. Assessment of self-injurious behaviour must take a bio-psycho-social approach, be person-centred and take account of up-to-date research on aetiology and intervention.

The importance of early intervention with a proactive approach to prevention (Oliver, 1993; Kahng et al., 2002) cannot be overemphasized. This should involve screening at all ages for behaviours that may evolve into self-injury, for mild forms of the behaviour, for minor illnesses that may precipitate it, and for environments that do not offer sufficient opportunities for other ways of behaviour to develop. Resources must be provided to insure behavioural assessments are rigorous and intervention programmes are implemented consistently. Medication should be used in a rational way that takes account of available neurochemical theories, and thorough psychiatric assessments and formulations.

Summary points

- Self-injurious behaviour is a term for a clinical problem that has a multiplicity of manifestations and possible causes.
- There is a need for consensus on definitions to facilitate international epidemiological research that is comparable and useful.
- Most aetiological theories are not supported by robust research.

- The importance of early intervention with a proactive approach to prevention cannot be overemphasized.
- Assessments and interventions must be multifactorial and multidisciplinary.
- Medication should be used in a way that takes account of available neurochemical theories and thorough psychiatric assessments and formulations, and involves monitoring with baseline behavioural assessment and follow-up.
- Resources must be provided to insure behavioural assessments are rigorous and intervention programmes are implemented consistently.

Acknowledgments

The authors wish to thank the National Association for the Mentally Handicapped of Ireland and the Irish Health Research Board for grants which partly supported this chapter. They are also grateful for the help of the Research Departments of the St John of God Brothers of Ireland and of the St Michael's House Services. Finally, they thank Dr Michael Mulcahy for his encouragement and guidance.

REFERENCES

Aman, M. G. (1993). Efficacy of psychotropic drugs for reducing self-injurious behaviour in the developmental disabilities. *Annals of Clinical Psychiatry*, **5**(3), 171–88.

Aman, M. G. & Madrid, A. (1999). Atypical antipsychotics in persons with developmental disabilities. *Mental Retardation & Developmental Disabilities Research Reviews*, **5**, 253–63.

American Psychiatric Association (1994). *Diagnostic and Statistical Manual of Mental Disorders*, 4th edition. Washington DC: Author.

Berkson, G., Tupa, M. & Sherman, L. (2001). Early development of stereotyped and self-injurious behaviours: 1. Incidence. *American Journal of Mental Retardation*, **106**, 539–47.

Bhargava, S. A., Putnam, P. E., Kocoshis, S. A., Rowe, M. & Hanchett, J. (1996). Rectal bleeding in Prader–Willi syndrome. *Paediatrics*, **97**(2), 265–7.

Bonell-Pascual, E., Hulie-Dickens, S., Hollins, S., Esterhuyzen, A. & Sedgwick, P. (1999). Bereavement and grief in adults with learning disabilities. A follow-up study. *British Journal of Psychiatry*, **175**, 348–51.

Borthwick-Duffy, S. A. (1994), Prevalance of destructive behaviours. In *Destructive Behaviour in Developmental Disabilities: Diagnosis, Treatment*, ed. T. Thompson & D. B. Gray, pp. 993–1023. Thousand Oaks, CA: Sage.

Bronfenbrenner, U. (1979). *The Ecology of Human Development: Experiments by Nature and Design*. Cambridge, MA: Harvard University Press.

Bryson, Y., Sakati, N., Nyhan, W. L. & Fisch, C. H. (1971). Self-mutilative behavior in the Cornelia de Lange syndrome. *American Journal of Mental Deficiency*, **76**, 319–24.

Carr, E. G. & Durand, V. M. (1985). Reducing behaviour problems through functional communication training. *Journal of Applied Behaviour Analysis*, **18**, 111–26.

Carr, E. G. & Smith, C. E. (1995). Biological setting events for self-injury. *Mental Retardation and Developmental Disabilities Research Reviews*, **1**(2), 94–8.

Chadsey-Rusch, J. & Sprague, R. L. (1989). Maladaptive behaviors associated with neuroleptic drug maintenance. *American Journal on Mental Retardation*, **93**, 607–17.

Clarke, D. J., Waters, J. & Corbett, J. A. (1989). Adults with Prader–Willi syndrome: abnormalities of sleep and behaviour. *Journal of the Royal Society of Medicine*, **82**, 21–4.

Deb, S., Thomas, M. & Bright, C. (2001). Mental disorder in adults with intellectual disability. 2: The rate of behaviour disorders among a community-based population aged between 16 and 64 years. *Journal of Intellectual Disability Research*, **45**(6), 506–14.

Emerson, E. (1990). Severe self-injurious behaviour: some of the challenges it presents. *Mental Handicap*, **18**, 92–8.

Emerson, E. (1992). Self-injurious behaviour: an overview of recent trends in epidemiological and behavioural research. *Mental Handicap Research*, **5**, 49–81.

Emerson, E., Felce, D., McGill, P. & Mansell, J. (1994). Introduction. In *Severe Learning Disabilities and Challenging Behaviours*, ed. E. Emerson, P. McGill & J. Mansell, pp. 3–16. London: Chapman & Hall.

Favazza, A. & Rosenthal, R. (1993). Diagnostic issues in self-mutilation. *Hospital and Community Psychiatry*, **44**(2), 134–40.

Fitzgerald, B., Morgan, J., Keene N. *et al.* (2000). An investigation into diet treatment for adults with previously untreated phenylketonuria and severe intellectual disability. *Journal of Intellectual Disability Research*, **44**(1), 53–9.

Foreman, D., Hall, S. & Oliver, C. (2001). Descriptive analysis of self-injurious behaviour and self-restraint. *Journal of Intellectual Disability Research*, **15**, 1–7.

Gardner, W. I. & Sovner, R. (1994). *Self-injurious Behaviours: Diagnosis and Treatment – A Multimodal Functional Approach*. Mountville, PA: VIDA Publishing.

Gillberg, C. & Coleman, M. (1992). Biochemistry. In *The Biology of the Autistic Syndromes*, 2nd edition, ed. C. Gillberg & M. Coleman, pp. 115–30. London: MacKeith Press.

Griffen, J., Williams, D., Stark, M., Altmeyer, B. & Mason, M. (1986). Self-injurious behavior: a state-wide prevalence survey of the extent and circumstances. *Applied Research in Mental Retardation*, **7**, 105–16.

Halliday, S. & Mackrell, K. (1998). Psychological interventions in self-injurious behaviour. *British Journal of Psychiatry*, **172**, 395–400.

Hemming, H. (1982). Mentally handicapped adults returned to large institutions after transfers to new small units. *British Journal of Mental Subnormality*, **28**, 13–18.

Hillery, J. & Mulcahy, M. (1997). Self-injurious behaviour in persons with a mental handicap: an epidemiological study in an Irish population. *The Irish Journal of Psychological Medicine*, **14**(1), 12–15.

Hollins, S. & Esterhuyzen, A. (1997). Bereavement and grief in adults with learning disability. *British Journal of Psychiatry*, **170**, 497–502.

Iwata, B. A., Dorsey, M. F., Slifer, K. J., Bauman, K. E. & Richman, G. S. (1994). Toward a functional analysis of self-injury. *Journal of Applied Behaviour Analysis*, **27**, 197–209.

Kahng, S., Iawata, B. A. & Lewin, A. B. (2002). Behavioural treatment of self-injury, 1964 to 2000. *American Journal on Mental Retardation*, **107**(3), 212–21.

King, B. H. (1993). Self-injury by people with mental retardation: a compulsive behavior hypothesis. *American Journal on Mental Retardation*, **98**(1), 93–112.

Lakin, K. C., Hill, B. K., Hauber, F. A., Bruininks, R. H. & Heal, I. W. (1983). New admissions and readmissions to a national sample of public residential facilities. *American Journal of Mental Deficiency*, **88**, 13–20.

La Vigna, G. W. & Donnellan, A. A. (1986). *Alternatives to Punishment: Solving Behaviour Problems with Non-aversive Therapies*. New York: Irvington.

Lesch, M. & Nyhan, W. L. (1964). A familial disorder of uric acid metabolism and central nervous system dysfunction. *American Journal of Medicine*, **36**, 561–70.

Lewis, M. H., Bodfish, J. W., Powell, S. B., Parker, D. E. & Golden, R. N. (1996). Clomipramine treatment for self-injurious behavior of individuals with mental retardation: a double-blind comparison with placebo. *American Journal on Mental Retardation*, **100**(6), 654–65.

Mace, C. F. & Mauk, J. E. (1995). Bio-behavioural diagnosis and treatment of self-injury. *Mental Retardation and Intellectual Disabilities Research Reviews*, **1**, 104–10.

Maurice, P. & Trudel, G. (1982). Self injurious behaviour; prevalence and relationships to environmental events (monograph.) In *Life-threatening Behavior*, ed. J. Hollis & C. Meyers, pp. 81–103. Washington, DC: AAMD.

McNaught, A. & Turk, J. (1993). Smith–Magenis syndrome mistaken for emotional abuse: a case report. Presentation at the Fourth Annual Meeting of the Society for the Study of Behavioural Phenotypes, Royal Society of Medicine, London.

Murphy, G. (1994). Understanding challenging behaviour. In *Severe Learning Disabilities and Challenging Behaviours: Designing High Quality Services*, ed. E. Emerson, P. Mc Gill & J. Mansell, pp. 37–68. London: Chapman & Hall.

O'Brien, G. (2003). The classification of problem behaviour in Diagnostic Criteria for Psychiatric Disorders for Use with Adults with Learning Disabilities/Mental Retardation (DC–LD). *Journal of Intellectual Disability Research*, **47** (Suppl. 1), S32–7.

Oliver, C. (1993). Self-injurious behaviour: from response to strategy. In *Research to Practice? Implications of Research on the Challenging Behaviour of People with Learning Disability*, ed. C. Kiernan, pp. 135–88. Clevedon: BILD Publications.

Oliver, C., Murphy, G. H. & Corbett, J. A. (1987). Self-injurious behaviour in people with mental handicap: a total population study. *Journal of Mental Deficiency Research*, **31**, 146–62.

Quine, L. & Pahl, J. (1985). Examining the causes of stress in families with mentally handicapped children. *British Journal of Social Work*, **15**, 501–17.

Reisman, J. (1993). Using a sensory integrative approach to treat self-injurious behaviour in an adult with profound mental retardation. *American Journal of Occupational Therapy*, **47**(5), 403–11.

Rojahn, J. (1986). Self-injurious and stereotypic behavior of non-institutionalised mentally retarded people. Prevalence and classification. *American Journal of Mental Deficiency*, **91**(3), 268–76.

Rojahn, J. (1994). Epidemiology and topographic taxonomy of self-injurious behaviour. In *Destructive Behaviour in Develomental Disabilities*, ed. T. Thompson & D. B. Gray, pp. 49–67. London: Sage Publications.

Ross, E. & Oliver, C. (2001). The relationship between levels of mood, interest and pleasure and 'challenging behaviour' in adults with severe and profound intellectual disability. *Journal of Intellectual Disability Research*, **46**, 191–7.

Roth, A. S., Ostrott, R. B. & Hoffman, R. E. (1996). Naltrexone as a treatment for repetitive self-injurious behaviour: an open-label trial. *Journal of Clinical Psychiatry*, **57**(6), 233–7.

Royal College of Psychiatrists (2001). *The Diagnostic Criteria for Psychiatric Disorders for Use with Adults with Learning Disabilities/Mental Retardation*. Occasional Paper 48, pp. 1–128. London: Gaskell Press.

Saloviita, T. (1988). *Self-injurious Behaviour in an Institution for Mentally Handicapped Persons. An Epidemiological Study*. Helsinki: Mental Handicap Research Unit.

Sandman, C. A., Barron, J. L., Chicz-DeMet, A. & DeMet, E. M. (1990). Plasma b-endorphin levels in patients with self-injurious behavior and stereotypy. *American Journal on Mental Retardation*, **95**(1), 84–92.

Sandman, C. A. & Hetrick, W. P. (1995). Opiate mechanisms in self-injury. *Mental Retardation and Developmental Disabilities Research Reviews*, **1**(2), 130–6.

Schroeder, S. R. (1996). Dopaminergic mechanisms in self-injury. *Psychology in Mental Retardation and Developmental Disabilities*, **22**(2), 10–13.

Schroeder, S. R., Hammock, R. G., Mulick, J. A. *et al.* (1995). Clinical trials of D1 and D2 dopamine modulating drugs and self-injury in mental retardation and developmental disabilities. *Mental Retardation and Developmental Disabilities Research Reviews*, **1**(2), 120–9.

Shlalock, R., Harper, R. & Genung, T. (1985). Community integration of mentally retarded adults: community placement and program success. *American Journal of Mental Deficiency*, **89**, 352–61.

Sutter, P., Mayeda, T., Call, T., Yanagi, G. & Yee, S. (1980). Comparison of successful and unsuccessful community-placed mentally retarded persons. *American Journal of Mental Deficiency*, **85**, 262–7.

Symons, F. J., Davis, M. L. & Thompson, T. (2000). Self-injurious behaviour and sleep disturbance in adults with developmental disabilities. *Research in Developmental Disabilities*, **21**, 115–23.

Symons, F. J., Sutton, K. A., Walker, C. & Bodfish, J. W. (2003). Altered diurnal pattern of salivary Substance P in adults with developmental disabilities and chronic self-injury. *American Journal on Mental Retardation*, **108**(1), 13–18.

Symons, F. J., Tapp, J., Wulfsberg, A. *et al.* (2001). Sequential analysis of the effects of naltrexone on the environmental mediation of self-injurious behaviour. *Experimental Clinical Psychopharmacology*, **9**(3), 269–76.

Taylor, D. V., Rush, D., Hetrick, W. P. & Sandman, C. A. (1993). Self-injurious behavior within the menstrual cycle of women with mental retardation. *American Journal on Mental Retardation*, **97**(6), 659–64.

Thompson, T., Egli, M., Symons, F. & Delaney, D. (1994). Neurobehavioural mechanisms of drug action in the developmental disabilities. In *Destructive Behaviour in Developmental Disabilities: Diagnosis and Treatment*, ed. T. Thompson & D. B. Gray, pp. 133–80. London: Sage Publications.

Tsiouris, J. A., Cohen, I. L., Patti, P. J. & Korosh, W. M. (2003). Treatment of previously undiagnosed psychiatric disorders in persons with developmental disabilities decreased or eliminated self-injurious behaviour. *Journal of Clinical Psychiatry*, **64**, 1081–90.

Turk, J. (1992). The fragile X syndrome. On the way to a behavioural phenotype. *British Journal of Psychiatry*, **160**, 24–35.

Wieseler, N. A., Hanson, R. H., Chamberlin, T. P. & Thompson, T. (1985). Functional taxonomy of stereotypic and self-injurious behavior. *Mental Retardation*, **23**(5), 230–4.

Wolfensberger, W. (1972). *Principles of Normalisation in Human Services*. Toronto: National Institute on Mental Retardation.

15

Mental health and epilepsy among adults with intellectual disabilities

Shoumitro Deb

Prevalence of epilepsy in people who have ID

Epilepsy is a tendency of occurrence of transient recurrent abnormal electrical discharges in the brain, affecting one or more of the following brain functions: motor, sensory, cognitive, speech, behavioural, emotional and psychological. Around 0.5% of the general population has epilepsy (Chadwick, 1994). A much higher proportion of people who have intellectual disabilities (ID) have epilepsy. Although the exact figure is not known, the reported prevalence of lifetime epilepsy among people who have ID (IQ < 70) varies between 14% and 24% (Rutter *et al.*, 1976; Forsgren *et al.*, 1990; Goulden *et al.*, 1991; McGrother *et al.*, 1996; Deb, 1997a). The prevalence rate depends on the age of the person, severity and cause of ID, and the presence and absence of associated neurological conditions. For example, the cumulative incidence of epilepsy was reported to be 9%, 11%, 13% and 15% among people with ID at age 5, 10, 15 and 22 years respectively (Goulden *et al.*, 1991).

The rate of epilepsy increases with the severity of ID. Steffenburg *et al.* (1996) found among 378 children with ID between age 6 and 13, that 15% of those with mild ID, as opposed to 45% of those with severe ID, had epilepsy. Similarly Shepherd and Hosking (1989) found 7% of children with mild to moderate ID, and 67% of those with severe ID, had epilepsy. The reported rate of epilepsy among people with profound ID (IQ < 20) varies between 50% (Michelucci *et al.*, 1989) and 82% (Suzuki *et al.*, 1991).

The rate of epilepsy rises if the ID is associated with any neurological disorder. For example, Goulden *et al.* (1991) found the cumulative incidence of epilepsy in people who had ID, but no associated neurological disability, was 2.6, 3.2, 3.9, and 5.2% at 5, 10, 15, and 22 years respectively; whereas among children with ID and cerebral palsy the cumulative risk was 28, 31, and 38% at age 5, 10, and 22 years respectively.

Psychiatric and Behavioural Disorders in Intellectual and Developmental Disabilities, ed. Nick Bouras and Geraldine Holt. Published by Cambridge University Press. © Cambridge University Press 2007.

There is a particular association between epilepsy and certain causes of ID. For example, epilepsy is reported among 5–10% of individuals who have Down syndrome, which is the most common chromosomal cause of ID (Stafstorm, 1999). Infantile spasm is the most common seizure type among children with Down syndrome. There is a further increase in the rate of epilepsy among people with Down syndrome later in their lives. It is reported that as many as 75% of older individuals with Down syndrome may develop epilepsy. This is not always believed to be associated with the increased rate of Alzheimer's disease that affects these people later in their lives. Although generalized tonic clonic seizures are reported to be the most common seizure type in late-onset epilepsy in people with Down syndrome, an increased incidence of myoclonic seizures is also observed. Interestingly the genes for both Unverricht–Lundborg disease, which causes a form of myoclonic seizure, and for the glutamate sub-unit GluR5 that may play a role in neuronal excitability, are localized at the distal long arm of chromosome 21, within the critical Down syndrome region (Lehesjoki *et al.*, 1991; Eubanks *et al.*, 1993) (cited in Stafstorm, 1999).

Different seizure types, especially generalized tonic clonic seizures, have been reported in about 25% of people with fragile X syndrome, which is a common inherited cause of ID. Seizures usually start at the onset of adolescence and the frequency tends to decrease with age. No direct relationship between seizure occurrence and the presence of autistic features is reported in people with fragile X syndrome (Wisniewski *et al.*, 1985). An EEG in children with fragile X syndrome is either normal or shows some non-specific abnormalities such as diffuse slowing of the background activities. However, a characteristic EEG similar to those seen in benign rolandic epilepsy is reported in a significant proportion of people who have fragile X syndrome (Stafstorm, 1999). There are also many rare conditions of ID in which a higher rate of epilepsy is reported. For example, epilepsy is reported in around 75% of people with Rett syndrome, 86% with Angelman syndrome, in a high proportion of people with Aicardi syndrome, about 50% of people with Lesch–Nyhan syndrome, about 30% of cases of Lowe syndrome, over 80% of cases of tuberous sclerosis and Sturge–Weber syndrome, and about 25% of cases of Rubenstein–Taybi syndrome (Deb & Ahmed, 2000).

Aetiologies of epilepsy and intellectual disabilities

Diagnosis of epilepsy syndrome depends on the combination of seizure types, age of onset, association with other clinical features, course of epilepsy and characteristic EEG abnormalities. Certain epilepsy syndromes such as West syndrome and Lennox–Gastaut syndrome are commonly associated with ID. Lennox–Gastaut syndrome usually starts between three and five years of age, involves multiple seizure types such as atypical absences, myoclonic, myoclonic-atonic (sudden falls) and axial tonic seizures, and shows characteristic EEG abnormalities in the form of diffuse spike-waves (2–3 hertz) while awake and bursts of 10-hertz rhythm during sleep. It is important to distinguish this syndrome from other childhood myoclonic seizures. This syndrome carries a poor prognosis in that complete recovery is unusual; ID is the rule, and a proportion (5%) die within 10 years. Seizure types may change in adulthood and include generalized tonic clonic, tonic, myoclonic, absence and partial seizures. This syndrome constitutes 5% of childhood epilepsies (Sillanpää, 1973), and Trevathan et al. (1997) reported Lennox–Gastaut syndrome among 17% of those with profound ID (cited in Sillanpää, 1999).

Malformation of cerebral cortical development (cerebral dysgenesis or dysplasias) (also known as neuronal migration disorders or NMDs) such as hemimegalencephaly, lissencephaly, pachygyria, polymicrogyria and heterotopia are important causes of ID and epilepsy. More than 25 syndromes associated with cerebral dysgenesis have been identified; most have a genetic basis (Dobyns & Truwit, 1995). Cerebral dysgenesis can also be seen as an isolated finding and not part of a genetic syndrome. These lesions can be focal or generalized and may affect one or both cerebral hemispheres. Li and colleagues (1995) found evidence of cerebral dysgenesis in MRI in 12% of adults with partial or secondary generalized epilepsy who attended a specialist epilepsy unit. Cerebral dysplasias also include neuroectodermal dysplasias such as tuberous sclerosis and Sturge–Weber disease, which are rare conditions but are usually associated with epilepsy. In the past, when evidence of cerebral dysgenesis primarily came from autopsy studies, it was thought that these conditions were only compatible with resistant epilepsy and severe ID. However, with the advancement of neuroimaging techniques, it has become apparent that even some people who do not have epilepsy and/or ID may show evidence of NMDs in MRI scans (Deb, 1997b). Although cerebral dysgenesis is often associated with resistant and partial seizures, neurosurgical interventions such as focal resection, hemispherectomy and corpus callosotomy may prove beneficial for some of these patients (Cataltepe & Comair, 1999; Holthausen et al., 1999; Roberts, 1999).

Diagnosis of epilepsy

The diagnosis of epilepsy depends on an eyewitness account of the seizures, examination of the person who has epilepsy, and investigations. Of these, a detailed eyewitness account is perhaps the most crucial component. Diagnosis of epilepsy, particularly the seizure type, can be difficult in people with ID, and therefore it is possible for clinicians to make both a false positive and a false negative diagnosis in a number of cases. Non-epileptic seizure disorders (pseudo-seizures) are known to be present in a proportion of the general population who have a diagnosis of epilepsy (Betts, 1990). Similarly, behavioural disorder could be misdiagnosed as an epileptic seizure in some people with ID (Coulter, 1993). On the other hand, partial and absence seizures could remain under-diagnosed in people with ID. It is imperative to gather a thorough description of the seizure activities from an eyewitness, including activities before and after the seizure.

A thorough examination of the person who has ID using standardized methods is necessary (see practice guideline by Deb *et al.*, 2001a or Deb & Iyer, 2005). Physical examination may detect organic factors that may cause or precipitate seizure disorders. A thorough assessment of the person's adaptive and maladaptive behaviour, and social circumstances is necessary to estimate the effect of epilepsy on their quality of life (Kerr *et al.*, 2001).

Investigations

The EEG is the main investigation in relation to the diagnosis of epilepsy. Other possible investigations include neuroimaging and specific investigations necessary to determine the cause of ID. It is also necessary to investigate any underlying physical condition that may be contributing to the epilepsy. Inter-ictal EEGs do not show any abnormality in a proportion of those who have epilepsy. In many people with ID it is difficult to perform an EEG. Also, in a high proportion of cases, abnormal EEGs in people with ID constitute non-specific abnormalities such as an excess of background slow activities, which could be a possible manifestation of underlying brain damage rather than specific epileptic changes (Deb, 1995; Deb & Joyce, 1999). A proportion of people with ID who manifest generalized seizures show focal epileptic changes in their EEG, indicating the possibility of secondary generalization of focal seizures in many people with ID. Video telemetry and 24-hour EEG recordings are also helpful in confirming a seizure diagnosis.

Structural neuroimaging such as CT and MRI are not necessary in most cases. The recent advances in MRI technology have made it possible to detect subtle focal brain malformation that was not possible before. This has led to successful neurosurgery for many patients who have epilepsy. The sensitivity of functional neuroimaging such as SPECT/PET (Single Photon Emission Computed Tomography/ Proton Emission Tomography) in detecting epileptic abnormality in the inter-ictal phase is low. The sensitivity increases if an ictal SPECT/PET can be performed. A combination of ictal and inter-ictal SPECT/PET is likely to detect abnormality in a high proportion of people with epilepsy. The usefulness of neuroimaging investigations in people with ID has not been explored. Magneto-encephalograph (MEG), which could be useful in the investigation of epilepsy, is not available in most centres.

Mental health and epilepsy

Mental health problems in the form of psychiatric disorders such as schizophrenia, personality disorders and depressive disorders; psychiatric symptoms such as depression and anxiety; and behaviour problems such as aggression and agitation can all be associated with epilepsy.

Mental health symptoms could be observed in the pre-ictal, ictal, post-ictal, and inter-ictal phases. Some people show a distinct pattern of change in mood and behaviour prior to having an epileptic seizure. This phase is called the 'prodrome' and can last from hours to days. During this period some people become agitated, anxious or depressed, or sometimes aggressive. The term 'working up to a fit' has been used to describe this prodromal phase. The exact mechanism that produces the prodrome is not known. This may be part of the ictal phenomenon, which may be associated with sub-clinical seizure activities. On the other hand, a change in mood itself may be a precipitating factor for an epileptic seizure. It is possible to take some measures during the prodrome, which may help to prevent the seizure. An 'aura', on the other hand, is a distinct focal ictal phenomenon, which can last for a few minutes leading up to the seizure. The seizures in these cases are secondarily generalized partial seizures. Certain psychological and behavioural symptoms can be manifested during an 'aura' including a feeling of 'butterflies in the stomach', anxiety, irritability, hallucinations and aggression.

In certain types of seizures, particularly complex partial seizures, certain psychological and behavioural symptoms may be manifested during the 'ictal' phase. These include confusion, hallucinations, anxiety, stereotyped behaviours and aggression. Some people show abnormal behaviour and mood immediately after a seizure in the post-ictal phase. Examples of abnormal behaviours are confusion, agitation and aggression. The aggression in the post-ictal phase is usually not goal-directed but random. Nevertheless it may inadvertently cause injury to others.

Inter-ictal psychopathology has been the subject of research over many years and the findings remain controversial. Overall, in the general population, there is an increase in psychopathology inter-ictally among people who have epilepsy, but the psychopathology usually consists of psychological symptoms such as depression and anxiety, which may have a greater preponderance among females. Depressive disorder is more common among people with epilepsy than in the general population. A relationship between schizophrenia and complex partial seizures has been reported. In the general population, the evidence remains equivocal for a relationship between aggression and epilepsy and between personality disorders and epilepsy. However, some have suggested that the personality changes in people with epilepsy have specific patterns that do not comply with the known classification of personality disorders within the existing psychiatric classification systems. Gastaut and Geschwind (Gastaut *et al.*, 1995; Geschwind, 1975) described a constellation of behaviours that are more commonly associated with epilepsy but particularly with complex partial seizure of temporal origin. These behaviours include a tendency towards excessive writing, over-religiosity, circumstantiality, stickiness, abnormal sexual inclinations, etc. (Bear & Fedio, 1977).

Although Rutter *et al.*'s (1976) study showed an increased rate of psychopathology among children with epilepsy and ID, subsequent studies have failed to show this (Lewis *et al.*, 2000). Among adults, the finding is more consistent. Apart from one exception (Lund, 1985), most studies failed to show an association between increased psychopathology and epilepsy among those who have ID.

Epilepsy-related factors such as the age of onset and duration of epilepsy, type and severity of epilepsy syndrome and seizures, type and locus of EEG changes, and the presence or absence of an underlying brain lesion can affect the mental health of a person who has epilepsy. Drug factors and psychosocial factors such as lack of social support, employment difficulties, social stigma, and an external locus of control can also affect mental health.

Psychiatric disorders

In the general population, post-ictal and inter-ictal psychoses have been reported. Psychoses in the context of epilepsy include bizarre delusions and prominent visual hallucinations in the presence of a relatively less impaired affective state and personality. In the general population, a phenomenon of forced normalization (Landolt, 1958) or an alternative psychosis (Tellenbach, 1965) has been described in which an inverse relationship between seizure frequency and psychotic features exists. Despite anecdotes, no study has explored this phenomenon systematically among people who have ID.

In a comparative study of adults with ID, with and without epilepsy, Deb and Hunter (1991) found a higher rate of psychoses (2.66%) among the epilepsy group as compared with the non-epilepsy group (0%) but this difference was not statistically significant. On the other hand, bipolar disorder was significantly less common among the epilepsy group (0%) than in the non-epilepsy group (4%). The rate of depressive and anxiety disorders did not differ between the two groups. The rate of depressive and anxiety symptoms were not compared. It is possible that psychosocial stressors are less influential in precipitating psychoses among people who have ID. However, the fact that the rate of psychoses among adults with ID and epilepsy is higher than that among adults with ID who do not have epilepsy goes against this hypothesis (Deb & Hunter, 1991). Some anti-epileptic drugs such as vigabatrin, topiramate and zonisimide are known to produce psychotic symptoms (Mitchell, 2004).

Personality disorders

Deb and Hunter (1991) found a similar rate of personality disorder by using the Standardized Assessment of Personality (SAP) scale between people with ID and epilepsy (20%) and those without epilepsy (19%). However, the rate of personality disorder according to the Temporal-Lobe (T-L) Personal Behaviour Inventory (Bear & Fideo, 1977), devised to reflect the instalation of behaviours described by Gestaut and Gwechwind (see previous page), was higher among the epilepsy (15/75) than in the non-epilepsy (8/75) group, although this was not a statistically significant difference. This was particularly so of the community-based group, those having epileptic attacks currently and those receiving more than one anti-epileptic medication. Aggressive disorder was the most common personality type according to the SAP scale and 'persistence and repetitiveness' was the most common type according to the T-L personality scale between both the epilepsy and non-epilepsy groups.

Behaviour disorders

The relationship between aggressive behaviour and epilepsy remains controversial (Geschwind, 1975). The answer to the question whether or not during a seizure, an individual is able to demonstrate co-ordinated goal-directed aggression to others, himself or property seems negative. The second issue relates to the question of whether people with epilepsy, as a group, manifest more aggression and other abnormal behaviours between seizures (inter-ictally) compared with those who do not have epilepsy. Despite many anecdotal reports in the literature and the media of violent outbursts by individuals with epilepsy, and the generally held view that inter-ictal aggression is more common among people with epilepsy, the evidence is lacking (see also Chapter 17 by Reese *et al.*). A non-surgical group of people with epilepsy had a much lower rate of aggression (4.8%; Rodin, 1973) relative to a neuro-surgical sample (36%; Serafetinides, 1965). Studies on prison populations show a higher prevalence of epilepsy than in the general population but no increase in violent or serious crimes among individuals with epilepsy. Some controlled studies have shown a higher rate of aggression among people with epilepsy than other types of illness or in healthy controls (Guerrant *et al.*, 1962; Cairns, 1974), others have failed to do so (Standage & Fenton, 1975). Most community-based studies did not find an increased rate of aggression among people with epilepsy (Kligman & Goldberg, 1975; Lishman, 1998).

There have been five controlled studies of behaviour disorders and psychopathology among adults with ID, with and without epilepsy (Espie *et al.*, 1989; Espie *et al.*, 1990; Deb, 1997c; Matson *et al.*, 1999; Chung & Cassidy, 2001). Overall, no significant difference is observed in the rate of behaviour disorders between the epilepsy and the non-epilepsy group. Further non-controlled studies have supported that finding (Deb & Joyce, 1999; Deb et al., 2001a; Espie et al., 2003a). As both epilepsy and behaviour disorders are common in people with ID (Deb et al., 2001b), Deb and Hunter (1991) hypothesized that the underlying brain damage that causes the ID is a stronger determinant of psychopathology than the epilepsy per se, particularly for behaviour disorders. They reported a significantly higher rate of behaviour disorders among the sub-group of those with epilepsy who showed generalized epileptiform EEG changes, who received one anti-epileptic drug at a time, and those who received carbamazepine. Similarly, they found a significantly lesser rate of behaviour disorders among the sub-group of people with epilepsy who had severe ID, sustained single seizure type, and showed only excessive slow background activities in the EEG.

Cognitive impairment

Cognitive impairment, particularly affecting memory and executive functions, are reported among people with epilepsy. In childhood repeated absence seizures can affect new learning. Underlying brain damage, for which the epilepsy is a manifestation, can also affect cognitive function. Some anti-epileptic drugs, particularly phenytoin and topiramate, can affect cognition. Although some childhood epilepsy syndromes may cause gradual deterioration in the overall cognitive function (sometimes associated with epileptic encephalopathy), the relationship between dementia and epilepsy remains unresolved. Although dementia can precipitate epilepsy, epilepsy per se is not known to cause dementia, unless it is caused by repeated head injury or an underlying neurodegenerative condition.

Quality of life

Like other chronic disorders, epilepsy tends to affect people's quality of life but in epilepsy an added dimension is the 'external locus of control', which means that people do not control the timing of their epileptic seizures. A considerable amount of social stigma still tends to isolate people with epilepsy from the wider society. A negative image of epilepsy also prevents many people with epilepsy from receiving appropriate social support. Some of the consequences of epilepsy include lack of freedom, and independence, disadvantage in the employment market, and financial penalty. Adverse effects of medication can also impair the quality of life of a person with epilepsy. McEwan and colleagues (2004) have shown that adolescents with epilepsy are concerned about 'peer acceptance', 'development of autonomy', 'school-related issues', 'epilepsy as part of me', 'future', 'medication issues', 'sense of uncertainty', 'seizures', and '(a lack of) knowledge of epilepsy'. Epilepsy can also cause concern among carers, which leads to an increased carer burden. Espie and colleagues (2003b) found that carers are concerned about seizures, treatment, caring and social impact.

Management of psychopathology in the presence of epilepsy

Despite a possible difference in the phenomenology of psychiatric disorders in the context of epilepsy, the management of these disorders is similar to those without epilepsy. However, caution should be used while using psychotropic drugs because both antipsychotics and antidepressants are known to precipitate epilepsy. Within the same class of medication, some drugs may be better than the others. Overall selective serotonin re-uptake inhibitors (SSRIs) seem less pro-convulsant than the older tricycle antidepressants. Among SSRIs, citalopram and paroxetine seem less pro-convulsant than sertraline. Newer non-SSRI antidepressants such as mirtazapine and nefazodone seem even less pro-convulsant than the SSRIs. Some antidepressants may show a paradoxical anti-epileptic effect. Like antidepressants, the newer atypical antipsychotics are seen as less pro-convulsant than the old generation of typical antipsychotics. Seizures are reported among 0.1% of risperidone, 0.2–0.9% of olanzapine, and 9 out of 1710 quetiapine treated patients. The pro-convulsant property of clozapine seems dose related; approximately 5% of people develop seizures when taking clozapine in a dose of 600 mg or over per day. Some benzodiazepines such as diazepam can paradoxically precipitate seizures; whereas other benzodiazepines such as clobazam have an anti-epileptic property. The epileptic effect of other drugs such as psychostimulants that may be used in people with ID is not known (Trimble, 2003).

The management of behaviour disorder among people with ID needs a careful initial assessment in the form of functional analysis of behaviour and involvement of a multidisciplinary team. The management need not necessarily be pharmacological and even if pharmacological treatment is used, it is often instituted along with other non-pharmacological interventions (see also Chapters 3 by O'Hara, 17 by Reese et al., and 18 by Benson and Havercamp). For some people better control of epilepsy per se will improve behaviour but in others this may make things worse because of possible 'forced normalization' or other effects such as the adverse effects of drugs. More complex dynamics such as diminished carer attention for the individual with improved seizure control or other psychological or social factors may make behaviour worse when epilepsy improves. Some anti-epileptic drugs also have indirect effects on behaviour in the form of mood stabilization or reducing the underlying level of anxiety and arousal. Although a discussion on the treatment of epilepsy is beyond the remit of this chapter, Table 15.1 highlights some important areas for consideration in relation to the treatment of epilepsy among people with

Table 15.1 Special considerations for the use of anti-epileptic drugs in people with intellectual disabilities.

1. Difficulty of diagnosis of epilepsy (both false positive and false negative diagnoses are possible).
2. Difficulty of diagnosing the seizure-type (because of difficulty of performing an EEG in some people with intellectual disabilities).
3. Common occurrence of multiple seizure-type.
4. Long duration of seizures.
5. A high proportion of treatment-resistant epilepsy (possibly because of underlying brain damage).
6. A higher sensitivity to cognitive and behavioural adverse effects of anti-epileptic drugs (many people with intellectual disabilities have concurrent mental health problems).
7. Likelihood of drug interactions (many people with intellectual disabilities receive antipsychotic and antidepressant drugs that are potentially epileptogenic).
8. Difficulty in detecting adverse effects of drugs (because of communication problems).

Possibility of central nervous system adverse effects of drugs being more pronounced in this population (because of pre-existing brain damage).

ID (Deb, 2000). The ultimate aim for the management of people with epilepsy and psychopathology must be an improvement in their quality of life and of their carers and not merely symptom reduction (Kerr *et al.*, 2001).

Conclusion

Between 14% and 24% of people who have ID have epilepsy. Approximately 7 to 15% of people with mild to moderate ID, 45 to 65% of those with severe ID, and 50 to 82% of those with profound ID are expected to have a lifetime history of epilepsy. The rate of epilepsy increases if there is an associated neurological disorder. Certain epilepsy syndromes such as the West syndrome and the Lennox–Gastaut syndrome are commonly associated with ID. Epilepsy is particularly common among people with fragile X syndrome, Rett syndrome, Angelman syndrome, Aicardi syndrome, Epiloia, NMDs, Down syndrome, Lesch–Nyhan syndrome, Lowe syndrome and Rubenstein–Taybi syndrome. Psychiatric symptoms may be manifested pre-ictally, ictally, post-ictally and inter-ictally. Psychiatric symptoms including behaviour disorders are not uncommon among people with ID and epilepsy. However, controlled studies have not shown any significant difference in the rate of psychiatric disorders among people with ID, with and without epilepsy. Epilepsy can cause considerable carer burden and affect a person's quality of life. Therefore, the ultimate aim for any management strategy should be improvement of quality of life and lessening of carer burden, and not just simple symptom reduction.

Summary points

- Epilepsy is common in people with ID, particularly those with severe ID.
- The rate of epilepsy increases in people with ID and neurological disorders.
- Certain forms of epilepsy are associated with genetic syndromes.
- Psychiatric symptoms are manifested in people with ID and epilepsy.
- It is unclear if people with ID and epilepsy have a higher rate of psychiatric disorders.

REFERENCES

Bear, D. M. & Fedio, P. (1977). Quantitative analysis of inter-ictal behaviour in temporal lobe epilepsy. *Archives of Neurology*, **34**, 454–67.

Betts, T. (1990). Pseudoseizures: Seizures that are not epilepsy. *Lancet*, **336**, 163–4.

Cairns, V. M. (1974). Epilepsy, personality and behaviour. In *Epilepsy: Proceedings of the Hans Berger Centenary Symposium*, ed. P. Harris and C. Maudsley. Edinburgh: Churchill Livingstone, pp. 256–68.

Cataltepe, O. & Comair, Y. G. (1999). Focal resection in the treatment of neuronal migrational disorders. In *The Epilepsies: Etiology and Prevention*, ed. Kotagal, P. & Lüders, H. O., San Diego, CA: Academic Press, pp. 87–92.

Chadwick, D. (1994). Epilepsy. *Journal of Neurology, Neurosurgery and Psychiatry*, **57**, 264–77.

Chung, M. C. & Cassidy, G. A. (2001). A preliminary report on the relationship between challenging behaviour and epilepsy in learning disability. *European Journal of Psychiatry*, **15**, 23–32.

Coulter, D. L. (1993). Epilepsy and mental retardation: an overview. *American Journal of Mental Retardation*, **98** (5), 1–11.

Deb, S. (1995). Electrophysiological correlates of psychopathology in individuals with mental retardation and epilepsy. *Journal of Intellectual Disability Research*, **39**, 129–35.

Deb, S. (1997a). Epilepsy and mental retardation. *Epilepsie Bulletin*, **25**, 91–94.

Deb, S. (1997b). Structural neuroimaging in mental retardation. *British Journal of Psychiatry*, **171**, 417–19.

Deb, S. (1997c). Mental disorder in adults with mental retardation and epilepsy. *Comprehensive Psychiatry*, **38**(3), 179–84.

Deb, S. (2000). Epidemiology and treatment of epilepsy in patients who are mentally retarded. *CNS Drugs*, **13**(2), 117–28.

Deb, S. & Ahmed, Z. (2000). Special conditions leading to mental retardation. In *New Oxford Textbook of Psychiatry*, ed. M. G. Gelder, N. Andreasen, J. J. Lopez-Ibor. Oxford: Oxford Press, pp. 1953–63.

Deb, S. & Hunter, D. (1991). Psychopathology of people with mental handicap and epilepsy. I. Maladaptive behaviour; II. Psychiatric illness; III. Personality disorder. *British Journal of Psychiatry*, **159**, 822–34.

Deb, S. & Iyer, A. (2005). Clinical interviews. In *Mood Disorders in People with Mental Retardation*, ed. P. Sturmey. New York: National Association for the Dually Diagnosed Press, pp. 159–73.

Deb, S. & Joyce, J. (1999). Characteristics of epilepsy in a population based cohort of adults with learning disability. *Irish Journal of Psychological Medicine*, **16** (1), 5–9.

Deb, S., Matthews, T., Holt, G. & Bouras N. (eds.) (2001a). *Practice Guidelines for the Assessment and Diagnosis of Mental Health Problems in Adults with Intellectual Disability*. London: Pavilion Press. www.estiacentre.org.

Deb, S., Thomas, M. & Bright, C. (2001b). Mental disorder in adults with intellectual disability. 2: The rate of behaviour disorders among a community-based population aged between 16–64 years. *Journal of Intellectual Disability Research*, **45** (6), 506–14.

Dobyns, W. B. & Truwit, C. L. (1995). Lissencephaly and other malformations of cortical development: 1995 update. *Neuropediatric*, **26**, 132–47.

Espie, C. A., Gillies, J. B. & Montgomery, J. M. (1989). Antiepileptic polypharmacy, psychosocial behaviour and locus of control orientation among mentally handicapped adults living in the community. *Journal of Mental Deficiency Research*, **34**, 351–60.

Espie, C. A., Gillies, J. B. & Montgomery, J. M. (1990). Antiepileptic polypharmacy, psychosocial behaviour and locus of control orientation among mentally handicapped adults living in the community. *Journal of Mental Deficiency Research*, **34**, 351–60.

Espie, C. A., Watkins, J., Curtice, L. *et al.* (2003a). Psychopathology in people with epilepsy and intellectual disability; an investigation of potential explanatory variables. *Journal of Neurology Neurosurgery and Psychiatry*, **74**, 1485–92.

Espie, C. A., Watkins, J., Duncan, R. *et al.* (2003b). Perspective on epilepsy in people with intellectual disabilities: comparison of family carer, staff carer and clinician score profiles on the Glasgow Epilepsy Outcome Scale (GEOS). *Seizure*, **12**, 195–202.

Eubanks, J. H., Puranam, R. S., Kleckner, N. *et al.* (1993). The gene encoding the glutamate receptor subunit GluR5 is located on human chromosome 21q21.1–22.1 in the vicinity of the gene for familial amyotrophic lateral sclerosis. *Proceedings of National Academy of Science, USA*, **90**, 178–82.

Forsgren, l., Edvinsson, S. O., Blomquist, H. K., Heijbel, J. & Sidenvall, R. (1990). Epilepsy in a population of mentally retarded children and adults. *Epilepsy Research*, **6** (3), 234–48.

Gastaut, H., Morrin, G. and Leserve, N. (1995). Etudes du compartment des epileptiques psychomoteur dans l'interval de leurs crises. *Annals of Medical Psychology*, **113**, 1–29.

Geschwind, N. (1975). The clinical setting of aggression in temporal lobe epilepsy. In *Neural Basis of Violence and Aggression*, ed. W. S. Fields and W. H. Sweet. St. Louis, MI: Warren H. Green, pp. 273–81.

Goulden, K. J., Shinnar, S., Koller, H., Katz, M. & Richardson, S. A. (1991). Epilepsy in children with mental retardation; a cohort study. *Epilepsia*, **32** (5), 690–7.

Guerrant, J., Anderson, W. W., Fischer, A. *et al.* (1962). *Personality in Epilepsy*, Springfield, IL: C. C. Thomas.

Holthausen, H., Tuxhorn, I., Pieper, T. *et al.* (1999). Hemispherectomy in the treatment of neuronal migrational disorders. In *The Epilepsies: Etiology and Prevention* ed. Kotagal, P. & Lüders, H. O. San Diego, CA: Academic Press, pp. 93–102.

Kerr, M., Scheepers, M., Besag, F. *et al.* (2001). Clinical guidelines for the management of epilepsy in adults with an intellectual disability. *Seizure*, **10**, 401–9.

Kligman, D. and Goldberg, D. A. (1975). Temporal lobe epilepsy and aggression. *Journal of Nervous and Mental Diseases*, **160**, 324–41.

Landolt, H. (1958). Some clinical electroencephalographical correlations in epileptic psychoses (twilight states). *Electroencephalography and Clinical Neurophysiology*, **5**, 121.

Lehesjoki, A.-E., Koskiniemi, M., Sistonen, P. *et al.* (1991). Localisation of a gene for progressive myoclonus epilepsy to chromosome 21q22. *Proceedings of National Academy of Science*, USA, **88**, 3696–9.

Lewis, J. N., Tonge, B. J., Mowat, D. R. *et al.* (2000). Epilepsy and associated psychopathology in young people with intellectual disabilities. *Journal of Paediatric and Child Health*, **36** (2), 172–5.

Li, L. M., Fish, D. R., Sisodiya, S. M. *et al.* (1995). High resolution magnetic resonance imaging in adults with partial or secondary generalised epilepsy attending a tertiary referral unit. *Journal of Neurology, Neurosurgery, and Psychiatry*, **59**, 384–7.

Lishman, W. A. (1998). *Organic Psychiatry – The Psychological Consequences of Cerebral Disorder.* Oxford: Blackwell Science.

Lund, J. (1985). Epilepsy and psychiatric disorder in the mentally retarded adults. *Acta Psychiatrica Scandinavica*, **72**, 557–62.

Matson, J., Bamburg, J. W., Mayville, E. A. & Khan, I. (1999). Seizure disorders in people with intellectual disability: an analysis of differences in social functioning, adaptive functioning and maladaptive behaviours. *Journal of Intellectual Disability Research*, **43**, 531–9.

McEwan, M. J., Espie, C. A., Metcalfe, J., Brodie, M. J. & Wilson, M. T. (2004). Quality of life and psychosocial development in adolescents with epilepsy: a qualitative investigation using focus group methods. *Seizure*, **13**, 15–31.

McGrother, C. W., Hauck, A., Bhaumik, S., Thorp, C. & Taub, N. (1996). Community care for adults with learning disability and their carers: needs and outcome from the Leicestershire register. *Journal of Intellectual Disability Research*, **40** (2), 183–90.

Michelucci, R., Forti, A., Rubboli, G. *et al.* (1989). Mental retardation and behavioural disturbances related to epilepsy: a review. *Brain Dysfunction*, **2** (1), 3–9.

Mitchell, A. J. (2004). Treatment in patients with epilepsy. In *Neuropsychiatry and Behavioural Neurology Explained.* Edinburgh: Saunders, pp. 329–36.

Roberts, D. W. (1999). Corpus callosotomy in the treatment of neuronal migrational disorders. In *The Epilepsies: Etiology and Prevention*, ed. Kotagal, P. & Lüders, H. O. San Diego, CA: Academic Press, pp. 103–12.

Rodin, E. A. (1973). Psychomotor epilepsy and aggressive behaviour. *Archives of General Psychiatry*, **28**, 210–13.

Rutter, M., Tizard, J., Yule, W., Graham, P. & Whitmore, K. (1976). Research report: Isle of Wight studies 1964–1974. *Psychological Medicine*, **6**, 313–32.

Serafetinides, E. A. (1965). Aggressiveness in temporal lobe epileptics and its relation to cerebral dysfunction and environmental factors. *Epilepsia*, **6**, 33–42.

Shepherd, C. & Hosking, G. (1989). Epilepsy in school children with intellectual impairment in Sheffield: the size and nature of the problem and its implications in service provision. *Journal of Mental Deficiency Research*, **33**, 511–14.

Sillanpää, M. (1973). Medico-social prognosis of children with epilepsy. Epidemiological study and analysis of 245 cases. *Acta Paediatrica Scandinavica*, **237**, 1–104.

Sillanpää, M. (1999). Definitions and epidemiology. In *Epilepsy and Mental Retardation*, ed. Sillanpää. M., Gram, L., Johannessen, S. I. & Tomson, T. Philadelphia, PA: Wrightson Biomedical Publishing Limited, pp. 1–6.

Stafstorm, C. E. (1999). Mechanisms of epilepsy in mental retardation: insight from Angelman syndrome, Down syndrome and Fragile X syndrome. In *Epilepsy and Mental Retardation*, ed. Sillanpää, M., Gram, L., Johannessen, S. I. & Tomson, T. Philadelphia, PA: Wrightson Biomedical Publishing Limited, pp. 7–40.

Standage, K. F. & Fenton, G. W. (1975). Psychiatric symptom profiles of patients with epilepsy: a controlled investigation. *Psychological Medicine*, **5**, 152–60.

Steffenburg, U., Hagberg, G. & Kyllerman, M. (1996). Characteristics of seizures in a population-based series of mentally retarded children with active epilepsy. *Epilepsia*, **37**, 850–6.

Suzuki, H., Aihara, M. & Sugai, K. (1991). Severely retarded children in a defined area of Japan: prevalence rate, associated disabilities and causes. *Brain and Development*, **23**(1), 4–8.

Tellenbach, H. (1965). Epilepsie als Anfallsleiden und als Psychose. Über alternative Psychosen paranider Prägung bei "forced Normalisierung" (Landolt) des Elektroenzephalogramms Epileptischer. *Der Nervenartz*, **36**, 190–202.

Trevathan, E., Murphy, C. C. & Yeargin-Allsopp, M. (1997). Prevalence and descriptive epidemiology of Lennox–Gastaut syndrome among Atlanta children. *Epilepsia*, **38**, 1283–8.

Trimble, M. R. (2003). On the use of psychotropic drugs in patients with learning disability and epilepsy. In *Learning Disability and Epilepsy: An Integrative Approach*, ed. Trimble, M. R. Guildford: Clarius Press Ltd., pp. 161–78.

Wisniewski, K. E., French, J. H., Fernando, S. *et al.* (1985). Fragile X syndrome: associated neurological abnormalities. *Annals of Neurology*, **18**, 665–9.

16

Neuroimaging and intellectual disabilities

Max Pickard and Dene Robertson

Introduction

Neuroimaging has become progressively more clinically available over the past twenty years. Magnetic resonance imaging (MRI) and computerized tomography (CT) have, in particular, become part of mental health practice. These techniques have had an important role in furthering our understanding of the biological and neurophysiological basis for developmental disorders.

In this chapter, we will:

1. Highlight some of the available techniques.
2. Illustrate how they have been used to study normal brain development.
3. Highlight the main research findings for important neurodevelopmental conditions (fragile X syndrome, Down syndrome, velo-cardio-facial syndrome, and autism).
4. Discuss how neuroimaging can be used in clinical practice.

Neuroimaging techniques

Computerized tomography (CT) scanning

X-ray CT was developed from pre-existing X-ray technology in the 1970s. It involves measuring X-ray attenuation of thin tissue slices from multiple angles, and combining this information to create images of slices through the body. Clinically, CT is the investigation of choice for certain acute brain investigations (e.g. haemorrhage or trauma). It demonstrates bone and bleeds with excellent detail, but has several disadvantages when compared with magnetic resonance imaging. For example, soft tissue contrast is inferior to MRI; CT is particularly poor at the visualization of some brain areas bordering thick bone (e.g. posterior fossa and inferior temporal lobes) and it exposes the patient to ionizing radiation.

Psychiatric and Behavioural Disorders in Intellectual and Developmental Disabilities, ed. Nick Bouras and Geraldine Holt. Published by Cambridge University Press. © Cambridge University Press 2007.

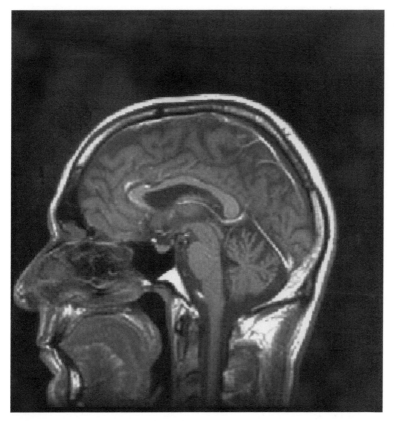

Fig. 16.1   MRI T1 weighted image: fluid appears dark and white matter is brighter than grey matter.

Magnetic resonance imaging (MRI)

The mechanism of action of MRI depends upon a property of biologically abundant atomic nuclei (e.g. ^{1}H, ^{31}P) with an uneven number of neutrons or protons called *spin*. The application of a powerful external magnetic field is applied which causes such nuclei to align with the field. A radio frequency burst is then applied which excites the nuclei into a higher energy state. The nuclei then emit the energy as a radio wave that can be detected by the MRI scanner. This process is known as *relaxation*.

There are two types of relaxation, known as T1 and T2. An MRI scanner can vary the applied radio frequency to give rise to predominantly T1 or T2 relaxation. The resulting MRI images are termed 'T1 weighted' or 'T2 weighted' respectively.

In T1 weighted images (Fig. 16.1), fluid appears dark, and white matter is brighter than grey matter. The T1 images are particularly useful at demonstrating neuro-anatomy. In T2 weighted images (Fig. 16.2), fluid appears bright, and grey matter brighter than white. The T2 images are particularly good at demonstrating brain oedema.

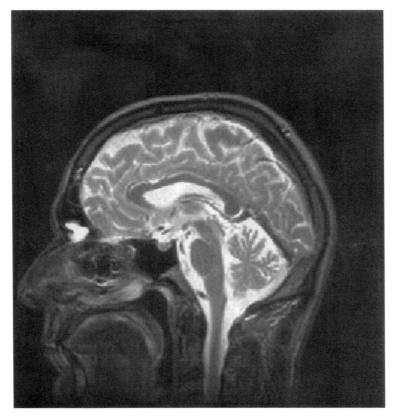

Fig. 16.2   MRI T2 weighted image: fluid appears bright and grey matter is brighter than white matter.

Overall, MRI offers outstanding soft tissue visualization, the ability to image the head in any plane, and importantly, a lack of any potentially harmful ionizing radiation. However, people undergoing MRI have to enter the narrow bore of the machine for a lengthy, noisy process during which they must remain still. Understandably, this may be particularly hard for a person with an intellectual disability (ID) (who may have a poor understanding of the process) and sedation may be required. In addition, because of the powerful magnetic field required for MRI, it cannot be used in people with metal implants (such as intracranial clips for aneurysms, cardiac pace makers, and cochlear implants). Suspicion that an implant might be present is a contra-indication to MRI scanning.

Magnetic resonance spectroscopy (MRS)

Magnetic resonance spectroscopy is a non-invasive technique that allows measurement of brain metabolites by measuring the spectra deriving from nuclei within particular chemical contexts.

Various important metabolites can be measured using MRS; for example, N-acetylaspartate (NAA) is a marker for neuronal density and may be reduced in conditions that cause neuronal death such as stroke (Bruhn *et al.*, 1989), tumour (Bruhn *et al.*, 1989), infections (Breiter *et al.*, 1994), and demyelinating diseases (Wolinsky *et al.*, 1990).

Positron emission tomography (PET)

Positron emission tomography requires the administration of radio-labelled compounds that emit positrons. These positrons give rise to the production of two photons when they collide with local electrons. These are detected by a system of photomultiplier tubes behind a collimator array and then used to form images.

Positron emission tomography is a flexible system, and various radiotracer compounds have been developed that have allowed imaging of receptor density/location, resting brain metabolism, and regional cerebral blood flow. In addition, changes in regional cerebral blood flow can be measured whilst a subject is performing a cognitive task. This enables investigation of (a) normal cognitive functioning, and (b) cognitive functioning in specific client groups.

Functional magnetic resonance imaging (fMRI)

The fMRI technique gives better image resolution than PET. It measures small signal changes related to changes in the concentration of deoxyhaemoglobin. As deoxyhaemoglobin is found at higher concentrations in metabolically active regions of the brain, and performing a cognitive task increases regional metabolic activity, fMRI allows identification of regions of brain involved with the cognitive task in question.

Normal brain development and ageing

Knowledge of normal brain development is essential in order to understand how brain structure and function may be modified in neurodevelopmental disorders.

Postmortem studies of the human brain demonstrate a quadrupling of brain size in the first decade, and very gradual decline thereafter (Debakan & Sadowsky, 1978). Myelination of neurones occurs at different rates in different locations of the brain. For example, the hippocampus does not become fully myelinated until the fourth decade of life, and does not have age-related cell loss until the fifth. In MRI studies it has been reported that white matter tracts are identifiable from one year of age, and that myelination continues into adolescence (e.g. Barkowich *et al.*, 1988; Christophe *et al.*, 1990; Holland *et al.*, 1986). White matter reaches a peak at around the age of 20 (Jernigan *et al.*, 1991a; Pfefferbaum *et al.*, 1994).

Table 16.1 Summary of neuroimaging techniques: advantages and disadvantages.

Imaging Technique	Advantages	Disadvantages
CT (Computerized tomography)	Good visualization of blood and fluids.	Exposure to ionizing radiation. Poor at soft tissue visualization. Poor visualization through thick bone.
MRI (Magnetic resonance imaging)	Excellent detail, particularly of soft tissue.	Cannot be used on clients with some implants (caution). Noisy, claustrophobic environment.
MRS (Magnetic resonance spectroscopy)	Measurement of concentration of metabolites in the CNS.	Relatively unavailable; primarily a research tool.
PET (Positron emission tomography)	Measurement of neuroreceptors, CNS metabolism, and cerebral blood flow.	Relatively unavailable; primarily a research tool.
fMRI (functional MRI)	High resolution of CNS activity.	Relatively unavailable; primarily a research tool.

It appears that age-related loss of brain tissue is mainly grey matter (Pfefferbaum et al., 1994, Resnick et al., 2003). As the brain ages, CSF (cerebro spinal fluid) also increases (Jernigan et al., 1991a; Jernigan et al., 1990; Jernigan et al., 1991b; Pfefferbaum et al., 1994). Age-related loss of brain tissue may vary from region to region; for example, the temporal lobes show less loss than the frontal lobes, with parieto-occipital regions relatively spared. (Resnick et al., 2000; DeCarli et al., 1994; Murphy et al., 1992).

Age-related changes may occur earlier in men than women (Kaye et al., 1992), although the progress of such changes may be faster in women once it occurs (Takeda & Matsuzawa, 1985). More recent MRI investigations have not been entirely consistent, although some have supported gender effects on brain imaging (e.g. Resnick et al., 2000).

Specific neurodevelopmental disorders

Autism

Autism has been the subject of much investigation as its aetiology remains elusive, although it is certainly a disorder of brain development. There has been a multitude of MRI studies of autism (for a comprehensive review see: Palmen and van Engeland, 2004). Generalized increase in brain volume has been a consistent finding, at least in males (Piven et al., 1995; Piven et al., 1996; Harden et al., 2001a), though it is not clear if this continues into adult life.

Cerebellar abnormalities are also a common research finding. Cerebellar hypoplasia has been reported (Courchesne *et al.*, 1988; Gafney *et al.*, 1987; Hashimoto *et al.*, 1995; Murakami *et al.*, 1989), though a more consistent finding is that of increased cerebellar volume (Herbert *et al.*, 2003; Sparks *et al.*, 2002; Harden *et al.*, 2001b; Piven *et al.* 1997a). Relative to controls, people with autism have reduced volume of the posterior regions of the corpus callosum (e.g. Saitoh *et al.*, 1995; Egaas *et al.*, 1995; Zilbovicius *et al.*, 1995), suggesting that people with autism may have deficits in inter-hemispheric communication.

Thus, although the specific nature of the structural findings in autism remains to a large extent unclear, the data are consistent with the hypothesis that people with autism have widespread abnormalities in brain development, and that these include deficits in inter-hemisphere connectivity. These may underlie the cognitive and social deficits seen in people with autism.

Fragile X syndrome (FRAX)

Fragile X syndrome is the commonest form of inherited ID. It is caused by an expansion of CGG triplet repeats (TRs) in the *fMR-1* gene on the X chromosome. Healthy normal subjects have up to approximately 50 TRs; pre-mutation carriers of FRAX have 50–200 TRs, and people with the full FRAX mutation have more than 200 TRs – causing inactivation of the *fMR-1* gene and consequently loss of gene expression (see also Chapter 12 by Hodapp and Dykens).

Developmental delay in those with FRAX varies considerably. Moreover, there are significant gender differences in the cognitive phenotype of FRAX. Most males with the FRAX full mutation have ID – usually in the moderate or severe range (Kemper *et al.*, 1986; Kemper *et al.*, 1988). The cognitive profile of relative strengths and weaknesses observed in FRAX females resembles that in FRAX males but is less severe and more variable (Freund & Reiss, 1991; Kemper *et al.*, 1986). In addition to an overall impairment of intelligence, people with FRAX have relatively greater deficits in attention, processing of sequential information, short-term memory, visual/spatial abilities, visual–motor coordination, and pragmatic language (Freund & Reiss, 1991; Kemper *et al.*, 1988; Sudhalter *et al.*, 1992; Sudhalter *et al.*, 1991). Thus, in FRAX some cognitive skills may be more susceptible to impairment than others, suggesting a possible selective role for the *fMR-1* gene's influence on brain development. This neuropsychological evidence for abnormal brain development in people with FRAX is supported by experimental evidence of changes in brain structure.

Structural MRI studies have reported deviations in the size of the cerebellar vermis, fourth ventricle, hippocampus and caudate volume which correlate with X activation ratio – the percentage of active X chromosomes carrying the FRAX mutation (Reiss *et al.*, 1995). Thus, specific cognitive difficulties and abnormalities in brain structure may result from relative lack of the gene product in brain areas normally having heavy *fMR-1* transcription.

Increased phenotypic expression of FRAX correlates with reduction in fragile X mental retardation protein (FMPR). Levels of FMPR are related to increased cortical activity during arithmetical tasks (Rivera *et al.*, 2002) and working memory tasks (Kwon *et al.*, 2001) in functional MRI experiments, suggesting that there is a gene-dosage dependent effect on brain development.

The behavioural phenotype of FRAX may include obsessional behaviours. Eliez *et al.* (2001) reported increased caudate nucleus volume in children with FRAX. The caudate nucleus has been implicated in the aetiology of obsessive-compulsive disorder, suggesting that caudate abnormalities may contribute to obsessive type behaviours in some children with FRAX.

Down syndrome (DS) and age-related change in the brain

People with DS have a high prevalence (and significant variation in severity) of ID and a high prevalence of age-related cognitive decline and Alzheimer's disease (Haxby, 1989; Shapiro *et al.*, 1989). However the neurobiological basis for this is unknown (see also Chapter 10 by Cooper and Holland).

A quantitative study of young adults with DS, using CT, reported decreased whole brain volume (Shapiro *et al.*, 1989). However, this may be accounted for by small stature and increased cranial cavity volume.

A volumetric MRI study of people with Down syndrome has reported decreased volume of frontal cortex and cerebellum, together with angulation of the brain stem. Also, there was less sulcal and gyral definition in the DS brains, together with abnormalities in the volume ratios of the hippocampus: parahippocampal gyrus and hippocampus: temporal cortex volumes (Kesslak *et al.*, 1994). Hippocampal area (even when corrected for head size) was significantly decreased, and was affected by ageing significantly more than in controls.

Tiepel *et al.* (2004) reported decreased grey matter in the medial temporal lobe and corpus callosum in non-demented adults with DS compared to normal controls. They suggest that the distribution and relative grey matter decrease may result from neuronal loss owing to underlying Alzheimer's disease pathology, which was not yet clinically manifest.

Velo-cardio-facial syndrome

Velo-cardio-facial syndrome (VCFS) is a genetic disorder caused by a deletion at chromosome 22q11. The size of the deletion varies, and the syndrome itself can present in a remarkably heterogeneous way, with consequences for both physical and mental health. The syndrome is of particular interest as it is strongly associated with ID (usually mild or borderline), psychotic disorders (10–30%), and other mental illness (Pulver *et al.*, 1994) (see also Chapter 12 by Hodapp and Dykens).

In a structural MRI study (van Amelsvoort *et al.*, 2001), people with VCFS had decreased cerebellar and right temporal grey matter volumes, and increased grey matter volumes in the left temporal lobe and parts of the frontal lobes compared with controls. In addition, regional decreases in white matter volume were reported in frontal lobes bilaterally, with excess white matter in the corpus callosum. Anatomical abnormalities of the septum pellucidum were also noted. Children with VCFS may have relatively greater deficits in white matter than grey matter volume (Eliez *et al.*, 2000; Kates *et al.*, 2001).

These findings are of interest in that they aid development of a convergent model of brain development in psychotic illnesses and ID (from genetic, neurobiological, anatomical, and functional perspectives). In Kates' sample, the most prominent cognitive deficits were in judgement of spatial orientation and phonological processing, which require temporal and parietal lobe processing, and then transmission of that information to the frontal lobe via cortico-cortical networks. Abnormalities of white matter in these areas may underlie disruption of the cortico-cortical transmission, which in turn gives rise to the neuropsychological deficits seen in VCFS. Such white matter abnormalities suggest that the chromosomal abnormality that causes VCFS (22q11 deletion) gives rise to neurodevelopmental abnormality in myelination.

Brain imaging in clinical practice

Magnetic resonance imaging scanning has significantly altered the risk/benefit ratio in considering who should undergo neuroimaging. Most importantly, there is no longer any need to subject the person to potentially harmful radiation. Excepting people with implants, who cannot be subject to high-intensity magnetic fields, and those who would find the tight enclosure of the scanner traumatic, MRI scanning is the structural neuroimaging investigation of choice.

There is an association between structural brain abnormalities and ID, which becomes stronger as the severity of ID increases. It is estimated that around one-third of people with ID have abnormalities that can be detected by structural neuroimaging (Deb, 1997; van Karnebeek *et al.*, 2005). However, these abnormalities are non-specific.

Significant traumatic brain injury during the developmental period may be apparent on neuroimaging. Perinatal CNS insults such as those that give rise to cerebral palsy have characteristic neuroimaging findings including smaller brain volume, dilated lateral ventricles and porencephalic cavities (Suvossa *et al.*, 1990). The cerebral dysgenesis caused by disorders of neuronal migration (which are often associated with epilepsy) also have characteristic appearances including macrogyria, polymicrogyria and heterotopias (Palmini *et al.*, 1991). However, whilst 'syndromal' causes of ID (as reviewed above), may give rise to characteristic neuroimaging findings when data from multiple cases are pooled together, such appearances are unlikely to be detected in an individual and do not yet have diagnostic utility. Van Karnebeek *et al.* (2005), in a review of the literature, concluded that there was only a 1.3% yield of positive diagnosis from neuroradiological investigations of people with a ID. Thus, neuroimaging only rarely has a role in determining the aetiology of ID. This is not surprising, as in many cases cause of ID remains unknown.

All clients who have or are at significant risk of progressive brain pathology should have baseline structural MRI for possible future comparison (should the clinical picture change). In the field of ID psychiatry, the most obvious candidates for neuroimaging are people with Down syndrome, where there is a high incidence of Alzheimer-type histological brain changes (and frank Alzheimer's disease) with increasing age. Given the difficulty of accurate diagnosis of Down syndrome-related dementia, it is our view that such baseline neuroimaging has a particularly important role to play. The age at which such routine scanning should be performed is debatable. Structural neuroimaging at age 35–40 years has the advantage of being likely to precede visible neuroimaging changes caused by the disease process, whilst not being so chronologically distant from such changes so as to impair the validity of comparison. More research is needed to properly evaluate the value of screening tools (neuroimaging, psychometric, and other) in the case of Down syndrome and dementia.

What of the person with ID who is not at increased risk of progressive brain pathology? Without a baseline measure it is difficult to differentiate new pathology from old. For example, it is common clinical experience for a structural brain scan from a person with ID to be reported as containing 'cortical atrophy'. However, without a baseline scan, it is impossible to establish whether such appearances are caused by cerebral dysgenesis (i.e. are neurodevelopmental in origin) or true atrophy (loss of tissue).

Aside from the value of neuroimaging in ID, there is also the value of neuroimaging in co-morbid mental illness to consider. As this book details, the level of psychiatric morbidity in the ID population is considerably above that in the non-ID population. Moreover, diagnosis is often more challenging. Neuroimaging is often used as part of generic psychiatric assessment, particularly for eliminating the possibility of an organic aetiology for psychiatric symptoms (such as an intracranial space occupying lesion). In people with ID, where the communication of the subtle symptoms of mental illness may be impaired, the use of neuroimaging to rule out organic pathology is at least as important as in the non-ID population. Further, accuracy of psychiatric diagnosis drops with increasing levels of ID, suggesting that the risk of missing an organic aetiology for mental illness is greater. Thus, the threshold for structural neuroimaging should be progressively lower the greater the degree of ID.

Neuroimaging has as yet highly limited value in the diagnosis of major mental illness. The most commonly cited changes in brain structure are those occurring in schizophrenia, and there is a large literature on this subject in non-ID populations. In a study of people who had schizophrenia and mild ID, Sanderson *et al.* (1999) reported decreased brain volume and larger ventricles compared with non-ID controls without schizophrenia. These structural changes were more closely related to those of people with schizophrenia but no ID than those of people with ID but no schizophrenia. These authors suggest that it is the schizophrenic disease process that leads to a co-morbid ID, rather than the presence of an ID per se that gives rise to the increased rate of psychotic disorders in this group.

Neuroimaging has been used in the investigation of behaviour outside of the realms of ID and of major mental illness. For example, structural and functional changes have been reported in prefrontal/subcortical brain regions of people who demonstrate violent behaviours, criminality, and sexual offending (Bassarath, 2001, for review). Similar brain regions are implicated in the aetiology of behavioural problems found in attention deficit hyperactivity disorder (Roth & Saykin, 2004 for a review). Further research is likely to shed additional light on the aetiology of other challenging behaviours, in people both with and without ID.

In a person who demonstrates behavioural abnormalities and has a structurally abnormal brain, it is often possible to hypothesize how the behaviour of the individual relates to the structure of the brain. Many clinicians, carers, clients and relatives find it helpful to know *why* an individual behaves in a particular way, where this is possible. Neuroimaging may also be useful in informing psychosocial treatment plans. For example, it may be unrealistic to design a treatment programme requiring a particular neuropsychological function when a person has structural abnormalities in the brain region that underlies it.

Conclusion

It is clear that when considering whether to proceed with structural neuroimaging, the clinician has to balance many clinical factors; these are summarized in Table 16.2. As with all investigations and interventions, the person's capacity to consent should be determined. In cases where capacity is not present, it is good practice to seek the views of the nearest relatives and members of the multidisciplinary team in order to determine the best interests of the client.

Table 16.2 Summary of clinical factors for consideration before the use of structural neuroimaging.

Factors for	Factors against
Focal neurological signs.	Normal physical and neurological examination.
Other investigations suggesting organic pathology; e.g. localized EEG abnormalities, raised serum prolactin, psychometric testing suggesting particular areas of cognitive deficit.	Normal investigations.
Pattern of symptoms not fitting into those of classical psychiatric illness.	Symptom profile has good fit with a psychiatric diagnosis.
Psychiatric symptoms suggestive of brain pathology (e.g. olfactory hallucinations, specific cognitive deficits).	Absence of such symptoms.
Evidence of change in level of cognitive abilities (from behaviour or psychometric testing).	No change in cognitive abilities.
Atypical age of presentation of neurological or psychiatric illness (e.g. schizophrenia presenting past the age of 40, late-onset epilepsy).	Normal age of presentation.
Medical or family history which raises risk of intracerebral pathology (e.g. cardiovascular or stroke risk, head injury, neurofibramotosis).	No risk factors for intracerebral pathology.
Suspected CNS pathology is potentially treatable (e.g. intracerebral tumour).	Suspected pathology would not be treatable (although diagnosis may inform prognosis and psychosocial management).
Procedure would be tolerated by client.	Procedure would not be tolerated, or would require sedation/general anaesthetic.
Patient is at high risk of a future progressive neurological disorder (e.g. Down syndrome and dementia).	No such risk.

Summary points

- Neuroimaging has become more available, refined, and clinically valuable.
- Neuroimaging also provides a valuable investigative tool for examination of environmental and genetic factors in brain development and ageing.
- However, neuroimaging remains a limited resource, and the decision about when to use is complex and multifactorial.
- People with an intellectual disability will often have morphometrically abnormal brains, which can be examined with neuroimaging.
- As with all investigations and interventions, capacity to consent must be assessed. If absent, an individual's best interests should guide the decision on whether to proceed with neuroimaging.

Acknowledgments

Our thanks to Declan Murphy, who was an author on this chapter in the first edition of this book.

REFERENCES

Barkowich, A. J., Kjos, B. O., Jackson, D. E. & Norman, D. (1988). Normal maturation of the neonatal and infant brain: MR imaging at 1.5T. *Neuroradiology*, **166**, 173–180.

Bassarath, L. (2001). Neuroimaging studies of antisocial behaviour. *Canadian Journal of Psychiatry*, **46**. 728–32.

Breiter, S. N., Arroyo, S., Mathews, V. P. *et al.* (1994). Proton, M. R. spectroscopy in patients with seizure disorders. *American Journal of Neuroradiology*, **15**, 373–84.

Bruhn, H., Frahm, J., Geyngell, M. L. *et al.* (1989). Non-invasive differentiation of tumours with use of localised H-1 MR spectroscopy in vivo: initial experience in patients with cerebral tumours. *Radiology*, **172**, 541–8.

Christophe, C., Muller, M. F., Baleriaux, D. *et al.* (1990). Mapping of normal brain maturation in infants on phase-sensitive inversion-recovery images. *Neuroradiology*, **32**, 173–8.

Courchesne, E., Yeung-Courchesne, R., Press, G., Hussein, J. R. & Jernigan, T. L. (1988). Hypoplasia of cerebellar vermal lobules V1 and V11 in autism. *New England Journal of Medicine*, **318**, 1349–54.

Deb, S. (1997). Structural neuroimaging in learning disability. *British Journal of Psychiatry*, **171**, 417–19.

Debakan, A. S. & Sadowsky, D. (1978). Changes in brain weights during the span of human life: relation of brain weights to body heights and body weights. *Annals of Neurology*, **4**, 345–356.

DeCarli, C. D., Murphy, D. G. M., Gillette, J. A. *et al.* (1994). Lack of age-related differences in temporal lobe volume of very healthy adults. *American Journal of Neuroradiology*, **15**, 689–96.

Egaas, B., Courchesne, E. & Saitoh, O. (1995). Reduced size of corpus callosum in autism. *Archives of Neurology*, **52**, 794–801.

Eliez, S., Blassey, C. M., Freund, L. S., Hastie, T. & Reiss, A. L. (2001). Brain anatomy, gender and IQ in children and adolescents with fragile X syndrome. *Brain*, **214**. 1610–18.

Eliez, S., White, C., Schmitt, E., Menon, V. & Reiss, A. (2000). Children and adolescents with velocardiofacial syndrome: a volumetric study. *American Journal of Psychiatry*, **157**, 409–15.

Freund, L. S. & Reiss, A. L. (1991). Cognitive profiles associated with Fra (X) syndrome in males and females. *American Journal of Medical Genetics*, **38**, 542–7.

Gafney, G. R., Tsai, L. Y., Kuperman, S. & Minchin, S. (1987). Cerebellar structure in autism. *American Journal of Diseases in Children*, **141**, 1330–2.

Harden, A. Y., Minshew, N. J., Mallikarjuhn, M. & Keveshan, M. S. (2001a). Brain volume in autism. *Journal of Child Neurology*, **16**, 421–4.

Harden, A. Y., Minshew, N. J., Mallikarjuhn, M. & Keveshan, M. S. (2001b). Posterior fossa magnetic resonance imaging in autism. *Journal of American Child and Adolescent Psychiatry*, **40**, 666–72.

Hashimoto, T., Tayama, M., Murakawa, K. *et al.* (1995). Development of the brainstem and cerebellum in autistic patients. *Journal of Autism and Developmental Disorders*, **25**, 1–18.

Haxby, J. V. (1989). Neuropsychological evaluation of adults with Down syndrome: patterns of selective impairment in non-demented old adults. *Journal of Mental Deficiency Research*, **33**, 193–210.

Herbert, M. R., Ziegler, D. A., Deutch, C. K. *et al.* (2003). Dissociations of cerebral cortex, subcortical and cerebral white matter volumes in autistic boys. *Brain*, **126**, 1182–92.

Holland, B. A., Haas, D. K., Norman, D., Brant-Zawadski, M. & Newton, T. H. (1986). MRI of normal brain maturation. *American Journal of Neuroradiology*, **7**, 201–8.

Jernigan, T. L., Archibald, S. L., Berhow, M. T. *et al.* (1991a). Cerebral structure on MRI, Part 1: Localization of age-related changes. *Biological Psychiatry*, **29**, 55–67.

Jernigan, T. L., Press, G. A. & Hesselink, J. R. (1990). Methods for measuring brain morphologic features on magnetic resonance images: Validation and normal aging. *Archives of Neurology*, **47**, 27–32.

Jernigan, T. L., Salmon, D., Butters, N. *et al.* (1991b). Cerebral structure on MRI, Part II: Specific changes in Alzheimer's and Huntington's diseases. *Biological Psychiatry*, **29**, 68–81.

Kates, W. R., Burnette, C. P., Jabs., E. W. *et al.* (2001). Regional cortical white matter reductions in velocardiofacial syndrome: A volumetric MRI analysis. *Society of Biological Psychiatry*, **49**, 677–84.

Kaye, J. A., DeCarli, C. D., Luxenberg, J. S. & Rapoport, S. I. (1992). The significance of age-related enlargement of the cerebral ventricles in healthy men and women measured by quantitative computed x-ray tomography. *Journal of the American Geriatric Society*, **40**, 225–31.

Kemper, M. B., Hagerman, R. J., Ahmad, R. S., Ahmad, R. S. & Mariner, R. (1986). Cognitive profiles and the spectrum of clinical manifestations in heterozygous fragile-X females. *American Journal of Medical Genetics*, **23**, 139–56.

Kemper, M. B., Hagerman, R. J. & Altshul-Stark, D. (1988). Cognitive profiles of boys with the fragile-X syndrome. *American Journal of Human Genetics*, **30**, 191–200.

Kesslak, J. P., Nagata, B. S., Lott, M. D. & Nalcoiglu, O. (1994). Magnetic resonance imaging analysis of brain age-related changes in the brains of individuals with Down's syndrome. *Neurology*, **44**, 1039–45.

Kwon, H., Menon, V., Eliez, S. *et al.* (2001). Functional neuroanatomy of visuo-spatial working memory in fragile X syndrome: relation to behavioural and molecular measures. *American Journal of Psychiatry*, **158**, 1040–51.

Murakami, J., Courchesne, E., Press, G., Yeung-Courchesne, R. & Hesselink, J. (1989). Reduced cerebellar hemisphere size and its relationship to vermal hypoplasia in autism. *Archives of Neurology*, **46**, 689–94.

Murphy, D. G. M., DeCarli, C. D., Schapiro, M. B., Rapoport, S. I. & Horwitz, B. (1992). Age-related differences in volumes of subcortical nuclei, brain matter, and cerebrospinal fluid in healthy men as measured with MRI. *Archives of Neurology*, **49**, 839–49.

Palmen, C. M. J. S, and van Engeland, H. (2004). Review on structural neuroimaging findings in autism. *Journal of Neural Transmission*, **111**, 903–29.

Palmini, A., Andermann, F., Olivier, A. *et al.* (1991). Focal neurnal migration disorders and intractable partial epilepsy: a study of 30 patients. *Annals of Neurology*, **30**, 741–9.

Pfefferbaum, A., Mathalon, D. H., Sullivan, E. V. *et al.* (1994). A quantitative magnetic resonance imaging study of changes in brain morphology from infancy to late adulthood. *Archives of Neurology*, **51**, 874–87.

Piven, J., Arndt, S., Bailey, J. & Andreasen, N. (1996). Regional brain enlargement in autism: a magnetic resonance imaging study. *Journal of American Child and Adolescent Psychiatry*, **35**, 530–6.

Piven, J., Arndt, S., Bailey, J. *et al.* (1995). An MRI study of brain size in autism. *American Journal of Psychiatry*, **152**, 1145–9.

Piven, J., Saliba, K., Bailey, J. & Arndt, S. (1997a). An MRI study of autism: the cerebellum revisited. *Neurology*, **49**, 546–51.

Pulver, A. E., Nestadt, G., Goldberg, R. *et al.* (1994). Psychotic illness in patients diagnosed with velo-cardio-facial syndrome and their relatives. *Journal of Nervous and Mental Disease*, **182**, 476–8.

Reiss, A. L., Abrams, M. T., Greenlaw, R., Freund, L. & Denckla, M. (1995). Neurodevelopmental effects of the FMR-1 full mutation in humans. *Nature Medicine*, **1**, 159–67.

Resnick, S. M., Goldszal, A. F., Davatszikos, C. *et al.* (2000). One year age changes in MRI brain volumes in older adults. *Cerebral Cortex*, **10**(5), 464–72.

Resnick, S. M., Pham, D. L., Kraut, M. A., Zonderman, A. B. & Davastzikos, C. (2003). Longitudinal magnetic resonance imaging studies of older adults: a shrinking brain. *Neuropsychologica*, **23**(8), 3259–301.

Rivera, S. M., Menon, V., White, C. D. *et al.* (2002). Functional brain activation during arithmetic processing in females with fragile X syndrome is related to FMR1 protein expression. *Human Brain Mapping*, **16**, 206–18.

Roth, R. M. & Saykin, A. J. (2004). Executive dysfunction in attention-deficit / hyperactivity disorder: cognitive and neuroimaging findings. *Psychiatric Clinics of North America*, **27**, 83–96.

Saitoh, O., Courchesne, E., Egaas, B., Lincoln, A. J. & Screibman, L. (1995). Cross-sectional area of the posterior hippocampus in autistic patients with cerebellar and corpus callosum abnormalities. *Neurology*, **45**, 317–24.

Sanderson, T. L., Best, J. J. K., Doody., G. A., Cunningham Owens, D. G. & Johnstone, E. C. (1999). Neuroanatomy of comorbid schizophrenia and learning disability: a controlled study. *The Lancet*, **354**, 1867–71.

Shapiro, M. B., Luxenberg, J., Kaye, J. *et al.* (1989). Serial quantitative CT analysis of brain morphometrics in adult Down Syndrome at different ages. *Neurology*, **39**, 1349–53.

Sparks, B. F., Friedman, F. D., Shaw, D. W. *et al.* (2002). Brain structural abnormalities in young children with autism spectrum disorder. *Neurology*, **59**, 184–92.

Sudhalter, V., Maranion, M. & Brooks, P. (1992). Expressive semantic deficit in the production language of males with fragile X syndrome. *American Journal of Medical Genetics*, **43** (1–2), 65–71.

Sudhalter, V., Scarborough, H. S. & Cohen, I. L. (1991). Syntactic delay and pragmatic deviance in the language of fragile X males. *American Journal of Medical Genetics*, **38**, 493–7.

Suvossa, J., Seidl, Z. & Faber, J. (1990). Hemiparesis of cerebral palsy in relation to epilepsy and mental retardation. *Developmental and Child Neurology*, **32**, 792–4.

Takeda, S. & Matsuzawa, T. (1985). Age-related brain atrophy: A study with computed tomography. *Journal of Gerentology*, **40**, 159–63.

Tiepel, S. J., Alexander, G. E., Schapiro, M. B. *et al.* (2004). Age-related cortical grey matter reductions in non-demented Down's syndrome adults determined by MRI with voxel-based morphometry. *Brain*, **127**(Pt 4), 811–24.

Van Amelsvoort, E., Daly, E., Robertson, D. *et al.* (2001). Structural brain abnormalities associated with deletion at chromosome 22q11: Quantative neuroimaging study of adults with velo-cardio-facial syndrome. *British Journal of Psychiatry*, **178**, 412–19.

Van Karnebeek, C. D., Jansweijer, M. C., Leenders, A. G., Offringa, M. & Hennekam, R. C. (2005). Diagnostic investigations in individuals with mental retardation: a systemic literature review of their usefulness. *European Journal of Human Genetics*, **13**(1), 6–25.

Wolinsky, J. S., Narayana, P. A. & Fenstermacher, M. J. (1990). Proton magnetic resonance spectroscopy in multiple sclerosis. *Neurology*, **40**, 1764–9.

Zilbovicius, M., Garrau, B., Samson, Y. *et al.* (1995). Delayed maturation of the frontal cortex in childhood autism. *American Journal of Psychiatry*, **152**, 248–52.

Part III

Treatment and therapeutic interventions

17

Treatment methods for destructive and aggressive behaviour in people with severe developmental and intellectual disabilities

R. Matthew Reese, Jessica Hellings and Stephen Schroeder

Introduction

People with severe developmental intellectual disabilities (ID) are increasingly being supported in community living programmes. Adequate community support involves effectively treating such behavioural difficulties as property destruction, aggression and self-injurious behaviour. The treatment of aggressive and destructive behaviour in these people has resulted in greater emphasis being placed on understanding the causes of such behaviours in any particular individual. Behavioural, medical and neuropsychiatric knowledge has developed rapidly, as have psychopharmacologic treatments. Progress is being made on integrating information from diverse fields such as genetics, neurology, medicine, and behavioural psychology (Schroeder et al., 2002). Effective team models are being developed to promote collaboration from medical and behavioural professions (Freeman et al., 2005; Koegel et al., 1996; Singh et al., 2002).

In this chapter we propose an integrated team approach for assessment and treatment of destructive and aggressive behaviour in people with severe ID. We will begin the chapter by first identifying some of the often-missed physical illnesses and neuropsychiatric conditions that can precipitate or worsen destructive and aggressive behaviour. The treating clinician is dependent on observations made in this regard by care givers of the person. Clinicians need to take a thorough medical, medication and neuropsychiatric history.

Second, behavioural assessment and treatment for destructive and aggressive behaviour are reviewed. We emphasize that researchers and clinicians using the behavioural approach are joining forces with medical and neuropsychiatric professionals in this field.

In the final section of this chapter, a model is proposed for effectively establishing treatment protocols for the individual who exhibits destructive and aggressive

Psychiatric and Behavioural Disorders in Intellectual and Developmental Disabilities, ed. Nick Bouras and Geraldine Holt. Published by Cambridge University Press. © Cambridge University Press 2007.

behaviour. The model is based on the work at the University of Kansas in establishing a state-wide system of Positive Behaviour Support (Freeman *et al.*, 2005).

Medical Perspective

Early assessment and treatment of underlying medical conditions is essential. Severe behaviour problems such as self-injury and aggression have been linked to pain (Breau *et al.*, 2003). Because people with severe ID are often non-verbal, they often cannot relate feelings of pain or illness. Fortunately, there has been increased attention to risk factors for pain (Breau *et al.*, 2004). Researchers have also explored non-verbal indications of pain or illness in people with severe ID (Zwakhalen *et al.*, 2004). Pain may cause significant problems if individuals are pressured to perform their usual tasks when feeling ill. The person may co-operate poorly with formal medical examinations. Thus, vigilance for acute, intermediate or chronic signs of pain and illness is essential so that diagnosis and treatment can be tailored to the underlying condition. Some, but by no means all, of the important clinical signs described below are examples of the authors' medical approach. These include intercurrent infections, allergies and medication side effects, which commonly occur but are often missed by caregivers and general clinicians.

Gastrointestinal disturbances are commonly overlooked, and may manifest as food refusal, self-induced vomiting, or the repeated discarding of food at mealtimes. Such disturbances, as well as appetite change, constipation or diarrhoea, may also be caused by medication side effects. Menstrual discomfort may contribute to severe behaviour problems (Carr *et al.*, 2003). Dental or periodontal disease may disturb eating. Eating disturbances may have an effect on problematic behaviour (Wacker *et al.*, 1996). The possibility of silent oesophageal or intestinal obstruction, such as caused by pica (eating of non-food items), or other missed abdominal crises underscores the need for specialist referral in any case that is not settling.

In the not infrequent case of intercurrent infections of the gastrointestinal, respiratory or genitourinary systems, flushing of the face associated with sweating or fever may be missed. Some detectable but often-missed physical signs of respiratory tract infections may include hoarseness, cough, or a nasal or ear discharge. Recurrent pulling or self-hitting of an ear, the head or face may occur in persons with infections of the ears, sinuses, nose or throat. Some individuals may insert objects into their ears in the presence of ear infections. Infections of the bladder or kidneys may present as a new onset of repeated day- or night-time wetting. The person may cry in pain when urinating or appear preoccupied with touching the genital region. Foul-smelling urine may be noted. Various dermatological problems may cause behavioural problems in association with generalized discomfort, persistent itching or irritation. Examples of conditions caused by infection include scabies, impetigo and fungal infections of skin folds (see also Chapter 5 by Lennox). Most medications can cause skin rash as an allergic reaction; in some cases, this may be caused by colouring dyes rather than the active drug.

Seasonal allergies such as hay fever may cause restlessness and behavioural agitation. Signs of allergies may include persistent redness, rubbing or running of the eyes and nose. Antihistamines and combination cold or allergy preparations used as treatments may also cause behavioural deterioration. Electrolyte and metabolic disturbances require correction, and this in turn may dramatically decrease associated behavioural problems. Examples of such disturbances include thyroid and parathyroid under-activity or over-activity, and pancreatic insulin-producing tumours. A low serum sodium affecting mental status may be owing to treatment with the anticonvulsant medication carbamazepine (Kastner *et al.*, 1992). Medication side effects may include aggression and can occur in association with medications of many classes. It is worth stating that a carefully taken, detailed treatment history is essential to identify any potential drug-related cause of the problem. In such cases, the behavioural deterioration may date to the time the drug was started or increased. Substituting the suspect medication, for example phenobarbital or phenytoin prescribed for epilepsy, with a newer antiseizure agent such as valproate may eliminate the aggression (Trimble, 1990) (see also Chapter 15 by Deb). The same principle applies to cough and cold medicines, antihypertensive preparations, especially those containing reserpine, hormone preparations such as the contraceptive pill, and many others. Benzodiazepines are recognized as causing behavioural disinhibition in this population and are generally avoided. Akathisia (agitation and motor restlessness) may occur in this population if the dose of antipsychotic medication is increased too rapidly, or in some individuals who are unable to tolerate the drug (Hellings *et al.*, 2006). Hunger related to impaired satiation caused by atypical antipsychotic drugs such as olanzepine, risperidone (Hellings *et al.*, 2001) or quetiapine may produce aggression related to food seeking. Antidepressants may produce agitation, especially in higher doses (see also Chapter 19 by King).

Genetic/neuropsychiatric perspective

There has been increased interest in behavioural phenotypes of various genetic disorders. Psychiatric conditions and destructive and aggressive behaviour may be part of the behavioural phenotype for particular genetic syndromes (see Chapter 12 by Hodapp and Dykens). People with any congenital ID syndrome, including Down syndrome, fragile X syndrome, Prader–Willi syndrome (Hellings & Warnock,

1994) and the rarer syndromes such as Rubinstein–Taybi syndrome (Hellings *et al.*, 2002), can present with aggressive or destructive behaviour related to medical or psychiatric illness, or to seizures related to that syndrome. Reese *et al.* (2006) have suggested how phenotypic characteristics may interact with specific types of environmental situations to increase the likelihood of aggressive and destructive behaviour.

With respect to neurological disorders, behavioural deterioration may occur during or between seizure episodes, or may be caused by side effects of certain anticonvulsant medications (Blumer, 1984; Trimble, 1990; Umbrick *et al.*, 1995).

Although the task is a more difficult one when the individual involved is non-verbal, it may be possible to diagnose and thus treat psychiatric conditions using DSM-IV or ICD-10 based criteria other than speech (Sovner & Fogelman, 1996). There has been increased research in examining and assessing how psychiatric conditions such as mood disorders are expressed in people with severe ID (Ross & Oliver, 2003) (see also Chapter 4 by Hemmings). For example, the manic-like signs of euphoria, irritability, over-activity, pacing, insomnia and hypersexuality, co-occurring with rapid flaring to aggression, may respond well to mood stabilizers such as valproate, lithium and gabapentin (Lowry, 1997; Hellings, 1999; Hellings *et al.*, 2005; Hellings *et al.*, 2006). Low-dose serotonin reuptake inhibitors such as sertraline or fluoxetine may prove useful in many cases, though controlled studies are needed (Hellings & Warnock, 1994; Hellings *et al.*, 1996). (A full discussion of the use of pharmacotherapeutic agents is provided in Chapter 19 by King.)

Behavioural perspective

The behavioural perspective assumes that problem behaviours such as destruction and aggression are learned, and are largely affected by environmental antecedents and consequences. A current trend in behavioural treatment is for practitioners to conduct a functional assessment of problem behaviours. This assessment refers to a collection of procedures that are used to assess the relationship between physiological and environmental events and problem behaviours. Functional assessment includes operationally defining the behaviour and measuring its frequency, intensity and duration. Functional assessment also involves examining the physiological and environmental variables that may relate to behaviour problems, and identifying the function, or any reinforcer for, challenging behaviours. The expansion of functional assessment methodology to examine medical and neuropsychiatric conditions, and how these conditions interface with learning appropriate and inappropriate behaviours, provides a link between medical and behavioural models (see also Chapter 18 by Benson and Havercamp). Recently, there has been interest in looking at quality-of-life variables that may affect problem behaviours. The next section of this chapter examines important environmental and physiological setting events, potential functions, and quality-of-life variables that may affect aggressive and destructive behaviours in people with severe ID.

Setting events

Setting events are conditions that precede and surround behaviour and affect the stimulus–response or response–consequence relationships (Kantor, 1959; Bijou & Baer, 1978; Wahler & Fox, 1981). Environmental setting conditions might include group size, population density, staff ratio, noise level, and room temperature (Reese & Leder, 1990). Biological setting events include illness, hunger, sleep, behavioural state, pain or psychiatric irritability (Didden *et al.*, 2002; Guess & Carr, 1991; Lowry, 1992; Rojahn *et al.*, 1993; Carr & Smith, 1995; Reese, 1997). Social setting events include unpredictable schedule changes, confrontational interchanges, and interaction styles (Horner *et al.*, 1996).

Consequence analysis

As noted above, the purpose of a functional assessment is to identify the re-inforcers for problem behaviours. There has been accumulating evidence that problem behaviours may have different functions, and that the same behaviour may have multiple functions in the same individual (Neef, 1994). Carr (1994) has described attention, escape, sensory reinforcement and obtaining tangible events as key potential functions for aggressive and destructive behaviours.

O'Neill *et al.* (1990) developed a matrix of possible functions of problem behaviours. The matrix included two broad categories: obtain or escape/avoid. In each of these categories, there is a subdivision of biological events, or external environmental events. Thus, the person may exhibit problem behaviours to obtain attention, tangible items, or sensory reinforcement. Similarly, the behaviours may be used to escape difficult tasks, demands, undesirable events, pain or undesirable sensory stimulation.

Identifying the functions and the potential reinforcers for the problem behaviour is important in developing treatment procedures. For example, Carr and Durand (1985) demonstrated that problem behaviours may have a communicative function, and that the individual may be better served by learning communicative strategies that could replace problem behaviours in obtaining reinforcement. An example is a young female with autism and severe epilepsy who was able to learn to say 'excuse me' to her mother to get her attention, rather than biting, scratching or choking her. There has been increased attention to the use of a procedure termed Functional Communication Training as a means of teaching functionally equivalent replacement skills (Hagopian *et al.*, 1998).

Quality-of-life analysis

Risley (1996) has described a level of analysis beyond what is in a functional assessment. He indicates that we consider life arrangement, and that some individuals need 'to get a life' as an effective treatment for their problem behaviours. Risley states that it is important to ask questions such as, 'How is the person doing overall, over time?' 'Is the person happy, satisfied and safe in their environment?' 'Does the person have a stable home, family, and friends in which to base his or her life and future?' 'Is the person productive and developing new interests, friends and skills over time?' One commonly used strategy is to hire a responsible high school or college student to take the teenager or young adult out to do preferred activities once or twice a week. The person's parents are advised to pay the individual as they would a sitter or respite worker.

Sprague and Horner (1995) and Kincaid (1996) propose similar analyses and suggest that person-centred planning needs to be a vital part of a positive behaviour support plan. There has been increasing evidence that improving quality of life (Lucyshyn et al., 2002) such as scheduling events that improve mood, interest and pleasure can be important treatment components.

Functional assessment methods

There are a number of direct and indirect methods to collect functional assessment data. One indirect method is to conduct a behavioural interview (Bailey & Pyles, 1989; O'Neill et al., 1990). The purpose of this interview is to obtain information regarding the topography of the behaviour problem, potential triggers, setting events, consequence events, and other variables that may be maintaining the behaviour. The interview may structure a more direct approach at observing the individual and the behaviour problems. Lennox and Miltenberger (1989) have pointed out some limitations of only using interviews. For example, the interview does not include direct observation to the behaviour and potential controlling variables. There may be faulty recollection of events, observer bias and observer expectations.

Another indirect method is to use behaviour rating scales, checklists and questionnaires. For example, answers to the 16-question Motivational Assessment Scale (Durand & Crimmins, 1988) can provide information about the potential functions or reinforcers that are maintaining the problem behaviour. Major drawbacks with these scales are reliability and validity (Sprague & Horner, 1995). Because of this, direct observation methods are often preferable to just using interviews and checklists. An observation method used to examine contextual variables that may be related to the behaviour problem is a scatter plot (Touchette et al., 1985). A scatter plot is a two-sided matrix with space for behaviour codes recorded across multiple times and days. The scatter plot is used to determine times in which the behaviour problem occurs at high and low frequencies. O'Neill *et al.* (1990) have developed one of the most sophisticated direct observation techniques. The data sheet involves a matrix in which episodes of the target problem behaviours are recorded. This matrix provides a scatter plot, and observers are asked to judge the function of the target behaviour.

Other direct observation techniques include using hand-held computers to examine relationships between antecedent conditions, consequences and problem behaviours (Mace & Lalli, 1991). The problem with this direct observation methodology, however, is that only correlational relationships between antecedent and consequence events and behaviour problems are provided. Manipulation of antecedent and consequent conditions, either in analogue situations (e.g. Iwata *et al.*, 1982) or natural situations (Mace & Lalli, 1991) may be necessary. However, the natural setting conditions for the behaviour problems may not be present in analogous situations (O'Reilly *et al.*, 1999).

Functional assessment and treatment

There are several steps to designing a treatment programme including improving quality of life to modify those environmental conditions that relate to problem behaviours, and teaching and reinforcing skills that serve the same function as the problem behaviours (Butterworth *et al.*, 1997; Holburn & Vietze, 2000). The next section provides a step-by-step, inter-disciplinary approach to the treatment of aggressive and destructive behaviour. Most of these suggestions are taken from the positive behaviour support literature, specifically the Kansas Institute on Positive Behaviour Support (Freeman *et al.*, 2005). Positive Behaviour Support is a comprehensive set of empirically validated strategies that are meant to redesign environments in such a way that a person's quality of life is improved and problem behaviours are prevented or inconsequential. There is also an emphasis on teaching new skills that make problem behaviours unnecessary. Positive Behaviour Support combines behavioural and biomedical sciences, validated procedures and systems change to enhance quality of life and reduce behaviour problems.

Biobehavioural assessment and treatment: a step-by-step approach

In the past, treatment of aggressive and destructive behaviours in people with severe ID has been addressed from either a behavioural or a medical point of view. Research involved either a medical or behavioural perspective, with little overlap (Gardner *et al.*, 1996). Adequate treatment requires an inter-disciplinary team approach with emphasis on data-based assessment and measuring the effects of treatment. The treatment team should consist of a behavioural psychologist, developmental physician, or neurologist and psychiatrist, as well as the individual's circle of support, all familiar with severe ID. Other team members who can contribute include those experienced in speech and language pathology, special education and occupational therapy.

Step one: diagnosis

Step one is a diagnostic task. For the developmental physician, and neurologist, this task includes assessment for medical and neurological disorders. The primary role of the psychiatrist is to assess the presence of possible treatable psychiatric disorders, as well as other illness. As with medical conditions, it is important to operationally define behaviours that suggest the person is experiencing psychiatric symptoms or physical distress.

The behavioural psychologist has a number of functions. One is to operationally define the target behaviours, as well as the psychiatric and associated symptoms such as mood, sleep, activity level, eating and sleeping patterns. The behavioural psychologist then begins to identify possible setting and antecedent conditions, as well as reinforcers for target behaviour, using interview and checklist data. With this information, the team sets up a data collection system. At the same time, client skills, particularly communication skills, are assessed. The inter-disciplinary team including the person's circle of support also assesses quality of life.

Step two: level-one interventions

Level-one interventions encompass several aspects. One aim is to improve the quality of life for the individual through beginning a person-centred plan. Quality of life interventions may involve arranging programme schedules so that there are frequent opportunities for choice, success and preferred activities. Interventions, also, involve improving the health status of the individual by treating illnesses or psychiatric disorders that may worsen aggressive and destructive behaviours.

Step three: re-assessment

As the team introduces level-one interventions, there is an ongoing functional assessment of setting conditions, behaviours, consequences and potential functions of behaviour. The inter-disciplinary team continues to assess the effects of quality of life changes on both appropriate and inappropriate behaviour, as well as health and affect.

Step four: level-two interventions

Level-two interventions involve changing specific environmental setting conditions that are shown to be related to the aggressive and destructive behaviours. By this point there has been ongoing data collection. Scatter plots of the target behaviours, which reflect times in which there are high probability and low probability of behaviour, may be of assistance. Activity schedules can be arranged to promote low probability of behaviour. Manipulations can be planned to examine the relationships between environmental conditions and aggressive and destructive behaviours, and functionally equivalent replacement skills can be taught.

Additionally, it is important to begin teaching coping skills. For example, if the behaviour occurs in situations in which there is a great deal of emotional agitation or fear, relaxation skills can be taught. If the behaviour occurs to escape or avoid the lack of predictability of transitions and changes in the programme schedule, a visual schedule can be set up, and the person may be taught to self-manage this schedule by putting representations (pictures) of activities that have been completed into a finished folder. Finally, level-two interventions may include the use of appropriate medications. Now that more data have been collected, there may be hypotheses about possible treatable psychiatric conditions.

Step five: re-assessment

It is important to continually assess treatment, particularly the contextual fit of the treatment procedures (Albin *et al.*, 1996). If the manipulation of setting events and the teaching of alternative responses are not successful, it may be necessary to use a micro-level type of behaviour analysis (Risley, 1996). Risley defines elements of this approach as the identification of powerful reinforcers and precise contingencies to shape new behaviour. These procedures are recommended as a final alternative because of the skill level that is required to carry them out (Risley, 1996), potential problems of contextual fit of these procedures in the natural environment (Albin *et al.*, 1996), and problems with generalization and maintenance (Horner *et al.*, 1988; Huguenin *et al.*, 1991).

Conclusion

Schroeder *et al.* (1997) indicate that severe behaviour problems in people with ID are often multiply caused. Fifteen years ago there was a paucity of research that was hypothesis-driven regarding the cause or treatment of aggressive and disruptive behaviour in this population. Today, there are a number of hypotheses to consider; however, few present an integrated developmental approach. An inter-disciplinary approach to research and treatment is needed. Behavioural researchers must take into account biological risk factors such as pain, sleep and psychiatric disorders.

Psychopharmacological researchers must begin conducting functional assessments. For example, Zarcone *et al.* (2004) suggested that psychotropic medications such as risperidone may affect some behavioural functions and not others. Lack of such an integrated approach will only increase the fragmentation process in medical and behavioural models. Schroeder *et al.* (1997) point out that a natural methodology for examining an integrated approach involves drug/behaviour interaction studies (Zarcone *et al.*, 2004). Such an integrated approach may also lead to useful models of prevention of destructive and aggressive behaviour by examining the interaction of biological and environmental risk factors (Chadwick *et al.*, 2000; McClintock *et al.*, 2003).

Summary points

- Treatment of severe aggressive and destructive behaviour in people with severe developmental disabilities and ID requires integration of biological and behavioural expertise.
- Medical conditions are often overlooked when treating severe destructive and aggressive behaviour.
- Effective treatment requires a multidisciplinary team approach.
- Functional assessment is a vital part of effective treatment.
- Examining and improving quality of life is a valuable tool for treatment.
- Integrating biological and behavioural information to identify risk factors will be important in preventing destructive and aggressive behaviour in people with severe ID.
- Drug–environment interaction studies may be a vehicle for integrating biological and environmental information.

Acknowledgments

This chapter and the preparation of the manuscript were supported by a National Institute of Child Health (NICH), as well as by a Maternal and Child Health (MCH) grant.

REFERENCES

Albin, R. W., Lucyshyn, J. M., Horner, R. H. & Flannery, K. B. (1996). Contextual fit for behaviour support plans: a model for 'Goodness of fit'. In *Positive Behavioral Support: Including People with Difficult Behavior in the Community*, ed. L. K. Koegel, R. L. Koegel & G. Dunlap, pp. 81–9. Baltimore: Paul H. Brooke.

Bailey, J. M. & Pyles, O. A. M. (1989). Behavioral diagnostics. In *The Treatment of Severe Behavior Disorders*, ed. E. Cipiani, pp. 85–107. Washington, DC: American Association on Mental Retardation.

Bijou, S. W. & Baer, D. M. (1978). *Behavior Analysis in Child Development*. Englewood Cliffs, NJ: Prentice-Hall.

Blumer, D. (1984). *Psychiatric Aspects of Epilepsy*. Washington, DC: American Psychiatric Press.

Breau, L. M., Camfield, C. S., McGrath, P. J. & Finley, G. A. (2004). Risk factors for pain in children with severe cognitive impairments. *Developmental Medicine and Child Neurology*, **46**, 364–71.

Breau, L. M., Camfield, C. S., Symons, F. J. *et al.* (2003). Relationship between pain and self-injurious behavior in non-verbal children with severe cognitive impairments. *Journal of Pediatrics*, **42**, 498–503.

Butterworth, J., Steere, D. & Whitney-Thomas, J., (1997). Using person-centered planning to address quality of life. In R. Schalock ed., *Quality of Life: Vol. II. Application to Persons with Disabilities*, pp. 5–23. Washington, DC: American Association on Mental Retardation.

Carr, E. G. (1994). Emerging themes in the functional analysis of problem behavior. *Journal of Applied Behavior Analysis*, **27**, 393–9.

Carr, E. G. & Durand, V. M. (1985). Reducing behavior problems through functional communication training. *Journal of Applied Behavior Analysis*, **18**, 111–26.

Carr, E. G. & Smith, C. (1995). Biological setting events for self-injury. *Mental Retardation and Developmental Disabilities Research Review*, **1**, 94–8.

Carr, E. G., Smith, C. E., Giacin, T. A., Whelan, B. M. & Pancari, J. (2003). Menstrual discomfort as a biological setting event for severe problem behavior: assessment and intervention. *American Journal on Mental Retardation*, **108**, 117–33.

Chadwick, O., Piroth, N., Walker, J., Bernand, S. & Taylor, E. (2000). Factors affecting the risk of behaviour problems in children with severe intellectual disability. *Journal of Intellectual Disability Research*, **44**, 108–123.

Didden, R., Korzilius, H., vanAperlo, B., VanOverloop, C. & deVries, M., (2002). Sleep problems and daytime problem behaviours in children with intellectual disability. *Journal of Intellectual Disability Research*, **46**, 537–47.

Durand, V. M. & Crimmins, D. B. (1988). Identifying the variables maintaining self-injurious behavior. *Journal of Autism and Developmental Disorders*, **18**, 99–117.

Freeman, R., Smith, C., Zarcone, J. *et al.* (2005). Building a statewide plan for embedding positive behavior support in human service organizations. *Journal of Positive Behavior Interventions*, **2**, 109–19.

Gardner, W. I., Graeber, J. C. & Cole, C. L. (1996). Behavior therapies: a multi-modal diagnostic and intervention model. In *Manual of Diagnosis and Professional Practice in Mental Retardation*, ed. J. Jacobson & J. A. Mulick, pp. 355–70. Washington, DC: APA Books.

Guess, D. & Carr, E. (1991). Emergence and maintenance of stereotype and self-injury. *American Journal on Mental Retardation*, **96**, 299–320.

Hagopian, L. P., Fisher, W. W., Sullivan, M. T., Acquisto, J. & LeBlanc, L. A. (1998). Effectiveness of functional communication training with and without extinction and punishment: A summary of 21 inpatient cases. *Journal of Applied Behavior Analysis*, **31**, 211–35.

Hellings, J. A. (1999). Psychopharmacology of mood disorders in persons with mental retardation and autism. *Mental Retardation and Developmental Disability Research Reviews*, **5**, 270–8.

Hellings, J. A., (2006). Much improved outcome with gabapentin–divalproex combination in adults with bipolar disorders and developmental disabilities. *Journal of Clinical Psychopharmacology*, **26**, 344–6.

Hellings, J. A., Hossain, S., Martin, J. K. & Baratang, R. (2002). Psychopathology, GABA, and the Rubinstein Syndrome: A review and case study. *American Journal of Genetics*, **114**, 190–5.

Hellings, J. A., Kelley, L. A., Gabrielli, W. F., Kilgore, E. & Shah, P. (1996). Sertraline response in adults with mental retardation and autistic disorder. *Journal of Clinical Psychiatry*, **57**, 333–6.

Hellings, J. A. & Warnock, J. K. (1994). Self-injurious behavior and serotonin in Prader–Willi syndrome. *Psychopharmacology Bulletin*, **2**, 245–50.

Hellings, J. A., Weckbaugh, R. N., Nickel, E. J. *et al.* (2005). A double-blind, placebo-controlled study of valproate for aggression in youth with pervasive developmental disorders. *Journal of Child and Adolescent Psychopharmacology*, **15**, 682–92.

Hellings, J. A., Zarcone, J. R., Crandall, K., Wallace, D., & Schroeder, S. R. (2001). Weight gain in a controlled study of children, adolescents and adults with mental retardation and autism. *Journal of Child and Adolescent Psychopharmacology*, **11**, 229–38.

Hellings, J. A., Zarcone, J. R., Reese, R. M. *et al.* (2006). A crossover study of risperidone in children, adolescents and adults with mental retardation. *Journal of Autism and Developmental Disorders*, **36**, 401–11.

Holburn, S. & Vietze, P. (2002). *Person Centered Planning: Research, Practice and Future Directions*. Baltimore, MD: Paul H. Brooks.

Horner, R. H., Dunlap, G. & Koegel, R. L. (1988). *Generalization and Maintenance*. Baltimore, MD: Paul H. Brooke.

Horner, R. H., Vaughn, B. J., Day, M. & Narde, W. R. (1996). The relationship between setting events and problem behavior: expanding our understanding of behavioral support. In *Positive Behavioral Support: Including People with Difficult Behavior in the Community*, ed. L. K. Koegel, R. L. Koegel & G. Dunlap, pp. 381–402. Baltimore, MD: Paul H. Brooke.

Huguenin, N. H., Weidenman, L. E. & Mulick, J. A. (1991). Programmed instruction. In *Handbook of Mental Retardation*, 2nd edn, ed. J. L. Matson & J. A. Mulick, pp. 451–67. Elmsford, NY: Pergamon Press.

Iwata, B., Dorsey, M., Slifer, K. *et al.* (1982). Toward a functional analysis of self-injury. *Analysis and Intervention in Developmental Disabilities*, **2**, 3–20.

Kantor, J. R. (1959). *Interbehavioral Psychology: A Sample of Scientific System Construction*. Chicago, IL: Principia.

Kastner, T., Friedman, D. L. & Pond, W. S. (1992). Carbamazepine-induced hyponatremia in patients with mental retardation. *American Journal of Mental Retardation*, **96**, 536–40.

Kincaid, D. (1996). Person-centered planning. In *Positive Behavioral Support: Including People with Difficult Behavior in the Community*, ed. L. K. Koegel, R. L. Koegel & G. Dunlap, pp. 425–38. Baltimore, MD: Paul H. Brookes.

Koegel, L. K., Koegel, R. C. & Dunlap, G. (eds.) (1996). *Positive Behavior Supports: Including People with Difficult Behavior in the Community*. Baltimore, MD: Paul H. Brookes.

Lennox, D. B. & Miltenberger, R. G. (1989). Conducting a functional assessment of problem behavior in applied settings. *Journal of the Association for People with Severe Handicaps*, **14**, 304–11.

Lowry, M. A. (1992). Assessment and treatment of mood disorders and associated behavior problems in adults with profound and severe mental retardation. Paper presented at American Psychological Association. Washington, DC.

Lowry, M. A. (1997). Unmasking mood disorders: recognizing and measuring symptomatic behaviors. *The Habilitative Mental Healthcare Newsletter*, **16**(1), 1–6.

Lucyshyn, J. M., Olson, D. L. & Horner, R. H. (2002). Building an ecology of support for a young woman with severe problem behaviors living in the community. In J. R. Scott, and Luanna H. Meyer, eds. *Behavioral Principles, Models, and Practices*. Baltimore, MD: Paul H. Brooks Publishing Co., pp. 269–89.

Mace, F. C. & Lalli, J. S. (1991). Linking descriptive and experimental analysis in the treatment of bizarre speech. *Journal of Applied Behavior Analysis*, **24**, 553–62.

McClintock, K., Hall, S. & Oliver, C. (2003). Risk markers associated with challenging behaviours in people with intellectual disabilities: a meta-analytic study. *Journal of Intellectual Disability Research*, **47**, 405–16.

Neef, N. A. (1994). Functional analysis approaches to behavior assessment and treatment. Special issue. *Journal of Applied Behavior Analysis*, 2, **27**, 195–420.

O'Neill, R. E., Horner, R. H., Albin, R. W., Storey, K. & Sprague, J. R. (1990). *Functional Analysis of Problem Behavior: A Practical Assessment Guide*. Pacific Grove, CA: Brooks/Cole.

O'Reilly, M. F., Lancioni, G. E. & Emerson, E. (1999). A systematic analysis of the influence of prior social context on aggression and self-injury within analogue analysis assessments. *Behavior Modification*, **23**, 578–96.

Reese, R. M. (1997). A biobehavioural analysis of self-injurious behavior in a person with profound handicaps. *Focus on Autism and Other Developmental Disabilities*, **12**(2), 87–94.

Reese, R. M. & Leder, D. (1990). An ecobehavioural setting event analysis of residential facilities for people with mental retardation. In *Ecobehavioral Analysis and Developmental Disabilities: The Twenty-First Century*, ed. S. R. Schroeder, pp. 82–93. New York: Springer-Verlag.

Reese, R. M., Richman, D. M., Belmont, J. M. & Morsey, P. (2006). Functional characteristics of disruptive behavior in developmentally disabled children with and without autism. *Journal of Autism and Developmental Disorders*, **35**, 419–28.

Risley, T. (1996). Get a life! Positive behavioral intervention for challenging behavior through life arrangement and life coaching. In *Positive Behavioral Support: Including People with Difficult Behavior in the Community*, ed. L. K. Koegel, R. L. Koegel & G. Dunlap, pp. 425–38. Baltimore, MD: Paul H. Brookes.

Rojahn, J., Borthwick-Duffy, S. A. & Jacobson, J. W. (1993). The association between psychiatric diagnosis and severe behavior problems in mental retardation. *Annual of Clinical Psychiatry*, **5**, 163–70.

Ross, E. & Oliver, C. (2003). The assessment of mood in adults who have severe or profound mental retardation. *Clinical Psychology Review*, **23**, 225–45.

Schroeder, S. R., Oster-granite, M. L. & Thompson, T. (2002). *Self-Injurious Behavior: Gene–Brain–Behavior Relationships*. Washington, DC: American Psychological Association.

Schroeder, S. R., Tessel, R. E., Loupe, P. & Stodgell, C. (1997). Severe behavioral problems in developmental disabilities. In *Handbook of Mental Deficiency*, 3rd edn, ed. W. E. MacLean, pp. 439–65. Hillsdale, NJ: Lawrence Erlbaum Associates.

Singh, N. N., Wahler, R. G., Sabaawi, M. *et al.* (2002). Mentoring treatment teams to integrate behavioral and psychopharmacological treatments in developmental disabilities. *Research in Developmental Disabilities*, **23**, 379–89.

Sovner, R. & Fogelman, S. (1996). Irritability and mental retardation. *Seminars in Clinical Neuropsychiatry*, **2**, 105–14.

Sprague, J. R. & Horner, R. H. (1995). Functional assessment and intervention in community settings. *Mental Retardation and Developmental Disabilities Research Review*, **1**, 89–93.

Touchette, P. E., MacDonald, R. F. & Langer, S. N. (1985). A scatterplot for identifying stimulus control of problem behavior. *Journal of Applied Behavior Analysis*, **23**, 343–51.

Trimble, M. (1990). Anti-convulsants in children and adolescents. *Journal of Child Adolescent Psychopharmacology*, **1**, 107–24.

Umbrick, D., Degree, F. A., Barr, W. B. *et al.* (1995). Post-ictal and chronic psychoses in patients with temporal lobe epilepsy. *American Journal of Psychiatry*, **152**, 224–31.

Wacker, D. P., Harding, J., Cooper, L. J. *et al.* (1996). The effects of meal schedule and quantity on problematic behavior. *Journal of Applied Behavior Analysis*, **29**, 79–87.

Wahler, R. G. & Fox, J. J. (1981). Setting events in applied behavior analysis: toward conceptual and methodological expansion. *Journal of Applied Behavior Analysis*, **14**, 327–38.

Zarcone, J. R., Lindauer, S. E., Morse, P. S. *et al.* (2004). Effects of risperidone on destructive behavior of persons with developmental disabilities: III. *Functional Analysis. American Journal on Mental Retardation*, **109**, 310–21.

Zwakhalen, S. M., VanDongen, K. A., Hamers, J. P. & Abu-Saad, H. H. (2004). Pain assessment in intellectually disabled people: non-verbal indications. *Journal of Advanced Nursing*, **45**, 236–45.

18

Behavioural approaches to treatment: principles and practices

Betsey A. Benson and Susan M. Havercamp

Introduction

Behavioural interventions have played a prominent role in the habilitation of persons with intellectual disabilities (ID) since the 1960s. Prior to the application of behavioural techniques, individuals with ID were often placed in institutions where they received custodial care and psychotropic drugs to manage disruptive behaviour. Behavioural techniques improved daily living skills and reduced the maladaptive behaviour of individuals of all ages and all levels of intellectual functioning (Matson, 1990). The results of behavioural interventions generated a positive outlook among professionals regarding the potential of individuals with ID to learn new behaviours and to become more independent.

One development in behavioural practices in recent years has been the emergence of an approach called Positive Behaviour Support (PBS) (Carr *et al.*, 2002). Positive Behaviour Support integrates behavioural analysis with person-centred philosophy by emphasizing the importance of co-ordinating with stakeholders and professionals, by promoting the value of proactive skill-building to prevent the recurrence of problem behaviour, and by incorporating strategies that are relevant to naturalistic, community-based settings (Carr *et al.*, 2002; Lucyshyn *et al.*, 2002). The approach reflects a general trend in the social sciences away from a focus on pathology to a positive model that stresses personal competence and environmental integrity (Carr *et al.*, 2002). An analysis of published research on PBS concluded that the approach is widely applicable to people with serious problem behaviour and that the field is growing rapidly, especially in the use of assessment and interventions focused on correcting environmental deficiencies. The authors found that PBS was effective in reducing problem behaviour in half to two-thirds of the cases and that success rates nearly doubled when the intervention was based on a prior

Psychiatric and Behavioural Disorders in Intellectual and Developmental Disabilities, ed. Nick Bouras and Geraldine Holt. Published by Cambridge University Press. © Cambridge University Press 2007.

functional assessment (Carr *et al.*, 1999). Some proponents of PBS claim that no aversive procedures should be used; however, a survey of professionals found that there is a considerable range of opinion on the matter (Michaels *et al.*, 2005). In addition, PBS has been criticized for emphasizing values over empirical results and for minimizing the training requirements of intervention specialists (Johnston *et al.*, 2006).

A complete review of behavioural interventions with persons who have intellectual and developmental disabilities is beyond the scope of this chapter; however, a number of excellent resources are available for further information (e.g. Emerson, 2001; Singh *et al.*, 1996). The chapter is divided into two main sections. First, behaviour principles and techniques are briefly described. Then, applications of behavioural techniques to diagnostic categories or problem behaviours are presented. No attempt is made here to address all behavioural techniques, but rather brief descriptions of those that are relevant to the practices section of the chapter are included. Further information can be found in basic texts of applied behaviour analysis and behaviour modification, such as Martin and Pear (2003) and Miltenberger (2001).

Principles

Several assumptions are made in adopting a behavioural approach to assessment and intervention. Most importantly, it is assumed that behaviour is primarily affected by the conditions existing in the person's environment, rather than by intra-psychic dynamics. The focus is on current behaviour and specific behaviour–environment interactions. Through these interactions, the individual learns how his or her behaviour affects the environment, including the behaviour of others such as parents, teachers, and staff. The goal of behavioural intervention is to change (either increase or decrease) one or more specific behaviours. For example, the goal may be to decrease hitting or to increase social skills.

The hallmarks of a behavioural approach to intervention are an operational definition of the target behaviour, behaviour analysis, and data collection as an ongoing part of assessment and intervention. Essential elements in the analysis of behaviour are defining the antecedent conditions and the consequences of the behaviour, as well as the setting or context in which the behaviour occurs. Behavioural interventions focus on systematically changing one or more of these elements. Treatment goals and specific strategies are described in detail in a *behaviour plan*. Once the plan is implemented, data continue to be recorded on the occurrence of the target behaviour and the use of the interventions, which indicate the effectiveness of the behaviour plan. The plan is modified, when appropriate, to achieve the desired effect on the target behaviour.

Co-ordinated approach: integration with carers and other disciplines

The critical role of family, teachers and staff members

The effectiveness of behavioural interventions depends in large part on the implementation by others, including family members and/or support staff (Lucyshyn *et al.*, 2002). Parents, teachers, staff, peers or the individual may carry out behavioural interventions. In many cases, the parents, teachers or staff members are asked to change *their* behaviour because such a change is expected to change the target individual's behaviour. To be effective, the behaviour plan must be carried out consistently. For this reason, implementation often involves training several carers in the details of the intervention (Reid & Green, 1990). In one study, parents were trained to identify and define problem behaviours, conduct a functional assessment, and design appropriate interventions (McNeill *et al.*, 2002).

The importance of involving family members to participate in behavioural interventions was highlighted in the publication Expert Consensus Guidelines Series: Treatment of Psychiatric and Behavioral Problems in Mental Retardation (Rush & Frances, 2000). Experts were asked to recommend psychosocial treatments for a variety of psychiatric disorders and behaviour problems. A striking finding was that for every diagnostic condition and problem behaviour, regardless of the severity of the problem or the level of the ID, the experts consistently recommended client and/or family education and behavioural training as first-line treatments. As defined in this report published by the American Association on Mental Retardation, client and/or family education involves helping clients and/or families understand more about behavioural and psychiatric problems and how to manage them.

Co-ordinating with other disciplines

In addition to enlisting the help of carers, it is important for the behaviourist to co-ordinate with other health professionals providing services to the client. Individuals with ID and co-occurring mental health or behavioural problems present a complex clinical picture. It is not unusual for individuals with ID to have seizure disorders and other chronic health conditions (Havercamp *et al.*, 2004; Hayden & Kim, 2002) (see also Chapter 15 by Deb). Consideration must be given to biological influences on the individual's behaviour, as well as the person's skills and needs, and their physical and social environment (Gardner *et al.*, 1996). The complexity of the clinical picture necessitates co-ordination among treating clinicians. A team approach is recommended where each professional providing services to the individual contributes to the team (American Academy of Child and Adolescent Psychiatry, 1999; Esbenson & Benson, 2003; Griffiths & Nugent, 1998; Kuhn & Matson, 2004) (see also Chapter 3 by O'Hara).

Assessment

Before behavioural interventions are implemented, a thorough medical, psychiatric, and functional assessment is needed. An inter-disciplinary team approach to assessment is recommended (Grey *et al.*, 2003).

Medical assessment

When an individual presents with mental health or behavioural problems, it is important to provide a thorough medical evaluation so that underlying health issues can be identified and treated. A medical review should include developmental and medical history, past aetiological assessments, and co-existing general medical disorders and their treatments. Because many individuals with ID have expressive language limitations, undiagnosed medical conditions are frequent in this population and may cause or exacerbate behavioural symptoms. Medical causes for an acute behavioural exacerbation must always be considered. For example, it is not uncommon for constipation, infection, or injury to precipitate behavioural problems (American Academy of Child and Adolescent Psychiatry, 1999) (see also Chapters 5 by Lennox and 17 by Reese *et al.*).

Psychiatric assessment

A thorough psychiatric evaluation is a necessary part of the assessment process. The purpose of this assessment should be to screen for psychiatric diagnoses and to evaluate ongoing psychological and pharmacological interventions. The psychiatric diagnostic evaluation of persons who have ID is basically the same as for persons without ID. The diagnostic approaches are modified, depending on the patient's cognitive level and communication skills. For persons who have mild ID and good verbal skills, the approach does not differ significantly from diagnosing persons with average cognitive skills. The poorer the communication skills, the greater the importance of information provided by carers familiar with the patient and direct behavioural observations (Deb *et al.*, 2001; Royal College of Psychiatrists, 2001) (see also Chapters 2 by Mohr & Costello and 3 by O'Hara).

A complete psychiatric evaluation should include a comprehensive history taken from the client and from several caregivers in different settings, an interview with the individual, direct observation of behaviour, medical history, medication and side effects evaluation (American Academy of Child and Adolescent Psychiatry, 1999; Rush & Frances, 2000). Medication side effects such as akathisia resulting from neuroleptics or disinhibition associated with sedative/hypnotic use can be expressed in aggressive and self-injurious behaviours (American Academy of Child and Adolescent Psychiatry, 1999).

Functional assessment

Functional assessment is a broad term encompassing a number of procedures for identifying the function of behaviour; that is, variables maintaining the occurrence of problem behaviour. Functional assessment procedures include functional analysis, recording antecedents and consequences of problem behaviour during naturalistic observation, structured behaviour interview, and completion of functional assessment rating scales.

Iwata *et al.* (1982) developed an assessment technology called *functional analysis*. This methodology was designed to assess functional relationships between problem behaviour and specific reinforcers. In this technique, the individual being assessed is repeatedly exposed to a series of analogue conditions to determine whether or not the behaviour is maintained by (1) sensory stimulation, (2) escape from demand, (3) social attention, or (4) tangible reinforcement (i.e. a preferred object). The frequency of problem behaviour – for example self-injury – is measured during each condition. When an individual's self-injury is most frequent during the 'escape from demand' condition, for example, this indicates that the behaviour is maintained by negative reinforcement by permitting the individual to escape from task demands. Iwata *et al.*'s results provided direct empirical evidence for the function of various sources of reinforcement in the maintenance of problem behaviour. Functional analysis has been found useful for prescribing specific treatments, even in a brief 90-minute outpatient setting (Asmus *et al.*, 2004; Derby *et al.*, 1992) (see also Chapter 14 by Hillery & Dodd).

Researchers have explored alternative approaches to obtaining functional assessment information. Functional hypotheses generated from naturalistic observations of antecedents and consequence of problem behaviour are largely consistent with those derived from experimental (analogue) functional analysis (Cunningham & O'Neill, 2000; Mace & Lalli, 1991), structured behaviour questionnaires (Ellingson *et al.*, 2000; Yarbrough & Carr, 2000), and functional assessment rating scales (Matson *et al.*, 1999; Matson *et al.* 2003; Paclawskyj *et al.*, 2000). For a review of functional assessment rating scales, see Sturmey (1994).

Functional analysis is widely used in clinical practice, applied settings (e.g. classrooms), and research (Crone & Horner, 2003; Dunlap & Kincaid, 2001; Ellis & Magee, 2004; Iwata *et al.*, 1994; O'Neill *et al.*, 1997; Sprague & Horner, 1995; Vollmer & Smith, 1996; Watson *et al.*, 1999). In some settings, functional assessment is required prior to the implementation of a systematic behavioural intervention

(Dunlap & Kincaid, 2001). In the United States, for example, federal legislation governing public schools (Individuals with Disabilities Education Act) requires a functional assessment for students whose placements are jeopardized due to problem behaviours.

Functional communication training

Problem behaviour may be considered a form of communication (Carr & Durand, 1985). For example, if an individual's self-injury is maintained by attention from others (positive reinforcement), the self-injury can be interpreted as a *request* for attention. The purpose of functional assessment is to determine the function that the behaviour serves for the individual. In functional communication training, an appropriate communication behaviour that is tailored to the function of the problem behaviour is taught as a substitute for the problem behaviour. For example, if it is determined that the function of Jenny's problem behaviour is attention, she can be taught a more appropriate means of obtaining attention (communication training). If her misbehaviour is then consistently ignored (extinction), Jenny will learn that the *only* way to get attention is to ask for it appropriately. We would expect her problem behaviour to be replaced by the communicative alternative. Appropriate communication is more likely to generalize to new environments and to be maintained for long periods of time (Bailey *et al.*, 2002; Durand, 1999; Durand & Carr, 1992).

Several factors have been identified that contribute to the success of functional communication training (Durand & Merges, 2001). First, the alternative communication behaviour should match the function of the problem behaviour. If the function of the problem behaviour is determined to be escape from demands, then the alternative communication should also achieve that outcome. Second, the communication alternative should be a more efficient response than the problem behaviour. To be more efficient, it will require less effort to reliably obtain the reinforcer and with no greater delay than the problem behaviour. If communicating 'I need help' does not reliably and efficiently lead to the desired assistance, then the problem behaviour is likely to persist. Third, the communication alternative should be acceptable and recognizable by others. Individuals in the environment need to be able to understand the communication and to respond to it consistently.

Comprehensive multimodal treatment packages that have proven most effective include functional communication training, choice making, and building tolerance for delay of reinforcement as well as biological or medical treatments (Carr & Carlson, 1993; Gardner & Graeber, 1993; Herzroni & Roth, 2003; Steed *et al.*, 1995).

Reinforcement

A reinforcer is an event that increases the probability that the response that directly precedes it will occur again (Singh *et al.*, 1996). For example, getting paid for walking the neighbour's dog increases the probability that one will agree to walk that dog in the future. In positive reinforcement, a behaviour results in the presentation of reinforcing stimuli (Miltenberger, 2001). When a request for a break is followed by cessation of work demands, for example, the communication behaviour may be negatively reinforced. Reinforcement is arguably the most powerful and most often used behavioural technique. The reinforcing value of an event varies from individual to individual and from time to time and therefore must be established empirically (Singh *et al.*, 1996).

Preference assessment

Determining what will function as a reinforcer for a given individual can be a difficult task, particularly if the person has difficulty making his/her preferences known (Ivancic & Bailey, 1996). A paired stimulus choice assessment procedure has been used to identify preferences for various stimuli among individuals with severe and profound ID (Fisher *et al.*, 1996; Piazza *et al.*, 1996). Stimuli are either placed in view of the client or are demonstrated by the therapist (for example hand clapping). Each stimulus in the assessment is paired with every other stimulus and approach responses to the stimuli are noted. An approach response is interpreted as evidence of a preference. The choice assessment procedure was found to be an effective way of predicting the relative reinforcing value of various stimuli for individuals with severe to profound disabilities (Lavie & Sturmey, 2002; Sturmey *et al.*, 2003a). Recently, Sturmey and colleagues developed the Choice Assessment Scale, a rating instrument to identify potential reinforcers for people with severe and profound ID (Sturmey *et al.*, 2003b).

Token economy

A token economy or token reinforcement system is often used as one component of a behaviour support programme. A token reinforcer is like money; it is something that can be exchanged for a desired object or activity at some future time. There are several advantages to using a token reinforcement system. Tokens are tangible and concrete; a person knows instantly when reinforcement is received. Tokens can be given immediately after the desired behaviour, even though the back-up reinforcer may be delivered at a much later time. Tokens allow the reinforcement to be broken into small segments; several tokens may be required to earn a valued reinforcer.

Examples of commonly used tokens include poker chips, milk bottle tops, points on a card, and stickers.

Matson (1982a) provided behavioural treatment involving a combination of techniques to three men with mild ID who displayed repetitive clothes checking or body checking. A procedure was instituted in which reinforcement was given for *not* performing the checking behaviour while the men completed work tasks. Tokens were provided for each minute out of 30 that the behaviour did not occur. The tokens could be exchanged later for snacks.

Behaviour shaping

If the desired response is not in the person's repertoire, it cannot be reinforced. One procedure that can be used to teach a new behaviour is *shaping*. Shaping of behaviour occurs when a reinforcer is provided for behaviour that is increasingly similar to the target desired behaviour. Reinforcement is then presented differentially for responses that more closely match the desired behaviour, or successive approximations, until the desired response is performed. Once the desired response occurs, it alone is reinforced to the exclusion of lesser approximations (Martin & Pear, 2003).

Extinction

When a previously reinforced behaviour is no longer reinforced, a process of extinction occurs in which the behaviour reduces in frequency. By design, any reinforcement programme also involves extinction because certain behaviours are reinforced while others are not (Singh *et al.*, 1996). Lovaas and Simmons (1969) found that for some children, self-injurious behaviour decreased from more than 2000 acts during the first session to no self-injurious acts in the tenth session once all sources of social reinforcement were removed. Magee and Ellis (2000) described an extinction burst where new target behaviours emerged as extinction was introduced sequentially across several problem behaviours. All target behaviours eventually decreased once extinction was applied systematically across all behaviours.

Self-management

Often, behaviour plans incorporate some aspect of self-management. With a self-management programme, the individual is taught three skills: self-monitoring, self-evaluation and self-reinforcement. The individual observes his or her own behaviour and records instances of target behaviours and desirable behaviours. The individual delivers reinforcement to him- or herself following self-evaluation of desirable behaviour, but not after target behaviours (Carr *et al.*, 1999). Video technology has proven to be a valuable tool in self-modelling and video feedback (Coyle & Cole, 2004; Embregts, 2003). Embregts (2003) used video feedback and self-management procedures to increase desired behaviour in children with ID and their staff members. Participants were video-taped during lunch and then shown segments of the tape and asked whether the observed behaviour was appropriate or inappropriate. The students could earn tokens for the identification of appropriate and inappropriate behaviours and were praised for appropriate behaviour. Staff members were praised and provided corrective feedback based on their video-taped responses to the students' behaviour. Rates of inappropriate target behaviours decreased for students with externalizing behaviour problems and appropriate target behaviours increased for students with internalizing behaviour problems. Both staff and students rated the video feedback and self-management strategies as very effective and pleasant. In another study, self-management procedures increased the rates of academically engaged behaviour and work completion in a 10-year-old girl with Down syndrome and mild ID in her fourth-grade classroom (Brooks *et al.*, 2003).

Punishment

Punishment is a procedure in which the target behaviour is followed by a consequence that decreases its future probability of occurrence. There are several behavioural procedures that can function as punishment including removal of reinforcement, verbal reprimands, withdrawal of privileges, and isolating the person from a reinforcing environment. Punishment procedures are to be used as a last resort, after reinforcement-only procedures are tried and found to be inadequate or when the problem behaviour presents a danger to self or others. When punishment is used to decrease problem behaviours, it is critical to use reinforcement procedures at the same time to develop appropriate behaviours, often functionally equivalent communicative replacement behaviour. In a meta-analysis of behavioural interventions, Scotti *et al.* (1991) concluded that while punishment procedures were effective in suppressing maladaptive behaviour, their effects were enhanced when combined with reinforcement procedures.

Response cost

Response cost procedures are frequently and successfully used to decrease rates of behaviour. Response cost procedures do not involve the addition of stimuli, which cause pain, illness, cold, or some other aversive condition. Rather, they involve the contingent removal of a preferred stimulus. Time-out and over-correction are forms of response cost. The addition of response cost to a reinforcement procedure resulted in a significant decrease in inappropriate vocalizations in an adult with autism (Falcomata *et al.*, 2004). In another study, the use of a token economy with a response-cost procedure successfully treated excessive inappropriate social behaviour in an adult with moderate ID (LeBlanc *et al.*, 2000).

Over-correction

Over-correction involves either repeatedly restoring a setting (or individual) to its previous state before the occurrence of an undesirable behaviour or the positive practice of behaviour that is incompatible with the undesired response (Singh *et al.*, 1996). For example, an individual who overturns a chair in a lounge area could be first manually guided and then instructed in the replacement and arrangement of *all* the chairs in the room. Cole *et al.* (2000) used positive practice over-correction to reduce stereotypic hand behaviour in adults with severe to profound ID.

Time-out

Time-out from positive reinforcement involves interrupting the reinforcement obtained by the individual, contingent on undesirable behaviour. Time-out can be exclusionary, in which the individual is removed from the setting for a period of time, or it can be non-exclusionary, in which the individual remains in the setting, but potential reinforcers are removed (Singh *et al.*, 1996). The absence of the problem behaviour is usually required to reinstate the previous reinforcing conditions. A combination of differential reinforcement and time-out has proven effective in treating a variety of behaviour problems in children (Alberto *et al.*, 2002; O'Conner *et al.*, 2003) and adults with ID (Toole *et al.*, 2003).

Contextual factors

Behaviour is not emitted in a vacuum. A large research literature has documented that the occurrence of problem behaviour is a function of both antecedents, such as task demands, and consequences, such as attention, escape from demands, and tangibles. This understanding is the basis of functional assessment. A behaviour is under stimulus control when its occurrence can be predicted by knowing whether or not a stimulus (a particular person, for example) is present in the environment (Cipani, 1990). When a behaviour is under stimulus control, there is a high probability that it will occur given that the stimulus is present.

In recent years, researchers have begun to explore the role of broader contextual influences on problem behaviour. These broader influences, or setting events, affect the impact of antecedents on behaviour. Setting events may include physical, social, and physiological factors including mental health status (Baker *et al.*, 2002). Carr *et al.* (2003) found that staff ratings of bad mood strongly predicted that problem behaviour would occur in the context of task demands, whereas a rating of good mood strongly predicted that problem behaviour would not occur in the same context. They further demonstrated that a mood induction procedure was effective in increasing the completed task steps following intervention. In addition, the occurrence of problem behaviour fell to a near zero level after mood induction. Recently, a contextual assessment inventory was developed to identify contextual variables relevant to problem behaviour in individuals with ID (McAtee *et al.*, 2004).

Further considerations

A few basic principles and procedures of behavioural interventions were described in this section. It is important to note, however, that many behavioural treatments involve combinations of techniques. For example, over-correction may be combined with a reinforcement procedure, or modelling may be used along with positive reinforcement of desired behaviour. In the Matson study (1982a) described earlier, behavioural treatment involving a combination of differential reinforcement was instituted in which reinforcement was given for *not* performing the checking behaviour while the men completed work tasks. Tokens were provided for each minute out of 30 that the behaviour did not occur. When clothes or body checking occurred, an over-correction procedure was used in which a set routine of hand and arm movements was repeated. Both self-reported anxiety and obsessive-compulsive behaviours decreased following treatment.

Although there are many behavioural interventions that could be incorporated into a behavioural treatment plan, a task force recommended that the selection of interventions proceed by choosing the *least restrictive, effective* technique from among those available to deal with that particular problem behaviour (Van Houten *et al.*, 1988). Further, an analysis of risks and benefits of treatment procedures should be conducted (Axelrod *et al.*, 1993).

Practices

Interpersonal skills

Social skills deficits are characteristic of people with ID owing to their adaptive behaviour deficits. Interpersonal skills are also of particular concern because of the association between poor social skills and psychopathology (Benson *et al.*, 1985). Social skills training is often one component of a multifaceted treatment package. A number of behaviourally based interventions that focus on improving social skills of persons with ID have been developed. Two notable programmes for improving social skills of adults with ID are Stacking the Deck (Foxx & McMorrow, 1983) and Home-of-Your-Own Cooperative Living Skills (Tassé *et al.*, 1997). Additional interventions are described in Benson and Valenti-Hein (2001).

Stacking the Deck (Foxx & McMorrow, 1983) is designed to be used with a board game. Players move their game pieces around the board by correctly answering questions of a social skills nature. The playing cards are organized by skill areas such as compliments, social interaction, politeness, criticism, social confrontation, and question and answers.

The Home-Of-Your-Own Cooperative Living Training Program (Tassé *et al.*, 1997) is a curriculum that incorporates behavioural techniques to improve skills required for sharing a residence. The skills are broadly defined as those that facilitate living and getting along with others and include borrowing and lending, sharing chores, respecting privacy, and resolving conflicts. The curriculum is designed to be used in groups of adults with ID during ten, one-hour sessions. The behavioural techniques used in each session include: instruction, discussion, modelling, role-playing (participant modelling), and feedback (positive reinforcement). The authors 'field-tested' and revised the curriculum over the course of two years based on their experience with fifteen different groups of over 100 individuals who had ID.

Relaxation training

Relaxation training is a group of anxiety-reduction techniques (Smith, 1985). The methods range from progressive muscle relaxation in which several muscle groups are individually tensed and relaxed (Bernstein & Borkovec, 1973) to imagery-based procedures and meditation. For each, the goal is to reduce tension and to produce a calm state in body and/or in mind. Relaxation training can be a primary intervention used to reduce general anxiety levels or it can be one part of a treatment 'package'. In systematic desensitization, a fearful client trained in relaxation skills imagines, or experiences in vivo, a series of anxiety-provoking situations starting with the least anxiety-provoking (Ollendick & Cerny, 1981). In anger management training (Benson, 1994), relaxation training is included to reduce arousal associated with anger-provoking situations.

Among the modifications used to enhance relaxation training for persons with ID are the use of simplified language, physical prompts and guidance, behaviour shaping of the response, biofeedback, and positive reinforcement for practice (Harvey, 1979). The addition of modelling and physical guidance to relaxation training helps individuals functioning with severe ID to discriminate between tense and relaxed states (Lindsay *et al.*, 1989). Adapting relaxation-training procedures for individuals with special needs is the subject of a manual (Cautela & Grodin, 1979) and a videotape (Grodin *et al.*, 1989).

Behavioural Relaxation Training (BRT; Poppen, 1998) was adapted for persons with ID. It has the advantage of being easy to learn and easily implemented in everyday situations. Behaviour Relaxation Training differs from progressive muscle relaxation training in that BRT does not require muscle contraction. Some persons with ID may be confused and have difficulty discriminating between tensed and relaxed states in progressive muscle relaxation. In addition, muscle contraction may be contraindicated for problems related to muscle tension such as tension headache. Another advantage of BRT is that it is easy for both trainer and trainee to monitor acquisition of target behaviour. This avoids what is known as 'the problem of privacy' in which the trainer attempts to teach discriminations of events to which he or she has no direct access. For example, it is impossible for the trainer to verify the trainee's thoughts during visual imagery or meditation exercises.

Behaviour Relaxation Training emphasizes motoric behaviour. The trainee is instructed to observe his or her overt body postures as well as the covert proprioceptive sensations and other feelings of relaxation that accompany them. Ten relaxed body positions are taught. Verbal definitions and 'labels' of relaxed postures are provided, and these may be covertly echoed by the trainee and used during practice on his or her own. Visceral behaviour, such as slowed breathing, and diaphragmatic breathing instruction also may be included in this training. Behavioural relaxation skills are quickly acquired (Lindsay & Baty, 1989) and effective in treating chronic headaches (Michultka *et al.*, 1988) improving performance on laboratory learning tasks (Lindsay & Morrison, 1996), improving concentration and decreasing rated anxiety, in adults with severe and profound ID (Lindsay *et al.*, 1994; Lindsay *et al.*, 1989).

Anxiety

Most published studies of behavioural approaches to treatment of anxiety and fear of persons with ID have dealt with specific phobias (Benson, 1990b; Jackson, 1983). A few examples are described here to illustrate behavioural approaches to reduce fears that interfered with community integration (see also Chapter 7 by Stavrakaki & Lunsky).

Specific phobia

Specific phobia was successfully treated in a young man with moderate ID, intermittent-explosive disorder, and cerebral palsy (Hagopian *et al.*, 2001). 'Patrick' was admitted to an inpatient unit for the assessment and treatment of severe behaviour problems including property destruction, aggression, and non-compliance with medical procedures. He was diagnosed with blood-injury-injection phobia, a type of specific phobia characterized by fear/avoidance of seeing blood, an injury, or receiving an injection. Patrick had a long history of avoidance, anxiety that frequently reached panic proportions, and severe inappropriate behaviour associated with medical procedures. These difficulties were highly resistant to outpatient treatment and prevented him from receiving adequate medical care for several years. On one occasion, when taken to the doctor's office, he destroyed a patient waiting room in an attempt to escape the situation. He had been diagnosed with severe kidney reflux and other medical problems; his extreme behaviour prevented regular monitoring of his health status. Treatment consisted of a graduated exposure procedure with modelling, non-contingent access to distracting and preferred items, and a 10-second reinforcement procedure for compliance. After six weeks of treatment, he voluntarily sat unrestrained to have his blood drawn. Exposure to the feared stimuli, while preventing avoidant behaviour and aversive events, is believed to result in both extinction of negatively reinforced avoidant behaviour as well as extinction of the association between the feared stimuli and the aversive event.

A teenage boy's severe dog phobia was treated with a behavioural intervention that included his mother's active participation (Newman & Adams, 2004). An individualized fear hierarchy was developed that was followed by graded exposure and relaxation training. The mother served as a model in the exposure sessions. Both mother and son reported a reduction in the son's anxiety level around dogs following treatment.

Post-traumatic stress disorder

Post-traumatic stress disorder (PTSD) is an anxiety disorder that may occur following an event that presents an actual or perceived threat of injury. The person's emotional response to the event includes intense fear; there are possible flashbacks to the event, as well as avoidance, sleep disturbances and other symptoms. People with ID are vulnerable to PTSD owing to the documented high rate of violence and abuse towards them (Sobsey, 1994). An effective intervention for PTSD involves exposure to the threatening stimuli, which allows the fear to extinguish. Lemmon and Mizes (2002) reported the use of exposure therapy with a woman with mild ID and PTSD following sexual assaults. The intervention included imaginal exposure to a hierarchy of anxiety-arousing cues that were associated with traumatic events and later in vivo exposure to trauma-related cues, such as the environments in which the assaults occurred. Following treatment, psychological distress and physiological reactivity were significantly reduced.

For individuals with ID who have difficulty expressing themselves, an act of refusal is one way to communicate. Some instances in which individuals are considered non-compliant could be owing to anxiety or fear concerning the activity

(Benson, 1990b). When non-compliance seems associated with a particular type of activity, rather than a general pattern of refusal, further inquiry is in order to determine if the avoidance is anxiety based.

Aggression

Disruptive behaviour in persons with ID is frequently defined as including aggression towards others, self-injury, and property destruction (Thompson & Gray, 1994). This group of behaviour problems is of great concern because of the potential for serious harm as well as because the behaviours interfere with attention, learning, and social and intellectual development. A brief discussion of interventions for disruptive behaviours is provided here. Additional information can be found in Benson and Aman (1999), Murphy (1997) and Gardner (2002) (see also Chapter 17 by Reese *et al.*).

Operant model of aggression

It has long been recognized that destructive behaviours are often learned because they are reinforced in some way (Carr, 1977; Ferster, 1961). For example, Carr proposed that self-injurious behaviour is learned, operant, and maintained by either positive social reinforcement or by the termination of an aversive stimulus (negative reinforcement). He also reviewed a self-stimulation hypothesis, which suggests that self-injurious behaviour may be a means of providing visual, tactile, or auditory sensory stimulation (Vollmer, 1994). Other researchers recognized the purposeful nature of other types of problem behaviour such as aggression (Sigafoos & Saggers, 1995), property destruction (Gardner & Cole, 1990), and stereotypy (Rojahn & Sisson, 1990) (see also Chapter 14 by Hillery & Dodd.)

Foxx (2003) summarized several case studies in which severe aggressive behaviour was successfully treated with behavioural interventions. Functional analysis was used to identify the determinants of the behaviours which were often multiple and complex. The comprehensive intervention programmes included punishment procedures, reinforcement, communication training, increased choice making and other approaches. Significant improvements in behaviour were maintained at long-term follow-up. The author contrasts the temporary restrictiveness and use of punishment for dangerous behaviour in the behavioural intervention to the prior years of ineffective treatment through restraint, seclusion, and large doses of psychotropic medications.

Anger management training

Anger management training is a self-management approach to dealing with aggressive behaviour. The goal of anger management training is to improve the self-control skills of the individual (Novaco, 1975). The cognitive-behavioural intervention was adapted for persons with mild to moderate ID. In an early study, groups of adults participated in a 12-week outpatient group in which the primary intervention was either relaxation training, self-instructional training, problem solving skills training, or a combination of the three interventions (Benson, 1994; Benson *et al.*, 1986). The techniques of training included lecture, discussion, modelling, role playing, feedback, and homework. Benson *et al.* (1986) reported improvements in supervisor ratings of behaviour, self-report, and role-play measures at post-test and follow-up, but no significant difference between the treatment groups. A no-treatment control group was not included in the study.

An anger management group intervention was contrasted with a waiting-list control group by Rose (2000) (see also Chapter 9 by Lindsay). Over a period of two years, groups of 5–9 adults participated in 16 treatment sessions; each participant was accompanied by a care worker. Reductions in self-reported anger and depression were obtained at follow-up evaluations six and 12 months later. The inclusion of the care worker was thought to aid the transfer of skills learned in the group to the outside environment and to manage some contextual cues that could be associated with anger arousal.

Substantial progress has been made in applying anger control treatment to offenders with ID who are confined to secure settings. In a publication that consolidated treatment results over a number of years, Lindsay *et al.* (2004) reported that 40 weekly group sessions were effective in reducing anger self-reports and anger responses during role play performance. The intervention included relaxation, problem solving, and stress inoculation through role play practice. Long-term follow-up revealed a generalization of treatment gains and a reduction in re-offending in comparison to waiting-list controls.

In individual anger control treatment, the intervention can be tailored to the needs of the individual to a greater degree than in a group intervention. Taylor *et al.* (2002) found that 18 sessions of individual anger control treatment was superior to routine care in reducing anger intensity of offenders. In a review of the anger control treatment studies to date, Taylor (2002) concluded that there is still room for improvement in the assessment and treatment of aggression in offenders with ID. Assessment tools need to be refined and treatment and control groups should be conducted across a range of settings.

Depression

The behavioural treatment of depression in persons with ID has focused on verbal statements and nonverbal behaviours occurring in social interactions (Benson, 1990a). A variety of behavioural techniques have been applied including self-management. Matson *et al.* (1979) worked with a man with borderline to mild

ID and a long history of depression. The intervention included modelling, praise (reinforcement), self-evaluation and self-reinforcement (self-management). The target behaviours were negative self-statements, suicide statements, and participation in activities. In individual training sessions, the man was praised for positive self-statements and he was asked to praise himself as well. If he made a negative self-statement, the therapist modelled an appropriate statement and the man rehearsed the modelled statement. Homework assignments were given that required tallying positive statements and noting participation in activities. Positive statements and participation in activities increased following the treatment. Using a similar intervention, Matson (1982b) reported the treatment of somatic complaints, negative self-statements, and grooming in four adults with ID and depression. Following a range of 10 to 35 individual sessions, the four participants improved in verbal and non-verbal behaviours and in self-reported depression.

The psychosocial treatment for depression in the general population has moved towards cognitive therapy as the standard. There have been some reports of successful cognitive behavioural therapy for depression in persons with ID (Lindsay et al., 1993). Following a review of a number of cognitive therapy interventions for persons with ID, Sturmey (2004) concluded that many include both behavioural and cognitive components, making it difficult to determine which elements are responsible for the reported improvement (see also Chapter 7 by Stavrakaki & Lunsky).

Psychosis

Behavioural techniques have been used to improve the social skills (Stephens et al., 1981) and decrease the inappropriate verbal behaviour of individuals diagnosed with psychotic disorders (Wilder et al., 2001). Dixon et al. (2001) described the functional assessment and successful treatment of inappropriate vocalizations (e.g. inappropriate sexual comments, illogical or irrational statements) in a man, 'Fernando', with moderate ID and a psychotic disorder not otherwise specified. The inappropriate verbal behaviour was attributed to auditory hallucinations symptomatic of his underlying psychotic disorder. Inappropriate verbal behaviour was defined as vocal utterances that were not relevant to the context or were sexually inappropriate, illogical placement of words within a sentence, or 'psychotic' statements (see also Chapter 8 by Clarke.)

A functional analysis of Fernando's inappropriate verbal behaviour was conducted alternating four conditions (attention, demand, alone and control) in a multi-element design. During the attention condition, the experimenter responded to Fernando's inappropriate verbal utterances with ten seconds of attention. During the demand condition, the experimenter presented Fernando with basic academic tasks. Each occurrence of inappropriate verbal behaviour produced ten seconds of escape from the tasks. During the alone condition, Fernando was in the room alone and observed via a one-way mirror. During the control condition, Fernando had access to his favourite activities (puzzles, markers and craft supplies). The experimenter delivered non-contingent attention every 30 seconds and provided no consequences for inappropriate behaviour. The results of the functional analysis suggested that inappropriate verbal behaviour was maintained by attention from others.

The intervention consisted of reinforcement (attention) contingent on appropriate verbal utterances. No attention was provided to Fernando following the emission of an inappropriate verbal statement. The intervention was alternated with a baseline condition where inappropriate behaviour produced attention and appropriate verbal behaviour was ignored. The treatment was associated with a decrease in the number of inappropriate utterances and a corresponding increase in appropriate utterances. These results were replicated across several contingency reversals, indicating that the treatment was effective in controlling the content of Fernando's verbal behaviour. The successful intervention to reduce inappropriate verbalizations associated with psychosis indicates that when psychiatric symptoms are functionally related to conditions in the environment, they can be altered through systematic changes in the consequences for the behaviour.

Conclusion

Behavioural interventions have in many ways succeeded in fulfilling their early promise to improve the independence and quality of life of individuals with ID. In addition, the emphasis on operational definitions of behaviour, systematic observation, and continuous data collection provides a methodology by which to evaluate the effects of interventions generally.

Remaining challenges include staff training in the functional analysis of behaviour and in implementation of behavioural treatment plans. Some evidence suggests that staff's immediate response to problem behaviour is counter to recommended behavioural approaches (Hastings, 1996). Thus, training must not only educate staff in specific procedures, but must overcome responses that appear 'natural' to workers in the setting. A significant effort in this regard was undertaken in the United States, where a comprehensive staff training programme in positive behaviour support was designed and implemented in the state of South Carolina (Reid & Parsons, 2004).

Several areas of behavioural treatment have been somewhat neglected. Tremendous attention has been focused on behavioural interventions for disruptive behaviours, while the treatment of anxiety, mood, and psychotic disorders has been relatively neglected. Positive results have been obtained, however, and await further application and refinement.

Greater emphasis on client involvement, whenever possible, in developing behaviour plans would be welcomed. Behavioural interventions that increase self-management skills are consistent with this philosophy. Self-management interventions have the potential to reduce demands on staff, teachers and family members in the long term.

The co-ordination of behavioural interventions with other approaches to treatment is also necessary. Psychiatric and behavioural interventions when co-ordinated with one another can maximize treatment outcomes. Evaluating the single and joint effects of these different treatments is a complex task that requires multidisciplinary co-operation.

Although behavioural interventions have had a short history, their impact has been enormous in raising expectations for what is possible for persons with ID. Behavioural treatments have the potential to teach new behaviours previously thought beyond the capability of individuals with ID. The effectiveness of behavioural interventions in reducing problem behaviour has opened doors to community integration and improved the quality of life of persons with ID.

Summary points

- A hallmark of the behavioural approach is a thorough assessment and continuous monitoring of target behaviours, replacement behaviours, and interventions.
- The effectiveness of behavioural interventions depends in large part on implementation by others, including family members, teachers and support staff. Training of implementers and the consistency of implementation of behavioural interventions are key factors in obtaining positive outcomes.
- Behavioural interventions have proven effective in the treatment of depression, psychosis and anxiety disorders, including specific phobias and post-traumatic stress disorder. Aggressive behaviour has been effectively reduced through behavioural interventions and, with anger control treatment, a combination of interventions to achieve self-control of anger.
- Integrating behavioural interventions with other treatment approaches requires multidisciplinary co-ordination. Further study is needed on optimal methods to implement and manage such efforts.

REFERENCES

Alberto, P., Heflin, L. J. & Andrews, D. (2002). Use of the time-out ribbon procedure during community-based instruction. *Behavior Modification*, **26**, 297–311.

American Academy of Child and Adolescent Psychiatry (1999). Practice parameters for the assessment and treatment of children, adolescents, and adults with mental retardation and comorbid mental disorders. American Academy of Child and Adolescent Psychiatry Working Group on Quality Issues. *Journal of the American Academy of Child and Adolescent Psychiatry*, **38**, 5–31.

Asmus, J. M., Ringdahl, J. E., Sellers, J. A. *et al.* (2004). Use of a short-term inpatient model to evaluate aberrant behavior: Outcome data summaries from 1996 to 2001. *Journal of Applied Behavior Analysis*, **37**, 283–304.

Axelrod, S., Spreat, S., Berry, B. & Moyer, L. (1993). A decision-making model for selecting the optimal treatment procedure. In R. Van Houten & S. Axelrod (eds.), *Behavior Analysis and Treatment* (pp. 183–202). New York: Plenum Press.

Bailey, J., McComas, J. J., Benavides, C. & Lovascz, C. (2002). Functional assessment in a residential setting: Identifying an effective communicative replacement response for aggressive behavior. *Journal of Developmental and Physical Disabilities*, **14**, 353–69.

Baker, D. J., Blumberg, E. R., Freeman, R. & Wieseler, N. A. (2002). Can psychiatric disorders be seen as establishing operations? Integrating applied behavior analysis and psychiatry. *Mental Health Aspects of Developmental Disabilities*, **5**, 118–24.

Benson, B. A. (1990a). Behavioral treatment of depression. In A. Dosen & F. J. Menolascino (eds.), *Depression in Mentally Retarded Children and Adults* (pp. 309–29). Leiden, Netherlands: Logon Publications.

Benson, B. A. (1990b). Emotional problems I: Anxiety disorders and depression. In J. L. Matson (ed.), *Handbook of Behavior Modification with the Mentally Retarded* (2nd edn, pp. 391–420). New York: Plenum Press.

Benson, B. A. (1994). Anger management training: a self-control programme for persons with mild mental retardation. In N. Bouras (ed.), *Mental Health in Mental Retardation* (pp. 224–32). Cambridge: Cambridge University Press.

Benson, B. A. & Aman, M. G. (1999). Disruptive behavior disorders in children with mental retardation. In H. C. Quay & A. E. Hogan (eds.), *Handbook of Disruptive Behavior Disorders* (pp. 559–78). New York: Plenum Press.

Benson, B. A., Reiss, S., Smith, D. C. & Laman, D. (1985). Psychosocial correlates of depression in mentally retarded adults: II. Poor social skills. *American Journal of Mental Deficiency*, **89**, 657–9.

Benson, B. A., Rice, C. J. & Miranti, S. V. (1986). Effects of anger management training with mentally retarded adults in group treatment. *Journal of Consulting and Clinical Psychology*, **54**, 728–9.

Benson, B. A. & Valenti-Hein, D. (2001). Cognitive and social learning treatments. In A. Dosen and K. Day (eds.), *The Treatment of Mental Illness and Behavior Disorders in Mentally Retarded Children and Adults* (pp. 101–18). Washington, DC: American Psychiatric Press.

Bernstein, D. A. & Borkovec, T. D. (1973). *Progressive Relaxation Training: A Manual for the Helping Professions*. Champaign, IL: Research Press.

Brooks, A., Todd, A. W., Tofflemoyer, S. & Horner, R. H. (2003). Use of functional assessment and a self-management system to increase academic engagement and work completion. *Journal of Positive Behavior Interventions*, **5**, 144–52.

Carr, E. G. (1977). The motivation of self-injurious behavior: A review of some hypotheses. *Psychological Bulletin*, **84**, 800–16.

Carr, E. G. & Carlson, J. I. (1993). Reduction of severe behavior problems in the community using a multicomponent treatment approach. *Journal of Applied Behavior Analysis*, **26**, 157–72.

Carr, E. G., Dunlap, G., Horner, R. H. *et al.* (2002). Positive behavior support: Evolution of an applied science. *Journal of Positive Behavior Interventions*, **4**, 4–16

Carr, E. G. & Durand, V. M. (1985). Reducing behavior problems through functional communication training. *Journal of Applied Behavior Analysis*, **18**, 111–26.

Carr, E. G., Horner, R. H., Turnbull, A. P. *et al.* (1999). *Positive Behavior Support for People with Developmental Disabilities: A Research Synthesis*, ed. D. Braddock. Washington, DC: American Association on Mental Retardation.

Carr, E. G., McLaughlin, D. M., Giacobbe-Grieco, T. & Smith, C. E. (2003). Using mood ratings and mood induction in assessment and intervention for severe problem behavior. *American Journal on Mental Retardation*, **108**, 32–55.

Cautela, J. R. & Grodin, J. (1979). *Relaxation: A Comprehensive Manual for Adults, Children, and Children with Special Needs*. Champaign, IL: Research Press.

Cipani, E. (1990). Principles of behavior modification. In J. L. Matson (ed.), *Handbook of Behavior Modification with the Mentally Retarded* (pp. 123–138). New York: Plenum Press.

Cole, G. A., Montgomery, R. W., Wilson, K. M. & Milan, M. A. (2000). Parametric analysis of over correction duration effects: Is longer really better than shorter? *Behavior Modification*, **24**, 359–78.

Coyle, C. & Cole, P. (2004). A videotaped self-modelling and self-monitoring treatment program to decrease off-task behaviour in children with autism. *Journal of Intellectual and Developmental Disability*, **29**, 3–15.

Crone, D. A. & Horner, R. H. (2003). *Building Positive Behavior Support Systems in Schools: Functional Behavioural Assessment*. New York: Guilford Press.

Cunningham, E. & O'Neill, R. E. (2000). Comparison of results of functional assessment and analysis methods with young children with autism. *Education and Training in Mental Retardation and Developmental Disabilities*, **35**, 406–14.

Deb, S., Matthews, T., Holt, G. & Bouras, N. (2001). *Practice Guidelines for the Assessment and Diagnosis of Mental Health Problems in Adults with Intellectual Disability*. Brighton: Pavilion.

Derby, K. M., Wacker, D. P., Sasso, G. M. *et al.* (1992). Brief functional assessment techniques to evaluate aberrant behavior in an outpatient setting: A summary of 79 cases. *Journal of Applied Behavior Analysis*, **25**, 713–21.

Dixon, M. R., Benedict, H. & Larson, T. (2001). Functional analysis and treatment of inappropriate verbal behavior. *Journal of Applied Behavior Analysis*, **34**, 361–3.

Dunlap, G. & Kincaid, D. (2001). The widening world of functional assessment: Comments on four manuals and beyond. *Journal of Applied Behavior Analysis*, **34**, 365–77.

Durand, V. M. (1999). Functional communication training using assistive devices: Recruiting natural communities of reinforcement. *Journal of Applied Behavior Analysis*, **32**, 247–67.

Durand, V. M. & Carr, E. G. (1992). An analysis of maintenance following functional communication training. *Journal of Applied Behavior Analysis*, **25**, 777–94.

Durand V. M. & Merges, E. (2001). Functional communication training: A contemporary behaviour analytic intervention for problem behaviors. *Focus on Autism and Other Developmental Disabilities*, **16**, 110–19, 136.

Ellingson, S. A., Miltenberger, R. G., Stricker, J., Galensky, T. L. & Garlinghouse, M. (2000). Functional assessment and intervention for challenging behaviors in the classroom by general classroom teachers. *Journal of Positive Behavior Interventions*, **2**, 85–97.

Ellis, J. & Magee, S. (2004). Modifications to basic functional analysis procedures in school settings: A selective review. *Behavioral Interventions*, **19**, 205–28.

Embregts, P. J. C. M. (2003). Using self-management, video feedback, and graphic feedback to improve social behavior of youth with mild mental retardation. *Education and Training in Developmental Disabilities*, **38**, 283–95.

Emerson, E. (2001). *Challenging Behaviour: Analysis and Intervention in People with Severe Intellectual Disabilities* (2nd edn). Cambridge: Cambridge University Press.

Esbenson, A. J. & Benson, B. A. (2003). Integrating behavioral, psychological and pharmacological treatment: A case study of an individual with borderline personality disorder and mental retardation. *Mental Health Aspects of Developmental Disabilities*, **6**, 107–13.

Falcomata, T. S., Roane, H. S., Hovanetz, A. N., Kettering, T. L & Keeney, K. M. (2004). An evaluation of response cost in the treatment of inappropriate vocalizations maintained by automatic reinforcement. *Journal of Applied Behavior Analysis*, **37**, 83–7.

Ferster, C. B. (1961). Positive reinforcement and behavioral deficits of autistic children. *Child Development*, **32**, 437–56.

Fisher, W. W., Piazza, C. C., Bowman, L. G. & Amari, A. (1996). Integrating caregiver report with a systematic choice assessment to enhance reinforcer identification. *American Journal on Mental Retardation*, **101**, 15–25.

Foxx, R. M. (2003). The treatment of dangerous behavior. *Behavioral Interventions*, **18**, 1–21.

Foxx, R. M. & McMorrow, M. J. (1983). *Stacking the Deck: A Social Skills Game for Adults with Developmental Disabilities*. Champaign, IL: Research Press.

Gardner, W. I. (ed.). (2002). *Aggression and Other Disruptive Behavioral Challenges*. Kingston, NY: National Association for the Dually Diagnosed Press.

Gardner, W. I. & Cole, C. L. (1990). Aggression and related conduct difficulties. In J. L. Matson (ed.). *Handbook of Behavior Modification with the Mentally Retarded* (2nd edn, pp. 225–1). New York: Plenum Press.

Gardner, W. I. & Graeber, J. L. (1993). Treatment of severe behavioral disorders in persons with mental retardation: A multimodal behavioral treatment model. In R. J. Fletcher & A. Dosen (eds.), *Mental Health Aspects of Mental Retardation: Progress in Assessment and Treatment* (pp. 45–69). New York: Lexington Books.

Gardner, W. I., Graeber, J. L & Cole, C. L. (1996). Behavior therapies: A multimodal diagnostic and intervention model. In J. W. Jacobson & J. A. Mulick (eds.), *Manual of Diagnosis and Professional Practice in Mental Retardation* (pp. 355–69). Washington, DC: American Psychological Association.

Grey, I. M., McClean, B. Kulkarni, L. & Hillery, J. (2003). Combining psychiatric and psychological approaches in the inpatient assessment of aggression in a client with moderate intellectual disability. *Irish Journal of Psychological Medicine*, **20**, 91–5.

Griffiths, D. M. & Nugent, J. A. (1998). Creating an integrated service system. In D. M. Griffiths, W. I. Gardner, and J. A. Nugent (eds.). *Behavioral Supports: Individual Centered Interventions – a Multimodal Functional Approach* (pp. 219–38). Kingston, NY: National Association for the Dually Diagnosed Press.

Grodin, J., Cautela, J. R. & Groden, G. (1989). *Relaxation Techniques for People with Special Needs: Breaking the Barriers.* [Video]. Champaign, IL: Research Press.

Hagopian, L. P., Crockett, J. L. & Keeney, K. M. (2001). Multicomponent treatment for blood-injury-injection phobia in a young man with mental retardation. *Research in Developmental Disabilities,* **22**, 141–9.

Harvey, J. R. (1979). The potential of relaxation training for the mentally retarded. *Mental Retardation,* **17**, 71–6.

Hastings, R. P. (1996). Staff strategies and explanations for intervening with challenging behaviours. *Journal of Intellectual Disability Research,* **40**, 166–75.

Havercamp, S. M., Scandlin, D. & Roth, M. (2004). Health disparities among adults with developmental disabilities, adults with other disabilities, and adults not reporting disability in North Carolina. *Public Health Reports,* **119**, 418–26.

Hayden, M. F. & Kim, S. H. (2002). Health status, health care utilization patterns, and health care outcomes of persons with intellectual disabilities: a review of the literature. *Policy Research Brief,* **13**, 1–18.

Herzroni, O. E. & Roth, T. (2003). Effects of a positive support approach to enhance communicative behaviors of children with mental retardation who have challenging behaviors. *Education and Training in Developmental Disabilities,* **38**, 95–105.

Ivancic, M. T. & Bailey, J. S. (1996). Current limits to reinforcer identification for some persons with profound multiple disabilities. *Research in Developmental Disabilities,* **17**, 77–92.

Iwata, B. A., Dorsey, M. F., Slifer, K. J., Bauman, K. E. & Richman, G. S. (1982). Toward a functional analysis of self-injury. *Analysis and Intervention in Developmental Disabilities,* **2**, 3–20.

Iwata, B. A., Pace, G. M., Dorsey, M. F. *et al.* (1994). The functions of self-injurious behavior: An experimental–epidemiological analysis. *Journal of Applied Behavior Analysis,* **27**, 215–40.

Jackson, H. J. (1983). Current trends in the treatment of phobias in autistic and mentally retarded persons. *Australia and New Zealand Journal of Developmental Disabilities,* **9**, 191–208.

Johnston, J. M., Foxx, R. M., Jacobson, J. W., Green, G. & Mulick, J. A. (2006). Positive Behaviour Support and Applied Behaviour Analysis. *The Behaviour Analyst,* **29**, 51–74.

Kuhn, D. E. & Matson, J. L. (2004). Assessment of feeding and mealtime behavior problems in persons with mental retardation. *Behavior Modification,* **28**, 638–48.

Lavie, T. & Sturmey, P. (2002). Training staff to conduct a paired-stimulus preference assessment. *Journal of Applied Behavior Analysis,* **35**, 209–11.

LeBlanc, L. A., Hagopian, L. P. & Maglieri, K. A. (2000). Use of token economy to eliminate excessive inappropriate social behavior in an adult with developmental disabilities. *Behavioral Interventions,* **15**, 135–43.

Lemmon, V. A. & Mizes, J. S. (2002). Effectiveness of exposure therapy: A case study of posttraumatic stress disorder and mental retardation. *Cognitive and Behavioral Practice,* **9**, 317–23.

Lindsay, W. R., Allan, R., Parry, C. *et al.* (2004). Anger and aggression in people with intellectual disabilities: Treatment and follow-up of consecutive referrals and a waiting list comparison. *Clinical Psychology and Psychotherapy,* **11**, 255–64.

Lindsay, W. R. & Baty, F. J. (1989). Group relaxation training with adults who are mentally handicapped. *Behavioural Psychotherapy,* **17**, 43–51.

Lindsay, W. R., Baty, F. J., Michie, A. M. & Richardson, I. (1989). A comparison of anxiety treatments with adults who have moderate and severe mental retardation. *Research in Developmental Disabilities*, **10**, 129–40.

Lindsay, W. R., Fee, M., Michie, A. & Heap, I. (1994). The effects of cue control relaxation on adults with severe mental retardation. *Research in Developmental Disabilities*, **15**, 425–37.

Lindsay, W. R., Fee, M. A. & Heap, I. (1994). The effects of cue control relaxation on adults with severe mental retardation. *Research in Developmental Disabilities*, **15**, 425–37.

Lindsay, W. R., Howells, L. & Pitcaithly, D. (1993). Cognitive therapy for depression with individuals with intellectual disabilities. *British Journal of Medical Psychology*, **66**, 133–41.

Lindsay, W. R. & Morrison, F. M. (1996). The effects of behavioural relaxation on cognitive performance in adults with severe intellectual disabilities. *Journal of Intellectual Disability Research*, **40**, 285–90.

Lovaas, I. O. & Simmons, J. Q. (1969). Manipulation of self-destruction in three retarded children. *Journal of Applied Behavior Analysis*, **2**, 143–57.

Lucyshyn, J., Dunlap, G. & Albin, R. W. (eds.). (2002). *Families and Positive Behavior Support: Addressing Problem Behavior in Family Contexts*. Baltimore, MD: Paul H. Brookes.

Mace, F. C. & Lalli, J. S. (1991). Linking descriptive and experimental analyses in the treatment of bizarre speech. *Journal of Applied Behavior Analysis*, **24**, 553–62.

Magee, S. K. & Ellis, J. (2000). Extinction effects during the assessment of multiple problem behaviors. *Journal of Applied Behavior Analysis*, **33**, 313–16.

Martin, G. & Pear, J. (2003). *Behavior Modification: What it is and How to Do it*. Upper Saddle River, NJ: Prentice-Hall.

Matson, J. L. (1982a). Treating obsessive-compulsive behavior in mentally retarded adults. *Behavior Modification*, **6**, 551–67.

Matson, J. L. (1982b). The treatment of behavioral characteristics of depression in the mentally retarded. *Behavior Therapy*, **13**, 209–18.

Matson, J. L. (1990). *Handbook of Behavior Modification with the Mentally Retarded* (2nd edn). New York: Plenum Press.

Matson, J. L., Bamburg, J. W., Cherry, K. E. & Paclawskyj, T. R. (1999). A validity study on the Questions About Behavioral Function (QABF) scale: Predicting treatment success for self-injury, aggression, and stereotypies. *Research in Developmental Disabilities*, **20**, 163–75.

Matson, J. L., Dettling, J. & Senatore, V. (1979). Treating depression of a mentally retarded adult. *British Journal of Mental Subnormality*, **16**, 86–8.

Matson, J. L., Kuhn, D. E., Dixon, D. R. *et al.* (2003). The development and factor structure of the Functional Assessment for multiple Causality (FACT). *Research in Developmental Disabilities*, **24**, 485–95.

McAtee, M., Carr, E. G. & Schulte, C. (2004). A contextual assessment inventory for problem behavior: Initial development. *Journal of Positive Behavior Interventions*, **6**, 148–65.

McNeill, S. L., Watson, T. S., Hennington, C. & Meeks, C. (2002). The effects of training parents in functional behavior assessment on problem identification, problem analysis, and intervention design. *Behavior Modification*, **26**, 499–515.

Michaels, C. A., Brown, F. & Mirabella, N. (2005). Personal paradigm shifts in PBS experts: Perceptions of treatment acceptability of decerative consequence-based behavioral procedures. *Journal of Positive Behavior Interventions*, **7**, 93–108.

Michultka, D. M., Poppen, R. L. & Blanchard, E. B. (1988). Relaxation training as a treatment for chronic headaches in an individual having severe developmental disabilities, *Biofeedback and Self Regulation*, **13**, 257–66.

Miltenberger, R. (2001). *Behavior modification: Principles and Procedures*. Pacific Grove, CA: Brooks/Cole.

Murphy, G. (1997). Understanding aggression in people with intellectual disabilities: lessons from other populations. *International Review of Research in Mental Retardation*, **21**, 33–67.

Newman, C. & Adams, K. (2004). Dog gone good: managing dog phobia in a teenage boy with a learning disability. *British Journal of Learning Disability*, **32**, 35–8.

Novaco, R. (1975). *Anger Control: The Development and Evaluation of an Experimental Treatment*. Lexington, MA: Lexington Books.

O'Conner, J. T., Sorenson-Burnworth, R. J., Rush, K. S. & Eidman, S. L. (2003). A mand analysis and levels treatment in an outpatient clinic. *Behavioral Interventions*, **18**, 139–50.

Ollendick, T. H. & Cerny, J. A. (1981). *Clinical Behavior Therapy with Children*. New York: Plenum Press.

O'Neill, R. E., Horner, R. H., Albin, R. W. *et al.* (1997). *Functional Assessment of Problem Behavior: A Practical Assessment Guide*. Pacific Grove, CA: Brooks/Cole.

Paclawskyj, T. R., Matson, J.L, Rush, K. S., Smalls, Y. & Vollmer, T. R. (2000). Questions About Behavioral Function (QABF): A behavioral checklist for functional assessment of aberrant behavior. *Research in Developmental Disabilities*, **21**, 223–29.

Piazza, C. C., Fisher, W. W., Hagopian, L. P., Bowman, L. G. & Toole, L. (1996). Using a choice assessment to predict reinforcer effectiveness. *Journal of Applied Behavior Analysis*, **29**, 1–9.

Poppen, R. (1998). *Behavioral Relaxation Training and Assessment* (2nd edn). Thousand Oaks, CA: Sage Publications.

Reid, D. H. & Green, C. W. (1990). Staff training. In J. L. Matson (ed.), *Handbook of Behavior Modification with the Mentally Retarded* (2nd edn, pp. 71–90). New York: Plenum Press.

Reid, D. H. & Parsons, M. B. (2004). *Positive Behavior Support Training Curriculum*. Washington, DC: American Association on Mental Retardation.

Rojahn, J. & Sisson, L. A. (1990). Stereotyped behavior. In J. L. Matson (ed.), *Handbook of Behavior Modification with the Mentally Retarded* (2nd edn, pp. 181–217). New York: Plenum Press.

Rose, J. (2000). Group interventions for anger in people with intellectual disabilities. *Research in Developmental Disabilities*, **21**, 171–81.

Royal College of Psychiatrists. (2001). *DC-LD Diagnostic Criteria for Psychiatric Disorders for Use with Adults with Learning Disabilities/Mental Retardation*. London: Gaskell.

Rush, A. J. & Frances, A. (2000). Expert consensus guideline series: Treatment of psychiatric and behavioral problems in mental retardation. *American Journal on Mental Retardation*, **105**, 159–228.

Scotti, J. R., Evans, I. M., Meyer, L. H. & Walker, P. (1991). A meta-analysis of intervention research with problem behavior: Treatment validity and standards of practice. *American Journal on Mental Retardation*, **96**, 233–56.

Sigafoos, J. & Saggers, E. (1995). A discrete-trial approach to the functional analysis of aggressive behaviour in two boys with autism. *Australia and New Zealand Journal of Developmental Disability*, **20**, 287–97.

Singh, N. N., Osborne, J. G. & Huguenin, N. H. (1996). Applied behavioral interventions. In J. W. Jacobson & J. A. Mulick (eds.), *Manual of Diagnosis and Professional Practice in Mental Retardation* (pp. 341–53). Washington, DC: American Psychological Association.

Smith, J. C. (1985). *Relaxation Dynamics: A Cognitive-Behavioral approach to Relaxation.* Champaign, IL: Research Press.

Sobsey, R. (1994). *Violence and Abuse in the Lives of People with Disabilities: The End of Silent Acceptance?* Baltimore, MD: Paul H. Brookes.

Sprague, J. R. & Horner, R. H. (1995). Functional assessment and intervention in community settings. *Mental Retardation and Developmental Disabilities Research Reviews*, **1**, 89–93.

Steed, S. E., Bigelow, K. M., Huynen, K. B. & Lutzker, J. R. (1995). The effects of planned activities training, low-demand schedule, and reinforcement sampling on adults with developmental disabilities who exhibit challenging behaviors. *Journal of Developmental and Physical Disabilities*, **7**, 303–16.

Stephens, R. M., Matson, J. L., Westmoreland, T. & Kulpa, J. (1981). Modification of psychotic speech with mentally retarded patients. *Journal of Mental Deficiency Research*, **25**, 187–97.

Sturmey, P. (1994). Assessing the functions of aberrant behaviors: A review of psychometric instruments. *Journal of Autism and Developmental Disorders*, **24**, 293–304.

Sturmey, P. (2004). Cognitive therapy with people with intellectual disabilities: A selective review and critique. *Clinical Psychology and Psychotherapy*, **11**, 222–32.

Sturmey, P., Lee, R., Reyer, H. & Robek, A. (2003a). Assessing preferences for staff: Some pilot data. *Behavioural and Cognitive Psychotherapy*, **31**, 103–7.

Sturmey, P., Matson, J. L. & Lott, J. D. (2003b). The internal consistency and factor structure of the Choice Assessment Scale. *Research in Developmental Disabilities*, **24**, 317–22.

Tassé, M. J., Havercamp, S. M. & Reiss, S. (1997). *Home-Of-Your-Own Cooperative Living Training Program.* Santa Barbara, CA: James Stanfield Publishing Company.

Taylor, J. L. (2002). A review of the assessment and treatment of anger and aggression in offenders with intellectual disability. *Journal of Intellectual Disability Research*, **46** (Suppl. 1), 57–73.

Taylor, J. L., Novaco, R. W., Gillmer, B. & Thorne, I. (2002). Cognitive-behavioural treatment of anger intensity among offenders with intellectual disabilities. *Journal of Applied Research in Intellectual Disabilities*, **15**, 151–65.

Thompson, T. & Gray, D. B. (eds.). (1994). *Destructive Behavior in Developmental Disabilities: Diagnosis and Treatment.* Thousand Oaks, CA: Sage Publications.

Toole, L. M., Bowman, L. G., Thomason, J. L., Hagopian, L. P. & Rush, K. S. (2003). Observed increases in positive affect during behavioural treatment. *Behavioral Interventions*, **18**, 35–42.

Van Houten, R., Axelrod, S., Bailey, J. S. *et al.* (1988). The right to effective behavioral treatment. *The Behavior Analyst*, **11**, 111–14.

Vollmer, T. R. (1994). The concept of automatic reinforcement: Implications for behavioral research in developmental disabilities. *Research in Developmental Disabilities*, **15**, 187–207.

Vollmer, T. R. & Smith, R. G. (1996). Some current themes in functional analysis research. *Research in Developmental Disabilities*, **17**, 229–49.

Watson, T. S., Ray, K. P., Turner, H. S. & Logan, P. (1999). Teacher implemented functional analysis and treatment: A method for linking assessment to intervention. *School Psychology Review*, **28**, 292–302.

Wilder, D. A., Masuda, A., O'Connor, C. & Haham, M. (2001). Brief functional analysis and treatment of bizarre vocalizations in an adult with schizophrenia. *Journal of Applied Behavior Analysis*, **34**, 65–8.

Yarbrough, S. C. & Carr, E. G. (2000). Some relationships between informant assessment and functional analysis of problem behavior. *American Journal on Mental Retardation*, **105**, 130–51.

19

Psychopharmacology in intellectual disabilities

Bryan King

Introduction

Little controversy surrounds the notion that persons with intellectual disabilities (ID) may engage in disruptive and challenging behaviours. One of the common referral queries to clinicians of people with ID – 'Is this a mental illness or just a problem behaviour?' – tends to stir up more discussion. At one extreme, attempts to understand maladaptive behaviours are merely descriptive and simply default to the ID itself. For example, aggression or self-injurious behaviour is said to be a product of the individual's cognitive disability and does not warrant a 'diagnosis'. At the same time, the degree to which an individual is held accountable for his behaviour is also placed into consideration, as is the appropriateness of pharmacotherapy, depending on the answer to the referral question.

At the other extreme, an attempt is made to identify a syndrome or disorder within which the behaviour in question can be understood – to cast the behaviour at issue as the manifestation of a physiological abnormality. For example, the self-injurious or aggressive behaviour may be viewed as a symptom of a mood disorder (see also Chapter 4 by Hemmings). Such attempts clearly carry therapeutic implications, and can be traced back to the origins of the psychiatry of ID.

Thus, Sir John Charles Bucknill (1858) observed that amongst the insane (including persons with ID then termed 'idiots'), 'one must recognize . . . [the] part of their conduct which they are unable to control, and which is neither more nor less than the expression of pathological states of the brain . . .' He went on to suggest that their 'insanity' was in large part responsible for the majority of the behavioural disturbances of significance, and hence 'this conduct must be resisted (e.g. treated) solely by physiological and pharmaceutical means; direct moral treatment

Psychiatric and Behavioural Disorders in Intellectual and Developmental Disabilities, ed. Nick Bouras and Geraldine Holt. Published by Cambridge University Press. © Cambridge University Press 2007.

is as much out of place as in inflammation of the heart, or of any other viscus' (p. 453).

Regarding our present medication interventions, the 'behaviour vs. diagnosis' question translates to whether one proposes to target a particular symptom or group of symptoms, or whether one is introducing a medication to address a specific disorder. These approaches, both 'dimensional' and 'categorical' may be received by individuals and care providers with varying degrees of enthusiasm, but these formulations are not mutually exclusive, and this chapter aims to address both.

While the aetiology and classification of maladaptive behaviour in people with ID is receiving deserved attention, our knowledge of brain–behaviour relationships at every level, from the molecular to the environmental, is exploding. This new knowledge may have the effect of stoking our excitement about new possibilities for therapeutic intervention. At the same time, it should be humbling to acknowledge how little we understand in terms of both what it is that we are treating and the complexities of our interventions.

Medications are blunt instruments. The 'therapeutic armamentarium' does not include 'smart bombs', but rather, molecules that distribute themselves throughout brain and body and which interact with relatively promiscuous neurotransmitter receptors or receptor subtypes to alter function. Side effects (collateral damage) are the expected consequence of this lack of specificity or of the downstream effects (fallout) of the intervention. Medications are not cognizant of the purpose for which they are utilized – for example, to treat psychosis or to treat hiccoughs, so to assume that a particular response to a drug confirms or rules out a diagnosis makes no more sense than to suggest that bombs only hurt bad people.

Medications can be wonderful. The history of medicine is filled with the life-saving effects that various medications have provided. As people we rely on medications to cure or manage our illnesses and to ease the burden of our infirmities. It is fair to say that we are positively predisposed to medication, and that we look forward to more and better medications with which to expand our ability to alleviate the burden of illness.

Against this backdrop, the use of medication in ID is seldom a neutral endeavour. Critics typically highlight a perceived lack of precision with respect to diagnosis, problems with the monitoring of effectiveness, and the risk of side effects that some recipients may not be able to understand or self-report. And, despite decades of drug treatment in this population, it is fair to assert, and perhaps difficult to reconcile, both that there remains a relative absence of data to inform optimal medication use, and that medication use is common.

Prevalence of psychotropic medication use

In his review of institutional treatment in the United States and Canada at the turn of the century, Tuke (1885) observes the use of hyocyamine ('Merck's white crystals'), extract of cannabis indica, digitalis, opium, bromide salts, chloral hydrate, paraldehyde, blood-letting and counter-irritation among the treatments used in the management of agitation in institutions which included individuals both with ID and with mental illness. With the advent of major tranquilizers came renewed enthusiasm for the treatment of behaviour problems in people with ID exemplified by LeVann's characterization of thioridazine as a drug with remarkable utility, 'virtually devoid of side-effects' (LeVann, 1961). Of course, this drug now carries a 'black box' warning for the possibility of causing sudden cardiac death, and there are many other side effects with which it has come to be associated.

As every new drug class has been developed over the years, potential uses for persons with ID have been explored. With an increased risk for the experience of mental disorders in this population, some individuals with ID continue to require the skilled application of 'medicinal treatment' (Bucknill & Tuke, 1858) or present-day psychopharmacologic treatment.

In their study of the prevalence of receipt of psychotropic medications for people with ID in residential settings, Robertson et al. (2000) observed that the use of psychotropic medication is commonplace, with up to 56% of individuals in the survey receiving a neuroleptic drug depending on their place of residence. Interestingly, they also found that while antidepressant receipt is more likely to be linked to symptoms of mental illness, the prescription of antipsychotic and anxiolytic medications is more often linked to problematic behaviour(s). Lewis and colleagues (2002) surveyed adults with ID living in community settings and noted that a third of the sample was receiving one or more psychotropic medications. Fully a third of the population did not have an identifiable diagnosis for which these medications were being prescribed. Expert consensus opinion is clear that, as like any therapeutic intervention, the use of psychotropic medications should follow, and should be informed by, a diagnostic hypothesis (Kalachnik et al., 1998; Szymanski and King, 1999; Anonymous, 2000).

Pharmacotherapy and aetiology of intellectual disabilities

With recent advances in the neurosciences and molecular biology in particular, hundreds of previously unidentified genetic causes of ID have been described. In some cases the underlying aetiology may be particularly important in considering treatments. For example, in phenylketonuria (PKU), attempts have been made to minimize or to attenuate behavioural disturbance, typically hyperactivity and impulsivity, by dietary modification. More recently as animal models of this disorder are developed and explored, it appears that dopaminergic abnormalities may play a particularly salient role in the expression of maladaptive behaviours and perhaps in the design of specific treatments. Thus, early intervention with dopamine agonists may ultimately play a unique role in the treatment of behavioural and cognitive disturbance associated with PKU (Diamond, 1996).

Abnormalities in serotonergic function have long been reported in Down syndrome. This hyposerotonemia led to trials of serotonin replacement with mixed results, but serotonergic drugs may yet hold particular relevance for persons with Down syndrome (Tu and Zellweger, 1965; Gedye, 1990; Hirayama *et al.*, 2004).

In Prader–Willi syndrome, serotonergic abnormalities are also being reported as are responses to serotonergic agents (Hellings and Warnock, 1994; Dykens and Shah, 2003). Taken together, support can easily be marshalled for the conclusion that the identification of the underlying cause of ID has become increasingly important in considering pharmacotherapy.

Although perhaps not a direct consequence of the underlying genetic abnormality, prevention of common medical consequences of a specific syndrome may also confer significant behavioural benefit, as well as even inform the pathogenesis of behavioural syndromes. Thus it is interesting to note that the anticonvulsant, vigabatrin, appeared to have a positive effect on autistic symptoms in young children with tuberous sclerosis complex (TSC) and infantile spasms. Jambaque *et al.* (2000) shared their experience with 13 children with TSC who received vigabatrin for treatment of refractory epilepsy. Half of the children (seven) had infantile spasms, and the remainder had partial seizures. In the former group, when treatment was initiated before two years of age, all subjects experienced the complete remission of spasms. All of these subjects had moderate to severe ID, with significant deficits in social interaction, and five of these subjects had autistic and hyperactive behaviour. However, there were dramatic improvements reported at the end of follow-up (3–5 yrs). The behavioural benefit of vigabatrin in the absence of epilepsy remains to be demonstrated, but in this context, perhaps similar to PKU, the aetiology of the ID may suggest important medical interventions that ultimately could have a positive effect on the developmental or behavioural trajectory.

Psychiatric disorders in ID

ID is a significant risk factor for psychopathology in general, and, as may be inferred from the description of causes above, this increased risk may derive from biological vulnerabilities as well as risks that accrue from the environment. Thus, the common co-occurrence of ID with other illness, for example epilepsy, may increase the risk of mental disturbance. Moreover, the treatments for epilepsy and other medical conditions may carry some 'behavioural toxicity' which can increase the likelihood of manifest mental illness. Phenobarbital has widely been reported to increase the risk of motoric hyperactivity and disinhibition in children and in individuals with developmental disorders (Devinsky, 1995), and topiramate may cause cognitive toxicity (Kockelmann *et al.*, 2004). Special conditions like these merely add to the potential explanations for mental illness in ID. Anxiety, mood, and thought disorders are prevalent as well.

Anxiety disorders

Anxiety disorders are common but likely underdiagnosed in the population with ID. Symptoms of anxiety disorders may include aggression, agitation, compulsive or repetitive behaviours and even self-injurious behaviour. Insomnia may also be a manifestation of anxiety. Symptoms of panic may be expressed as agitation, screaming, crying or clinging – which might even suggest delusional or paranoid behaviour to some observers.

Treatment of anxiety disorders

As for the population in general, many different medications have been explored in the treatment of anxiety. Antidepressants, anxiolytics, beta blockers and antipsychotics appear to form the mainstay of treatment in persons with ID – which is to say that virtually any medication class may be considered for this purpose. In addition to exerting a primary anxiolytic effect, successful medication treatment may also improve an individual's accessibility to traditional educational and behavioural therapeutic interventions. As yet there are, however, no systematic clinical trials of the pharmacological treatment of anxiety for people with ID. As for anxiety disorders in the general population, serotonin reuptake inhibitors (SSRI) including citalopram, escitalopram, paroxetine, fluoxetine, fluvoxamine and sertraline may be useful in persons with ID. However, there are some individuals with ID, particularly a sub-group of individuals with disorders in the autism spectrum, who appear to exhibit extraordinary sensitivity to drugs of this and other classes. This sensitivity can present with activation or disinhibition – an increase in target symptoms at doses of medication that might otherwise appear quite low.

While it may be of particular relevance for the SSRIs, it is worth noting that metabolic interactions with cytochrome P-450 enzyme systems may affect the plasma levels of concurrent medications, and thus individuals with ID may require relatively unique dosing strategies. Thus, in some populations where 30 to 40% of persons have epilepsy and/or as many as 70% may have some other medical condition of significance (King *et al.*, 1994), drug interactions become an increasingly important consideration.

Buspirone is another serotonergic agent that may be of benefit for some persons with ID. Buspirone is a partial agonist at the $5\text{-}HT_{1A}$ receptor subtype, and its effects (e.g. whether there is a net increase or decrease in serotonergic activity) may vary as a function of the endogenous serotonergic 'tone' in the recipient. Ratey et al. (1989) reported the use of buspirone in an open trial in persons with diagnosed anxiety disorders manifest by aggressive and self-injurious behaviours. Typical doses at which responses were evident ranged from 15 to 45 mg daily. In another open trial by King and Davanzo (1996), it appeared that non-responders to buspirone remained so even as the medication dose was increased beyond the levels used by Ratey and colleagues. A study from Verhoeven and Tuinier (1996) also explored buspirone in the treatment of anxiety and was quite positive – suggesting that this agent should be among those considered in treating this population. Moreover, specific advantages include a relatively benign side-effect profile, most notably the absence of motor or cognitive toxicities at therapeutic doses (Ratey et al., 1989). Our recent experience with this agent has led us to consider its use particularly in individuals who have demonstrated behavioural activation or disinhibition with the SSRIs. In this context, the drug may simply be better tolerated, or its partial agonism may have a unique role in modulating an 'overactive' system.

Beta-adrenergic antagonists have also been reported to be of use in the population with ID. Ratey and colleagues were led to explore this class of drugs based upon their perception that many individuals with ID appear to have a low frustration tolerance (Ratey and Gordon, 1993). At doses of propranolol upwards of 1000 mg per day, the mechanism of action of this drug might arguably become less selective for adrenergic systems and perhaps similar to that for buspirone as a partial serotonin $5\text{-}HT_{1A}$ agonist.

Data on the use of anticonvulsant medications – for example, valproic acid and carbamazepine, in the treatment of anxiety disorders in people with ID are limited. Because of reports that valproic acid may decrease symptoms of flashbacks, hyperarousal and hyper-reactivity in the context of post-traumatic stress disorder (Clark et al., 1999), it may be useful in a person who has failed other treatments. The same may be true for carbamazepine, which also has been reported helpful in the context of post-traumatic stress disorder in the general population (Sutherland and Davidson, 1994).

Although benzodiazepines are commonly prescribed for short periods in treatment for anxiety in the general population, there are unique concerns when used in the context of ID, particularly regarding the possibility of increased confusion, cognitive impairment, unsteadiness and paradoxical excitement (Kalachnik et al., 2002). Barron and Sandman (1985) reported paradoxical excitement associated with benzodiazepines, which occurred in upwards of 35% of individuals from an institutionalized population. Nevertheless, drugs like lorazepam, alprazolam, and clonazepam are widely used for the treatment of acute anxiety, particularly that associated with procedures like dental visits and blood tests. As with persons without ID, benzodiazepines should be considered alongside other drugs, particularly for acute management of anxiety. It is probably prudent, however, to test the response to one of these agents at a time and place and setting where disinhibition and agitation could be managed – and not to risk making a difficult situation worse by assuming the drug will be well tolerated when it is initially administered (e.g. for a transatlantic flight).

Though not the subject of studies specifically looking at their effectiveness in the treatment of anxiety, antipsychotics have been widely used in the context of mental disorders in people with ID and are indeed the most commonly prescribed class of psychotropic drugs in this population (Aman, 1993; Baumeister et al., 1998). Though potentially very effective in attenuating anxiety, concerns about the long-term side effects of these drugs would typically prompt considering alternatives like serotonin reuptake inhibitors and other antidepressants prior to antipsychotics. Since anxiety disorders are often chronic conditions, clinicians should hesitate to commit an individual with ID to a long-term trial of antipsychotic agents in the absence of convincing evidence of effectiveness and periodic attempts to confirm the ongoing need for such medication (Kalachnik et al., 1998).

Mood disorders

(See Chapter 7 by Stavrakaki and Lunsky.) Special considerations in the use of antidepressant medication must take into account the frequency of co-occurring medical conditions in this population. Thus, tricyclic antidepressants must be used with the knowledge that the risks of lowering seizure threshold are significant (Trimble, 1984). Cardiac anomalies are common in some ID syndromes, and the anticholinergic side effects of tricyclic antidepressants may be particularly significant for some persons – for example, those with Down syndrome. Individuals with ID may require lower levels of antidepressant drug than their 'neurotypical' peers and, as noted earlier, disinhibition or behavioural activation has been described even with typical antidepressant doses of the serotonin reuptake inhibitors (Racusin et al., 1999).

Verhoeven et al. (2001) in the Netherlands examined the effect of the serotonin reuptake inhibitor, citalopram, on depression in an open prospective trial of adults with ID of mixed aetiologies. For 12 of the 20 subjects treated with doses from 20 to 40 mg of citalopram, moderate to marked improvement was observed in measures of affect, motivation, motor activity (including aggression, self-injury, irritability), and vegetative (sleep/appetite) symptoms. Improvement was maintained for over one year. Side effects were reported to be minimal, and included the possible new onset of epilepsy in one subject, and dose-related behavioural disinhibition in another.

The same group was also positively impressed with the effect of citalopram for depression in an adult with 4p− syndrome (Verhoeven *et al.*, 2002). Masi *et al.* (1997) treated 7 adolescents with mild ID with paroxetine and observed significant improvement in the absence of treatment-limiting side effects.

Psychosis

Antipsychotic medications (neuroleptics) have long been used, arguably overused, in persons with ID. Antipsychotics continue to be the most widely prescribed class of psychotropic medication, even more commonly prescribed than anticonvulsant drugs. Yet the incidence of diagnosed psychotic disorders does not approach the frequency that might be inferred from the use of this class of agent. It is likely not the case that this is merely a manifestation of poor clinical care, as the same finding holds for the general population. At some point the atypical antipsychotics may come to be regarded less for their antipsychotic effects and more for their apparent impact on mood and self-regulatory disturbances. In any case, their pharmacology is complex and it should not be assumed that their broad use reflects poor clinical care.

Individuals with ID are at greater risk of developing tardive dyskinesia than the general population (Bodfish *et al.*, 1996; Sachdev, 1992). On the other hand, spontaneous abnormal involuntary movements are not uncommon in this population (Bodfish *et al.*, 1996) and confound interpreting rates of antipsychotic-induced tardive dyskinesia. The growing availability of atypical antipsychotic drugs and their use in persons with ID is clearly enhanced by the reduced risk for tardive dyskinesia and extrapyramidal symptoms as well as cognitive toxicity. They do not come without side effects however. Weight gain and metabolic disturbances may in fact be of greater consequence than abnormal involuntary movements for some persons (Hellings *et al.*, 2001).

Prescriptions for the atypicals have dramatically outpaced and replaced those for the first generation (e.g. haloperidol, thioridazine, chlorpromazine) antipsychotic drugs. Friedlander *et al.* (2001) observed that risperidone and olanzapine were the most frequently prescribed of the atypicals in their clinic. The evidence supporting expanded indications for risperidone, including behavioural disturbances in persons with ID, continues to be elaborated (Schweitzer, 2001; Van Bellinghen and De Troch, 2001; Turgay *et al.*, 2002; Buitelaar *et al.*, 2001; Zarcone *et al.*, 2001; Aman *et al.*, 2002). In a randomized, placebo-controlled cross-over trial of risperidone on aberrant behaviour in 20 individuals with ID of mixed aetiology, with a response definition of a 50% reduction in mean Aberrant Behaviour Checklist total scores, half of the subjects responded to risperidone (Zarcone *et al.*, 2001). Weight gain

(84% of subjects) and sedation (40% of subjects) were common side effects. Cohen *et al.* (2001) have shown that weight gain in this context may not relate to dose, and calorie restriction may not be sufficient to result in weight loss.

Although experience is still growing, experience with the atypicals thus far is generally encouraging with respect to their side-effect profiles in persons with ID. Advokat *et al.* (2000) used the Matson Evaluation of Drug Side Effects (MEDS) scale to assess 51 institutionalized adults with ID. Subjects were divided into three groups on the basis of their receipt of typical (thioridazine, chlorpromazine, haloperidol) or atypical antipsychotics (risperidone or olanzapine) or no psychotropic medication at all. The scores on their side-effects scale were significantly higher in the group receiving typical antipsychotics in comparison to the other two groups. Moreover, the scores in the atypical antipsychotic and no psychotropic groups were essentially equivalent.

Attempts to taper and discontinue antipsychotic drugs in persons long exposed to them continue to be justified in light of the Ahmed *et al.* (2000) findings. In this study, non-psychotic subjects, most of whom had received antipsychotics for over five years, were assigned to receive either a taper to discontinuation over four months, or maintenance of their drug regimen. A third of the subjects assigned to discontinuation were able to tolerate the complete withdrawal of their antipsychotics with this strategy. Another fifth were able to be maintained at a dose that was half of their starting dose. Compared with the control group, drug reduction was not associated with an increase in maladaptive behaviour.

While highlighting the importance of establishing the minimum effective dose (Kalachnik *et al.*, 1998), this study is also helpful with respect to pace of reductions for which there is no consensus in the literature. One should taper at a rate that is clinically meaningful, while at the same time taking care to limit any withdrawal-emergent effects. Ahmed *et al.*'s approach demonstrates that some individuals who have received medication chronically for over three years may still be completely withdrawn without incident in just four months.

Attention deficit hyperactivity disorder

Rates of attention deficit hyperactivity disorder (ADHD) in people with ID are higher than for the general population, but most treatment studies of this disorder have specifically excluded children with cognitive disability (Pearson *et al.*, 2004).

Despite reports of paradoxical responses to stimulant medications in persons with ID, with higher than expected rates of emergent motor tics and emotional lability (Handen *et al.*, 1991, 1992), a growing body of literature supports the use of stimulant drugs for the treatment of ADHD in the context of ID (Handen *et al.*, 1992, 1994; Aman *et al.*, 1993; Johnson *et al.*, 1994; Pearson *et al.*, 2004). A problem awaiting clarification concerns the likelihood of a response to stimulants in relation to the severity of cognitive disability. For example, Handen *et al.* (1992) studied children with mild to moderate ID and ADHD. The study was a double-blind, placebo-controlled cross-over design in which methylphenidate was administered twice daily at 0.3 and 0.6 mg/kg. Of the 14 children, nine were responders, and of those remaining, three subjects showed improved behaviour ratings on both placebo and active drug. Aman *et al.* (1993) also examined the effect of a morning dose of methylphenidate (0.4 mg (kg/day)) in a double-blind, placebo-controlled cross-over comparison with fenfluramine (up to 1.5 mg (kg/day)). All children had an IQ below 75, Conners' hyperactivity indices in the 90th percentile, and DSM-IIIR diagnoses of ADHD. Both drugs outperformed placebo, with an advantage to methylphenidate. However, none of the subjects with IQ below 45 improved, a finding consistent with earlier work (Aman *et al.*, 1991). On the other hand, while Handen and colleagues (1994) also confirmed the effectiveness of methylphenidate in children with ID, their data do not support the finding that IQ was a negative predictor of response. Children with lower IQ actually showed more improvement in work output in the methylphenidate condition.

Agarwal *et al.* (2001) observe that problems of impulsivity, disinhibition, and behavioural difficulties in the context of hyperkinesis often pose significant problems for parents and teachers. These investigators performed a randomized controlled trial of the alpha-2 agonist, clonidine, for symptoms of hyperactivity and impulsivity in children with ID ranging from mild to severe. In total, ten children were treated with clonidine (4, 6, and 8 micrograms daily) in a cross-over design. Clonidine significantly improved hyperactivity, impulsivity, and inattention in a dose-dependent manner with the highest dose being most effective. Although half of the children became drowsy on the clonidine, this problem seemed to diminish over time.

Santosh and Baird (1999) also have favourable experience with clonidine for ADHD with hyperarousal, aggression, and tics. Conversely, they have observed more frequent side effects of sleep and appetite disturbance, seizures, tics, and even haematological side effects and hair loss associated with stimulants in this population.

Impulse control and behavioural disorders

Aggression and self-injurious behaviour (SIB) can occur in a variety of disorders and are thus non-specific from a psychiatric diagnostic perspective. Where these behaviours are concerned, the clinician must consider the presence or absence of a number of factors to arrive at the presumptive diagnosis that should inform the choice of potential medication interventions. These factors include the chronicity of the behaviour, whether it may serve a communicative function, whether it is invariant in its topography (e.g. hitting only the left ear suggesting an ear infection), whether it is situational, whether it is associated with regression from a previous level of function, whether there are appetitive changes or changes in mood that correlate with its onset, and so on. Every effort should be aimed at treating the underlying cause of SIB or aggression, not merely to address the behaviour in isolation (see also Chapters 14 by Hillery and Dodd and 17 by Reese *et al.*). Tsiouris *et al.* (2003) rather pointedly demonstrated the importance of this process with the successful treatment of SIB, using a variety of medication strategies, guided by psychiatric diagnoses in a sample of 26 children and adults with ID whose behaviour had not responded to prior treatment.

Notwithstanding such demonstrations of the importance of diagnosis, there will be some persons – for example, those with the diagnosis of stereotyped movement disorder with SIB, for whom the symptom is essentially the diagnosis. Pharmacological interventions in these situations draw more heavily upon studies that have been aimed at specifically attenuating SIB. These studies derive from observations that dopaminergic, serotonergic, and opioidergic mechanisms can influence the expression or maintenance of stereotypy and even SIB in some animal models (Schroeder *et al.*, 2001).

Thus there is evidence to support the use of dopamine antagonists in SIB and aggression, both in theory and in practice (Aman, 1993). For thioridazine in particular, at least 11 studies since 1959, totalling over 1000 children and adults with ID, have been published, suggesting that SIB and aggression may improve. Of these studies, five were double-blind, placebo-controlled trials. Typical doses were less than 300 mg/day, with daily doses as low as 15 mg/day being reported for some children. Thioridazine is seldom used these days because of its potential for delaying cardiac conduction, but positive reports can also be found for most other antipsychotics in this population. Although suggested by some, there is no convincing evidence that the mechanism of therapeutic action of antipsychotics in SIB or aggression is merely to suppress behaviour generally through a non-specific sedating effect. Most would view such an outcome as clearly undesirable in an individual with pre-existing cognitive disability, and many of the earliest reports specifically noted the absence of sedation.

Clearly, subsequent experience with these agents has revealed their potential for lasting side effects like tardive dyskinesia, and enthusiasm for antipsychotic use in this population should be tempered. Recent interest in atypical antipsychotics for SIB and aggression has grown however, and positive reports (reminiscent of the initial experience with haloperidol, chlorpromazine, and thioridazine in this population) do exist to support consideration of risperidone, olanzapine, clozapine, and sulpiride. For example, McDonough *et al.* (2000) reported the use of olanzapine in the treatment of SIB in seven adults with ID residing in an institutional setting. In this open, prospective trial, each of the subjects was characterized as having a 'stereotypic subtype' of self-injury. Olanzapine was added to existing antipsychotics in each case, and measures of SIB frequency and severity were recorded for 17 weeks. In total, three subjects responded.

Hammock *et al.* (2001) presented the cases of two individuals with profound ID whose self-injury had been refractory to multiple medication trials, including risperidone, but who responded to clozapine at daily doses of 200 mg.

Based upon pre-clinical data, drugs, which selectively antagonize D_1 receptor function, when they become available, may carry unique potential for attenuation of repetitive SIB (King, 2002; Turner and Lewis, 2002).

A sub-group of persons with SIB also exhibit self-restraining behaviours – for example, binding their extremities in their clothing, or seeking out self-protective devices like helmets or gloves. Such behaviour might indicate an ego-dystonic quality of self-injury, and suggests the possibility of SIB as a compulsive or 'driven' phenomenon (King, 1993). In the Prader–Willi Syndrome, obsessive-compulsive disorder occurs more commonly than in the general population, and compulsive skin picking may improve along with other compulsive behaviours with an SSRI (Hellings and Warnock, 1994). Given these findings, trials of serotonin re-uptake inhibitors are increasingly common among individuals with SIB. Favourable experiences have been reported for fluoxetine, paroxetine, fluvoxamine, sertraline, trazodone, and clomipramine in this regard. However, of these agents, only clomipramine has been shown to be useful in controlled studies (Lewis *et al.*, 1996). Owing to its effect of lowering seizure threshold, clomipramine is generally not a first-line treatment for compulsive SIB in individuals frequently co-morbid for epilepsy. On the other hand, anticonvulsant levels must be closely monitored with the addition of an SSRI. Individuals whose behaviour worsens with an SSRI may still benefit from this class of drug but reintroduction should be at a greatly reduced dosage.

Some individuals who self-injure appear to have altered pain sensitivity as was suggested nearly a century ago (Ireland, 1898). This observation, coupled with data indicating that opioid antagonists can reduce stereotyped movements and self-injury in animal models, and the knowledge that opioids may influence dopaminergic function, has fuelled interest in this class of drugs. Naltrexone is the opioid antagonist most widely used for SIB, based upon a literature that is quite evenly mixed between positive and neutral – there is surprisingly little evidence of naltrexone actually contributing to negative responses. Typical doses range from 0.5 to 2.0 mg (kg/day) in children and up to 200 mg/day in adults. In a study examining the effect of naltrexone on drug-induced self-biting behaviour in an animal model, King and colleagues (1993) found that a dose of 0.01 mg/kg of naltrexone was consistently effective in attenuating SIB, but that this effect was lost as doses were increased. Thus, lower doses may deserve consideration for some individuals who do not respond to conventional doses. On balance, naltrexone appears to be well tolerated in persons with ID; sedation is the side effect most likely to be observed.

A growing appreciation exists for the therapeutic utility of drugs acting at glutamate receptor subtypes. Glutamatergic and dopaminergic interactions in the neostriatum are the focus of research on the pathogenesis of a host of neuropsychiatric illnesses including schizophrenia, obsessive-compulsive disorder, SIB and aggression. Dextromethorphan is a cough suppressant that binds to the NMDA (N-methyl-D-aspartate) receptor, and was reported by Welch and Sovner (1992) to have dramatically improved SIB in a 25-year-old with congenital rubella syndrome. The benefit persisted for 16 months of continued treatment. Perhaps ominously, no follow-up studies have been reported with this drug in SIB. Lamotrigine is an anticonvulsant drug that also appears to indirectly antagonize glutamate through reducing its release. A case report suggests that lamotrigine may also be useful in reducing self-injury in the context of a stereotyped movement disorder (Davanzo and King, 1996). More recently, Crawford and colleagues (2001) presented an open-label, randomized, parallel group, multicentre add-on study comparing the (non-glutamatergic) anticonvulsant gabapentin with lamotrigine in 109 patients with ID and treatment-resistant, focal epilepsy. Both drugs were equally well tolerated and each achieved similar improvement in seizure frequency. Gabapentin may have had an edge with respect to some behavioural indices, denoted by the investigators as communication, co-operation, and restlessness, but lamotrigine also was credited with improving challenging behaviour.

On the other hand, in a controlled trial of lamotrigine for challenging behaviour in children with autism, Belsito et al. (2001) could not observe any advantage for lamotrigine over placebo. Moreover, Beran and Gibson (1998) identified several cases of distinct behavioural worsening, primarily aggression, associated with lamotrigine treatment.

Amantadine is another NMDA receptor antagonist that has been explored in the treatment of behavioural disturbance in ID. King and colleagues (2001) observed a very impressive reduction in impulsive and aggressive behaviour in a small series of children with severe behaviour disturbance treated openly in an inpatient setting. The structurally related drug, memantine, is likely to receive attention in this regard as well.

Amongst other drugs that have been described in managing SIB include adrenergics, primarily beta-adrenergic antagonists, lithium, and anticonvulsants. Interestingly, in at least two reported cases, SIB dramatically improved with the withdrawal of phenobarbital. The potential behavioural 'toxicity' of this and any drug should not be overlooked in designing treatment strategies for persons with ID. Medical co-morbidity is the rule in individuals with ID, and the importance of identifying and treating underlying medical problems, or refining that treatment, cannot be overstated.

Sleep disturbance

Sleep disturbance is a surprisingly little studied but often significant problem for some persons with ID (Gail Williams *et al.*, 2004). Although sedating antidepressants appear to be used with some frequency in clinical practice, melatonin is the best studied medication for the treatment of insomnia in children with disabilities.

Coppola *et al.* (2004) performed a randomized, controlled cross-over study in which melatonin was given to children, adolescents, and young adults at doses up to 9 mg daily. Sleep onset was improved in the active treatment group. Jan (2000) also observed a positive experience with melatonin prescribed openly to children with moderate to severe ID of mixed aetiologies. Hours of sleep, nocturnal awakenings, sleep onset, and early morning awakening were all improved in this series. Similarly, Pillar *et al.* (2000) administered a single 3 mg dose of melatonin, but monitored sleep efficiency as well as activity (wrist actigraph) in their sample of children with severe ID. Sleep was significantly improved with melatonin, and two of the subjects continued to receive the medication for 18 months following the completion of the study. The authors conclude that melatonin deserves broader consideration for the treatment of children with ID and disturbed circadian rhythm of sleep.

Conclusion

Pharmacotherapy continues to be widely used for the treatment of both symptoms and syndromes of emotional and behavioural disturbance in persons with ID. Because of the complexity of the clinical situations for individuals with ID, and because of the myriad of vastly different directions that can be pursued with individual psychotropic medications, it should be clear that medication should be guided by a complete diagnostic assessment aiming for multidisciplinary care. Antipsychotic medications are the most common of the classes of medication typically prescribed, for a variety of indications. In some circumstances it is clear that attempts to establish a minimum effective dose may lead to the successful discontinuation of these drugs. In general, evidence is accumulating to support the shift from typical to atypical antipsychotic agents in this population.

Summary points

- The rational or appropriate use of psychopharmacological treatment will be advanced by our growing knowledge of the causes of ID, greater attention to diagnosis and outcome measures in clinical trials, and greater attention to this population.
- New drugs are also being developed with greater selectivity, and our knowledge of how drugs work is also growing.
- Pharmacotherapy should be part of a multimodal and multidisciplinary approach to treatment.

Acknowledgment

The author wishes to thank Aziz Soomro, M.D., for technical assistance in the preparation of this chapter.

REFERENCES

Advokat, C. D., Mayville, E. A. & Matson, J. L. Side effect profiles of atypical antipsychotics, typical antipsychotics, or no psychotropic medications in persons with mental retardation. *Research in Developmental Disabilities*. **21**(1):75–84, 2000.

Agarwal, V., Sitholey, P., Kumar, S. & Prasad, M., Double-blind, placebo-controlled trial of clonidine in hyperactive children with mental retardation. *Mental Retardation*. **39**(4):259–67, 2001.

Ahmed, Z., Fraser, W., Kerr, M. P. *et al.* Reducing antipsychotic medication in people with a learning disability. *British Journal of Psychiatry*. **176**:42–6, 2000.

Aman, M. G. Efficacy of psychotropic drugs for reducing self-injurious behavior in the developmental disabilities. *Annals of Clinical Psychiatry*. **5**:171–188, 1993.

Aman, M. G., De Smedt, G., Derivan, A., Lyons, B. F & Findling, R. L. Risperidone Disruptive Behavior Study Group. Double-blind, placebo-controlled study of risperidone for the treatment of disruptive behaviors in children with subaverage intelligence. *American Journal of Psychiatry*. **159**(8):1337–46, 2002.

Aman, M. G., Kern, R. A., McGhee, D. E. & Arnold, L. E. Fenfluramine and methylphenidate in children with mental retardation and ADHD: clinical and side effects. *Journal of the American Academy of Child & Adolescent Psychiatry*. **32**(4):851–9, 1993.

Aman, M. G., Marks, R. E., Turbott, S. H., Wilsher, C. P. & Merry, S. N. Clinical effects of methylphenidate and thioridazine in intellectually subaverage children. *Journal of the American Academy of Child & Adolescent Psychiatry*. **30**(2):246–56, 1991.

Anonymous. Expert Consensus Guideline Series: Treatment of psychiatric and behavioral problems in mental retardation. *American Journal of Mental Retardation*. **105**(3):159–226, 2000.

Barron, J. & Sandman, C. A. Paradoxical excitement to sedative-hypnotics in mentally retarded clients. *American Journal of Mental Deficiency*. **90**(2):124–9, 1985.

Baumeister, A. A., Sevin, J. A. & King, B. H. Neuroleptics. In *Psychotropic Medications and Developmental Disabilities: The International Consensus Handbook*, ed. Reiss, S. & Aman, M., Columbus, OH: Ohio State University Nisonger Center, pp. 133–50, 1998.

Belsito, K. M., Law, P. A., Kirk, K. S., Landa, R. J. & Zimmerman, A. W. Lamotrigine therapy for autistic disorder: a randomized, double-blind, placebo-controlled trial. *Journal of Autism & Developmental Disorders*. **31**(2):175–81, 2001.

Beran, R. G. & Gibson, R. J. Aggressive behavior in intellectually challenged patients with epilepsy treated with lamotrigine. *Epilepsia*. **39**(3):280–2, 1998.

Bodfish, J. W., Newell, K. M., Sprague, R. L., Harper, V. N. & Lewis M. H. Dyskinetic movement disorder among adults with mental retardation: phenomenology and co-occurrence with stereotypy. *American Journal of Mental Retardation*, **101**:118–29, 1996.

Bucknill, J. C. & Tuke, D. H. (1858). A manual of psychological medicine: containing the history, nosology, description, statistics, diagnosis, pathology, and treatment of insanity, with an appendix of cases. Philadelphia, PA: Blanchard and Lea, 1858.

Buitelaar, J. K., van der Gaag, R. J., Cohen-Kettenis, P. & Melman, C. T. A randomized controlled trial of risperidone in the treatment of aggression in hospitalized adolescents with subaverage cognitive abilities. *Journal of Clinical Psychiatry*. **62**(4):239–48, 2001.

Clark, R. D., Canive, J. M., Calais, L. A., Qualls, C. R. & Tuason, V. B. Divalproex in post-traumatic stress disorder: an open-label clinical trial. *Journal of Traumatic Stress*. **12**(2):395–401, 1999.

Cohen, S., Glazewski, R., Khan, S. & Khan, A. Weight gain with risperidone among patients with mental retardation: effect of calorie restriction. *Journal of Clinical Psychiatry*. **62**(2):114–16, 2001.

Coppola, G., Iervolino, G., Mastrosimone, M., La Torre, G., Ruiu, F. & Pascotto A. Melatonin in wake–sleep disorders in children, adolescents and young adults with mental retardation with or without epilepsy: a double-blind, cross-over, placebo-controlled trial. *Brain & Development*. **26**(6):373–6, 2004.

Crawford, P., Brown, S. & Kerr M. Parke Davis Clinical Trials Group. A randomized open-label study of gabapentin and lamotrigine in adults with learning disability and resistant epilepsy. *Seizure*. **10**(2):107–15, 2001.

Davanzo, P. A. & King, B. H. Open trial of lamotrigine in the treatment of self-injurious behavior in an adolescent with profound mental retardation. *Journal of Child and Adolescent Psychopharmacology*. **6**:273–9, 1996.

Devinsky, O. Cognitive and behavioral effects of antiepileptic drugs. *Epilepsia*. **36** (Suppl. 2):S46–65, 1995.

Diamond, A. Evidence for the importance of dopamine for prefrontal cortex functions early in life. Philosophical Transactions of the Royal Society of London. Series B: Biological Sciences. **351**:1483–93, 1996.

Dykens, E. & Shah, B. Psychiatric disorders in Prader–Willi syndrome: epidemiology and management. *CNS Drugs*. **17**(3):167–78, 2003.

Friedlander, R., Lazar, S. & Klancnik, J. Atypical antipsychotic use in treating adolescents and young adults with developmental disabilities. *Canadian Journal of Psychiatry*. **46**(8):741–5, 2001.

Gail Williams, P., Sears, L. L. & Allard, A. Sleep problems in children with autism. *Journal of Sleep Research*. **13**(3):265–8, 2004.

Gedye, A. Dietary increase in serotonin reduces self-injurious behaviour in a Down syndrome adult. *Journal of Mental Deficiency Research*. **34**:195–203, 1990.

Hammock, R., Levine, W. R. & Schroeder S. Brief report: effects of clozapine on self-injurious behaviour of two risperidone nonresponders with mental retardation. *Journal of Autism & Developmental Disorders*. **31**(1):109–13, 2001.

Handen, B. J., Breaux, A. M., Janosky, J. *et al.* Effects and noneffects of methylphenidate in children with mental retardation and ADHD. *Journal of the American Academy of Child and Adolescent Psychiatry*. **31**:455–61, 1992.

Handen, B. L., Feldman, A., Goslingi, A. M. & McAuliffe, S. Adverse side effects of methylphenidate among mentally retarded children with ADHD. *Journal of the American Academy of Child and Adolescent Psychiatry*. **30**:241–5, 1991.

Handen, B. L., Janosky, J., McAuliffe, S., Breaux, A. M. & Feldman H. Prediction of response to methylphenidate among children with ADHD and mental retardation. *Journal of the American Academy of Child and Adolescent Psychiatry*, **33**:1185–93, 1994.

Hellings, J. A. & Warnock, J. K. Self-injurious behaviour and serotonin in Prader–Willi syndrome. *Psychopharmacology Bulletin*. **30**:245–50, 1994.

Hellings, J. A., Zarcone, J. R., Crandall, K., Wallace, D. & Schroeder S. R. Weight gain in a controlled study of risperidone in children, adolescents and adults with mental retardation and autism. *Journal of Child & Adolescent Psychopharmacology*. **11**(3):229–38, 2001.

Hirayama, T., Kobayashi, T., Fujita, T. & Fujino, O. Two cases of adult Down syndrome treated with selective serotonin re-uptake inhibitor for behaviour disorders. *No to Hattatsu [Brain & Development]*. **36**(5):391–4, 2004.

Ireland, W. W. Mental Affections of Children, Idiocy, Imbecility and Insanity. Oxford: Churchill, 1898.

Jambaque, I., Chiron, C., Dumas, C., Mumford, J. & Dulac, O. Mental and behavioural outcome of infantile epilepsy treated by vigabatrin in tuberous sclerosis patients. *Epilepsy Research*. **38**(2–3):151–60, 2000.

Jan, M. M. Melatonin for the treatment of handicapped children with severe sleep disorders. *Pediatric Neurology*. **23**(3):229–32, 2000.

Johnson, C. R., Handen, B. L. Lubetsky, M. J. & Sacco, K. A. Efficacy of methylphenidate and behavioral intervention on classroom behavior in children with ADHD and mental retardation. *Behavior Modification*. **18**(4):470–87, 1994.

Kalachnik, J. E., Hanzel, T. E., Sevenich, R. & Harder, S. R. Benzodiazepine behavioural side effects: review and implications for individuals with mental retardation. *American Journal of Mental Retardation*. **107**(5):376–410, 2002.

Kalachnik, J. E., Leventhal, B. L., James, D. H. *et al.* Guidelines for the use of psychotropic medication. In Reiss, S. & Aman, M. G. (eds.), *Psychotropic Medications and Developmental*

Disabilities: The International Consensus Handbook. Columbus, OH: Ohio State University, pp. 45–72, 1998.

King, B. H. Pemoline and other dopaminergic models of self-biting behavior. In Schroeder, S. R. & Oster-Granite, M. L. (eds.), *Self-injurious Behavior: Gene-Brain-Behavior Relationships.* Washington, DC: American Psychological Association, pp. 181–89, 2002.

King, B. H. Self-injury by people with mental retardation: a compulsive behavior hypothesis. *American Journal of Mental Retardation.* **98**(1):93–112, 1993.

King, B. H., DeAntonio, C., McCracken, J. T., Forness, S. R. & Ackerland, V. Psychiatric consultation in severe and profound mental retardation. *American Journal of Psychiatry*, **151**:1802–8, 1994.

King, B. H. & Davanzo, P. A. Buspirone treatment of aggression and self-injury in autistic and non autistic persons with severe mental retardation. *Developmental Brain Dysfunction.* **9**:22–31, 1996.

King, B. H. & Wright, D. M., Snape, M. & Dourish, C. T. Case series: amantadine open-label treatment of impulsive and aggressive behavior in hospitalized children with developmental disabilities. *Journal of the American Academy of Child & Adolescent Psychiatry.* **40**(6):654–7, 2001.

Kockelmann, E., Elger, C. E. & Helmstaedter, C. Cognitive profile of topiramate as compared with lamotrigine in epilepsy patients on antiepileptic drug polytherapy: relationships to blood serum levels and co-medication. *Epilepsy & Behaviour.* **5**(5):716–21, 2004.

LeVann, L. J. Thioridazine (Mellaril): A psycho-sedative virtually free of side-effects. *Alberta Medical Bulletin*, **26**:144–7, 1961.

Lewis, M. H., Bodfish, J. W., Powell, S. B., Parker, D. E. & Golden, R. N. Clomipramine treatment for self-injurious behaviour of individuals with mental retardation: a double-blind comparison with placebo. *American Journal of Mental Retardation.* **100**:654–65, 1996.

Lewis, M. A., Lewis, C. E. Leake, B., King, B. H. & Lindemann, R. The quality of health care for adults with developmental disabilities. *Public Health Reports.* **117**(2):174–84, 2002.

Masi, G., Marcheschi, M. & Pfanner, P. Paroxetine in depressed adolescents with intellectual disability: an open label study. *Journal of Intellectual Disability Research.* **41**(Pt 3):268–72, 1997.

McDonough, M., Hillery, J. & Kennedy N. Olanzapine for chronic, stereotypic self-injurious behaviour: a pilot study in seven adults with intellectual disability. *Journal of Intellectual Disability Research.* **44**(Pt 6):677–84, 2000.

Pearson, D. A., Santos, C. W., Casat, C. D. *et al.* Treatment effects of methylphenidate on cognitive functioning in children with mental retardation and ADHD. *Journal of the American Academy of Child & Adolescent Psychiatry.* **43**(6):677–85, 2004.

Pillar, G., Shahar, E., Peled, N., Ravid, S., Lavie, P. & Etzioni, A. Melatonin improves sleep-wake patterns in psychomotor retarded children. *Pediatric Neurology.* **23**(3):225–8, 2000.

Racusin, R., Kovner-Kline, K. & King, B. H. Selective serotonin reuptake inhibitors in intellectual disability. *Mental Retardation & Developmental Disabilities Research Reviews.* **5**(4): 264–9, 1999.

Ratey, J. J. & Gordon, A. The psychopharmacology of aggression: toward a new day. *Psychopharmacology Bulletin*, **29**:65–73, 1993.

Ratey, J. J., Sovner, R., Mikkelsen, E. & Chmielinski, H. E. Buspirone therapy for maladaptive behaviour and anxiety in developmentally disabled persons. *Journal of Clinical Psychiatry.* **50**:382–4, 1989.

Robertson, J., Emerson, E. Gregory, N. *et al.* A. Receipt of psychotropic medication by people with intellectual disability in residential settings. *Journal of Intellectual Disability Research.* **44** (Pt 6):666–76, 2000.

Sachdev, P. Drug-induced movement disorders in institutionalised adults with mental retardation: clinical characteristics and risk factors. *Australian and New Zealand Journal of Psychiatry.* **26**:242–8, 1992.

Santosh, P. J. & Baird, G. Psychopharmacotherapy in children and adults with intellectual disability. *Lancet.* **354**(9174):233–42, 1999.

Schroeder, S. R., Oster-Granite, M. L., Berkson, G. *et al.* Self-injurious behavior: gene–brain–behavior relationships. *Mental Retardation & Developmental Disabilities Research Reviews.* **7**(1):3–12, 2001.

Schweitzer, I. Does risperidone have a place in the treatment of nonschizophrenic patients? *International Clinical Psychopharmacology.* **16**(1):1–19, 2001.

Sutherland, S. M. & Davidson, J. R. Pharmacotherapy for post-traumatic stress disorder. *Psychiatric Clinics of North America.* **17**:409–23, 1994.

Szymanski, L. & King, B. H. Practice parameters for the assessment and treatment of children, adolescents, and adults with mental retardation and comorbid mental disorders. American Academy of Child and Adolescent Psychiatry Working Group on Quality Issues. *Journal of the American Academy of Child & Adolescent Psychiatry.* **38** (Suppl. 12):5–31, 1999.

Trimble, M. R. Epilepsy, antidepressants, and the role of nomifensine. *Journal of Clinical Psychiatry.* **45**(4 Pt 2):39–42, 1984.

Tsiouris, J. A., Cohen, I. L., Patti, P. J. & Korosh, W. M. Treatment of previously undiagnosed psychiatric disorders in persons with developmental disabilities decreased or eliminated self-injurious behaviour. *Journal of Clinical Psychiatry.* **64**(9):1081–90, 2003.

Tu, J. B. & Zellweger, H. Blood-serotonin deficiency in Down syndrome. *Lancet.* **2**(7415):715–16, 1965.

Tuke, D. H. The Insane in the United States and Canada. London: H. K. Lewis. (1885).

Turgay, A., Binder, C., Snyder, R. & Fisman, S. Long-term safety and efficacy of risperidone for the treatment of disruptive behavior disorders in children with subaverage IQs. *Pediatrics.* **110**(3):e34, 2002.

Turner, C. A. & Lewis, M. H. Dopaminergic mechanisms in self-injurious behavior and related disorders. In: Schroeder, S. R. & Oster-Granite, M. L. (eds.), Self-injurious Behavior: Gene–Brain–Behavior Relationships. Washington, DC: American Psychological Association. pp. 165–179, 2002.

Van Bellinghen, M. & De Troch, C. Risperidone in the treatment of behavioral disturbances in children and adolescents with borderline intellectual functioning: a double-blind, placebo-controlled pilot trial. *Journal of Child & Adolescent Psychopharmacology.* **11**(1):5–13, 2001.

Verhoeven, W. M., Moog, U., Wagemans, A. M., Tuinier, S. & Wolf-Hirschhorn (4p-) syndrome in a near adult with major depression; successful treatment with citalopram. *Genetic Counseling.* **13**(3):297–301, 2002.

Verhoeven, W. M. & Tuinier, S. The effect of buspirone on challenging behaviour in mentally retarded patients: an open prospective multiple-case study. *Journal of Intellectual Disability Research.* **40**:502–8, 1996.

Verhoeven, W. M., Veendrik-Meekes, M. J., Jacobs G. A., van den Berg, Y. W. & Tuinier, S. Citalopram in mentally retarded patients with depression: a long-term clinical investigation. *European Psychiatry: The Journal of the Association of European Psychiatrists.* **16**(2):104–8, 2001.

Welch, L. & Sovner, R. The treatment of a chronic organic mental disorder with dextromethorphan in a man with severe mental retardation. *British Journal of Psychiatry.* **161**:118–20, 1992.

Zarcone, J. R., Hellings, J. A., Crandall, K. *et al.* Effects of risperidone on aberrant behavior of persons with developmental disabilities: I. A double-blind crossover study using multiple measures. *American Journal of Mental Retardation.* **106**(6):525–38, 2001.

20

Psychosocial interventions for people with intellectual disabilities

Dave Dagnan

Introduction

Psychosocial interventions have been described and evaluated with respect to a range of physical and mental health difficulties for people without intellectual disabilities (e.g. National Institute for Clinical Excellence, 2002) and are considered essential parts of the delivery of mental health services to people with severe mental health problems (Department of Health, 2001). The range of interventions described as 'psychosocial' is very broad, suggesting that the term is often used for any intervention that is not primarily medical. Currently, the only review of psychosocial intervention for people with intellectual disabilities (ID) and mental health problems identifies individual cognitive therapy as the main focus for psychosocial intervention (Hatton, 2002). Given the breadth of interventions that can be considered as psychosocial it is useful to consider the interventions taking place with the individual, in their immediate social environment, or within the wider social context and also to consider the structure of services that deliver such interventions.

- Psychosocial interventions with the individual include supportive educational interventions, programmes that address the individual's perspective on their illness and its management; skills training in areas such as independent daily living, social skills, and skills to enable the individual to enter work or leisure settings, and problem or symptom-focused therapies.
- Psychosocial intervention can take place within the immediate social context of the person – for example, using family interventions which help the family understand the nature of the difficulties that their family member experiences.
- Psychosocial interventions can take place within the broader social context of the person through provision of supported housing or supported employment.

Psychiatric and Behavioural Disorders in Intellectual and Developmental Disabilities, ed. Nick Bouras and Geraldine Holt. Published by Cambridge University Press. © Cambridge University Press 2007.

- Psychosocial intervention has also been defined as including the service provision structure through which interventions are delivered. Intensive case management systems have been reported within the service structures as essential elements of the psychosocial management of people with psychosis, and the comprehensive delivery of such approaches has been described in team perspectives including assertive outreach (National Institute for Clinical Excellence, 2002).

Many of the intervention areas identified above have been substantially researched within the general ID literature, for example there are a number of studies that demonstrate psychological and social benefits from intervention in social areas such as supported employment (e.g. Forrester-Jones *et al.*, 2004) or residential provision (Perry & Felce, 2003). However, there is little evidence that is specific to people with ID and severe mental health problems. Similarly family and paid carer training and support interventions have been described for those supporting people with ID (Hastings & Beck, 2004; Innstrand *et al.*, 2004), although the use of educational and symptom management and monitoring approaches as used with families of people with severe mental health problems have not been reported in the ID literature.

A small number of studies have reported the provision of psychosocial interventions for people with ID and severe mental health problems through structured team-based approaches. For example Hassiotis *et al.* (2003) describes assertive outreach teams for people with ID developed within specialist ID services. One of the examples of assertive outreach teams given by Hassiotis and colleagues is reported as providing a broad range of psychosocial interventions including skills assessment and teaching, psychological support such as cognitive behavioural therapy, help with access to education and employment, and relapse prevention. There is no formal evaluation of the assertive outreach approach or of the individual interventions reported in this paper. However, Hassiotis *et al.* (2001) does report on the potential importance of intensive case management (often a key part of psychosocial packages). From a larger randomized trial of intensive case management she reports on a sub-group of people with borderline ID. She identifies that this group responded significantly better to intensive care management than people without ID, experiencing reductions in total days in hospital, total numbers of admission, total costs and needs. However, in general there is little discussion of the provision and impact of co-ordinated psychosocial intervention within the ID field. In fact the multi-component and locally developed nature of community services for people with ID services has been suggested as a barrier to evaluation of such services (Oliver *et al.*, 2002). Martin *et al.* (2005) in an exploratory randomized controlled trial found no statistically significant differences between assertive and standard community treatment in ID in terms of the level of unmet needs, carer burden, functioning and quality of life. Both treatment methods decreased level of unmet needs and carer burden, and increased functioning. However, they pointed out that the fidelity of both treatment methods needed further development, as it was also possible that the two treatment arms were too similar to show the expected differences, as people with ID are usually receiving some form of regular support from social services, support staff and carers. Similar findings were also reported by Oliver *et al.* (2005).

Clearly, in this area there are a number of well-established interventions that have well-established evidence bases for people without disabilities; there is an obvious need to report and evaluate the delivery and adaptation of these approaches to people with ID and mental health problems.

The most frequently reported psychosocial interventions for people with ID and mental health problems are of individuals using either behavioural, cognitive behavioural or psychodynamic frameworks. Other chapters in this book report on the use of behavioural and psychodynamic approaches (see also Chapters 18 by Benson & Havercamp and 21 by Parkes & Hollins). Therefore this chapter will concentrate on discussion of cognitive therapy with individuals with ID.

Cognitive therapy

Dagnan and Chadwick (1997) identify two approaches to cognitive therapy that have been applied to people with ID; they identify these as 'deficit' and 'distortion' approaches. The deficit approach is based upon the premise that psychological and emotional distress is caused by poor cognitive skills, with self-talk seen as either absent or poorly structured. The distortion approach sees emotions and behaviour as mediated by cognition but suggests that the view of the world that shapes the emotional response is in some way distorted, unhelpful, or irrational. The deficit approaches have the best evidence base in the ID field (Dagnan & Chadwick, 1997). Interventions based upon these approaches have been applied to skill development and vocational compliance for people with ID (Harchik *et al.*, 1992). Clearly, these are important areas of psychosocial intervention; however, such interventions have typically had broad developmental goals rather than being seen as supportive treatments as part of the management of mental health problems. When these approaches have been applied to symptomatic treatment of mental health problems it has been for presentations that can be easily formulated from a skill deficit perspective such as anxiety or anger, where treatments involve the acquisition of appropriate self-management skills such as relaxation, positive self-talk and problem solving (Lindsay *et al.*, 1997; Rose *et al.*, 2000).

The distortion model of cognitive therapy emphasizes the development of individual meaning; people are seen as engaging in self-talk but the content of the self-talk is seen as unhelpful or irrational. There is increasing interest in such therapeutic models (Kroese *et al.*, 1997; Dagnan & Lindsay, 2004). A number of comprehensive reviews of the cognitive area and the difficulties with its evidence base have been published (Dagnan & Lindsay, 2004; Beail, 2003; Sturmey, 2004).

Assessment

Cognitive therapy is a process through which individual meanings are addressed; thus, self-report is necessary to demonstrate change in these areas. There is considerable research on self-report measures for people with ID (Finlay & Lyons, 2001). There are a number of examples of self-report measures that have been used in therapeutic research with people with ID; measures developed for people without disabilities have been used in both adapted and original forms (e.g. Nezu *et al.*, 1995; Dagnan & Sandhu, 1999) and measures have also been specifically developed for people with ID (Cuthill *et al.*, 2003). The conclusions drawn from the assessment literature in this area is that the level of psychometric and clinical development of such scales does not match that of scales used for people without ID, and that this has resulted in a wide variation in the scales used in the small number of studies reporting cognitive behavioural interventions (Dagnan & Lindsay, 2004).

Assessment will often also be necessary to determine the presence of skills that might be helpful for people with ID to most effectively engage in cognitive therapy. Thus, in considering cognitive therapy for people with ID it is necessary to determine whether the person's cognitive profile (for example, limitations in memory, abstract reasoning, attention etc.) will require adaptation of the therapeutic approach (Dagnan & Chadwick, 1997; Dagnan *et al.*, 2000). Using this information a therapist can either adjust their therapeutic approach to ensure that the person's strengths are incorporated into the therapeutic interaction, or use particular types of therapy that are better suited to the person's cognitive abilities, or apply developmental and training approaches to ensure that the person is more able to make use of the therapeutic approach. It is notable that current literature on cognitive therapy does not give detailed accounts of therapeutic process, and the degree of adaptation reported in published studies varies considerably. There are some accounts that suggest that relatively simple adaptations of therapy process and structure might sometimes be required (Lindsay *et al.*, 1993; Haddock *et al.*, 2004), whilst other accounts suggest more substantial adaptations may be needed (Rose *et al.*, 2000). The use of comprehensive assessment will allow a systematic approach to determining the degree and nature of adaptation to therapy that is required, and research in the area of therapy process will be very important in understanding how adaptation works in making therapy effective for people with ID.

Outcomes

Currently the evidence base for cognitive therapy used with people with ID is limited (Beail, 2003; Sturmey, 2004). It is widely acknowledged that there are few reported randomized controlled trial designs; those that are published are purely in the area of group interventions for anger (Taylor *et al.*, 2002). There is also a growing literature base on the use of cognitive approaches with people with ID who have offended. For example, Lindsay *et al.* (1999) reported a cognitive treatment for four adolescent sex offenders. The techniques included eliciting cognitions consistent with sexual offending and repeated challenging of these cognitions through the use of scenarios illustrating potential offending situations and problem-solving techniques (see also Chapter 9 by Lindsay and Chapter 7 by Stavrakaki and Lunsky). For depression there are a number of behavioural interventions reported (Lindsay & Olley, 1998), but again a limited number of single-case design studies using cognitive approaches (e.g. Lindsay *et al.*, 1993; Dagnan & Chadwick, 1997). Anxiety treatments have also tended to be predominantly behavioural and predominantly involving people with phobias and obsessive-compulsive problems (Lindsay & Olley 1998). More recently Lindsay *et al.* (1997) reported two successful case studies employing Beck's cognitive therapy for anxiety, and Lindsay (1999) reports a cohort of 15 individuals with clinically significant levels of anxiety: treatment took place over an average of 23 sessions and resulted in a statistically significant reduction in self-report measures of anxiety; improvements were maintained at six-month follow-up. For areas such as psychosis there is beginning case series literature describing interventions with people with ID, using protocols developed for people without disabilities (Haddock *et al.*, 2004). In overviewing the outcome literature, it is notable that the reported interventions for people with ID lack the specificity or sophistication of interventions that exist for people without disabilities. For example, Wells (1997) reports a series of distinct models and interventions for a range of distinct anxiety presentations; these have not yet been described or evaluated for people with ID.

Cognitive models of distress

A number of researchers have begun to recognize that there is a tension between the individual model of therapy and social models of the experience of disability (e.g. Dagnan & Waring, 2004). Social models identify disability as created by social structures or through social construction; such models identify people with ID as stigmatized and disempowered (Shakespeare & Watson, 1997). Interventions based upon such models have been significantly responsible for the changes in service structure that have occurred in Britain in the past 40 years. Cognitive models within ID services increasingly acknowledge the impact of social experience on people with ID and their cognitive structures. A number of researchers have begun to develop a cognitive perspective that emphasizes the effects of negative social construction and stigmatization (Jahoda *et al.*, 2001). Dagnan and Waring (2004) suggest that when stigmatization and negative social construction are recognized by a person with ID this will have a profound impact upon a person's psychological well-being. Core cognitive experiences such as negative self-evaluation and negative social comparison might then be expected as a direct consequence of the long-term experience of discrimination and social isolation. A truly psychosocial intervention may use such a model and encourages the therapist and team to formulate the individual's presentation within their social context and to acknowledge the social processes that shaped their fundamental evaluations, attributions and meanings concerning their world. Thus, based upon an individual formulation, psychosocial interventions may be co-ordinated to provide individualized opportunities in work and leisure, to enable support and intervention with family and immediate social contexts, as well as to inform therapeutic work with the individual.

Conclusion

Psychosocial interventions are considered a powerful part of the core interventions for people without ID with a range of mental health problems. Many interventions reported for people with ID and their environments are clearly psychosocial; however, there is little literature that discusses their application to mental health problems and very little literature that presents the comprehensive and co-ordinated application of such approaches in order to manage severe mental health problems. As people with ID begin to receive services from mainstream mental health services it is important that co-ordinated psychosocial interventions are made available to people with ID and severe mental heath problems, and that these interventions are properly evaluated.

Summary points

- Psychosocial intervention refers to a broad range of non-medical interventions with the individual and their immediate and wider social context, for which there is significant evidence of effectiveness when applied to people who do not have ID.
- Psychosocial interventions are part of the required framework of services for people with mental health problems. People with ID should be enabled to receive such services from within mainstream services where possible.
- There is empirical evidence of the general importance of psychosocial factors to people with ID but this evidence is generally not specific to mental health problems.

- There is a beginning literature that considers the service structures for mental health services to people with ID. This is starting to consider the structures through which psychosocial intervention might be delivered.
- The most widely reported areas of psychosocial intervention for people with ID and mental health problems are individual interventions within behavioural, cognitive behavioural and psychodynamic frameworks.
- The evidence base for cognitive therapy is relatively weak, although there is beginning to develop sufficient conceptual and outcome data to suggest that such interventions should be made routinely available to people with ID.
- The value base of ID services has always stressed the importance of the social environment on the quality of lives of people with ID. Psychosocial interventions are entirely consistent with this value base.

REFERENCES

Beail, N. (2003). What works for people with mental retardation? Critical commentary on cognitive behavioral and psychodynamic psychotherapy research. *Mental Retardation*, **41**, 468–72.

Cuthill, F. M., Espie, C. & Cooper, S. A. (2003). Development and psychometric properties of the Glasgow Depression Scale for people with a learning disability: individual and carer supplement versions. *The British Journal of Psychiatry*, **182**, 347–53.

Dagnan, D. & Chadwick, P. (1997). Cognitive behaviour therapy for people with learning disabilities: assessment and intervention. In Kroese, B., Dagnan, D. & Loumidis, K. (eds.), *Cognitive Behaviour Therapy for People with Learning Disabilities*. London: Routledge.

Dagnan, D. Chadwick, P. & Proudlove, J. (2000). Towards an assessment of suitability of people with mental retardation for cognitive therapy. *Cognitive Therapy and Research*, **24**, 627–36.

Dagnan, D. & Lindsay, W. R. (2004). Cognitive therapy with people with learning disabilities: In E. Emerson & C. Hatton, T. Parmenter & T. Thompson (eds.), *International Handbook of Research and Evaluation in Intellectual Disabilities*. Chichester: J. Wiley & Sons.

Dagnan, D. & Sandhu, S. (1999). Social comparison, self-esteem and depression in people with learning disabilities. *Journal of Intellectual Disability Research*, **43**, 372–79.

Dagnan, D. & Waring, M. (2004). Linking stigma to psychological distress: A social-cognitive model of the experience of people with learning disabilities. *Clinical Psychology and Psychotherapy*, **11**, 247–54.

Department of Health (2001). *The Mental Health Policy Implementation Guide*. London: Department of Health.

Forrester-Jones, R., Jones, S. & Heason, S., Di'Terlizzi, M. (2004). Supported employment: A route to social networks. *Journal of Applied Research in Intellectual Disabilities*, **17**, 199–208.

Findlay, W. M. L. & Lyons, E. (2001). Methodological issues in interviewing and using self-report questionnaires with people with mental retardation. *Psychological Assessment*, **13**, 319–35.

Haddock, G., Lobban, F., Hatton, C. & Carsons, R. (2004). Cognitive-behaviour therapy for people with psychosis and mild intellectual disabilities: a case series. *Clinical Psychology & Psychotherapy*, **11**, 282–98.

Harchik, A. E., Sherman, J. A. & Sheldon, J. B. (1992). The use of self-management procedures by people with developmental disabilities: a brief review. *Research in Developmental Disabilities*, **13**, 211–27.

Hassiotis, A., Tyrer, P. & Oliver, P. (2003). Psychiatric assertive outreach and learning disability services. *Advances in Psychiatric Treatment*, **9**, 368–73.

Hassiotis, A., Ukoumunne, O. C., Byford, S. *et al.* (2001). Intellectual functioning and outcome of patients with severe psychotic illness randomized to intensive case management: report from the UK 700 case management trial. *British Journal of Psychiatry*, **178**, 168–71.

Hastings, R. P. & Beck, A. (2004). Practitioner review: stress intervention for parents of children with intellectual disabilities. *Child Psychology and Psychiatry*, **45**, 1338–49.

Hatton, C. (2002). Psychosocial interventions for adults with intellectual disabilities and mental health problems: A review. *Journal of Mental Health*, **11**, 357–73.

Innstrand, S. T., Espnes, G. A. & Mykletun, R. (2004). Job stress, burnout and job satisfaction: an intervention study for staff working with people with intellectual disabilities. *Journal of Applied Research in Intellectual Disbailities*, **17**, 119–26.

Jahoda, A., Trower, P. & Pert, C. (2001). Contingent reinforcement or defending the self? A review of evolving models of aggression in people with mild learning disabilities. *British Journal of Medical Psychology*, **74**, 305–21.

Kroese, B., Dagnan, D. & Loumidis, K. (eds.) (1997). *Cognitive Behaviour Therapy for People with Learning Disabilities*. London: Routledge.

Lindsay, W. R. (1999). Cognitive therapy. *The Psychologist*, **12**, 238–41.

Lindsay, W. R., Howells, L. & Pitcaithly, D. (1993). Cognitive therapy for depression with individuals with intellectual disabilities. *British Journal of Medical Psychology*, **66**, 135–41.

Lindsay, W. R., Neilson, C. & Lawrenson, H. (1997). Cognitive behaviour therapy for anxiety in people with learning disabilities. In Kroese, B. S., Dagnan, D. & Loumidis, K. (eds), *Cognitive Behaviour Therapy for People with Learning Disabilities*. London: Routledge.

Lindsay, W. R. & Olley, S. (1998). Psychological treatment for anxiety and depression for people with learning disabilities. In Fraser, W., Sines, D. & Kerr, M. (eds.), *Hallas' the Care of People with Intellectual Disabilities, 9th Edn*. Oxford: Butterworth Heinemann.

Lindsay, W. R., Olley, S., Baillie, N. & Smith, A. H. W. (1999). The treatment of adolescent sex offenders with intellectual disability. *Mental Retardation*, **37**, 320–33.

Martin, G., Costello, H., Leese, M. *et al.* (2005). An exploratory study of assertive community treatment for people with intellectual disability and psychiatric disorders: conceptual, clinical, and service Issues. *Journal of Intellectual Disability Research*, **49**, 516–24.

National Institute for Clinical Excellence (2002). *Schizophrenia: Core Interventions in the Treatment and Management of Schizophrenia in Primary and Secondary Care*. Clinical Guideline 1. London: NICE.

Nezu, C. M., Nezu, A. M., Rothenburg, J. L., DelliCarpini, L. & Groag, I. (1995). Depression in adults with mild mental retardation: are cognitive variables involved? *Cognitive Therapy & Research*, **19**, 227–39.

Oliver P. C., Piachaud, J., Done, J., Regan, A., Cooray, S. & Tyrer, P. (2002). Difficulties in conducting a randomized controlled trial of health service interventions in intellectual disability: implications for evidence-based practice. *Journal of Intellectual Disbnaility Research*, **46**, 340–5.

Oliver, P. C., Piachaud, J., Tyrer, P. *et al.* (2005). Randomized controlled trials of assertive community treatment in intellectual disability. *Journal of Intellectual Disability Research*, **49**, 507–15.

Perry, J. & Felce, D. (2003). Quality of life outcomes for people with intellectual disabilities living in staffed community housing services: A stratified random sample of statutory, voluntary and private agency provision. *Journal of Applied Research in Intellectual Disabilities*, **16**, 11–28.

Rose, J., West, C. & Clifford, D. (2000). Group interventions for anger in people with intellectual disabilities. *Research in Developmental Disabilities*, **21**, 171–81.

Shakespeare, T. & Watson, N. (1997). Defending the social model. *Disability & Society*, **12**, 293–300.

Sturmey, P. (2004). Cognitive therapy with people with intellectual disabilities. A selective review and critique. *Clinical Psychology and Psychotherapy*, **11**, 222–32.

Taylor, J. L., Novaco, R. W., Gillmer, B. & Thorne, I. (2002). Cognitive-behavioural treatment of anger intensity among offenders with intellectual disabilities. *Journal of Applied Research in Intellectual Disabilities*, **15**, 151–65.

Wells, A. (1997). *Cognitive Therapy of Anxiety Disorders: A Practice Manual and Conceptual Guide.* Chichester: John Wiley & Sons.

21

Psychodynamic approaches to people with intellectual disabilities: individuals, groups/systems and families

Georgina Parkes and Sheila Hollins

Introduction

There have been many barriers preventing people with intellectual disabilities (ID) from accessing psychodynamic treatments. Therapists, notably Freud in the early 1900s and later Carl Rogers in the 1960s, believed that people with ID were unsuitable for psychodynamic therapies, as they did not have the intelligence seen as a prerequisite for this mode of treatment. There were also assumptions that people with ID were immune to emotional distress or did not understand emotional pain and suffering, and so were not affected by it. Until relatively recently, treatments have tended to be social (e.g. institutionalization), behavioural, or pharmacological, despite the growing trend towards more talking treatments in the non-ID population.

What is psychodynamic psychotherapy?

The term psychotherapy includes any type of talking therapy. The Department of Health's review of strategic policy on National Health Service psychotherapy services in 1996, advised that every mental health professional should be able to offer supportive and psycho-educational therapy as part of a combined package of care. This should include engaging the person sufficiently so that they return for follow up, asking exploratory questions if they don't understand, and listening to their difficulties.

Essentially, any type of treatment that involves talking to the person – either individually or in a group, as part of a care network or family – can be approached psychodynamically. However, the policy review placed psychodynamic or psychoanalytic therapy as a type C therapy, a formal psychotherapy practised by or under the supervision of a specialist practitioner trained in a particular school

Psychiatric and Behavioural Disorders in Intellectual and Developmental Disabilities, ed. Nick Bouras and Geraldine Holt. Published by Cambridge University Press. © Cambridge University Press 2007.

of formal psychotherapeutic work. This is undertaken by two kinds of people: those who have specialized after a broader training, which includes clinical psychologists and those psychiatrists and psychiatric nurses whose trainings have encompassed this; and those who have trained from the outset in a single theoretical framework. Formal psychodynamic therapy usually takes place at the same time and place every week, maintaining a consistency of setting as much as possible. This approach looks for personal meaning in the presenting symptoms and behaviours and uses the person's mental representations of early life experiences and the way they see themselves in the world to search for that meaning. The aim is to increase the person's understanding of their thoughts, feelings and behaviour.

The relationship between therapist and service user and the therapist's counter-transference feelings are the main tools with which to understand the person's experience, the interpretation of which can lead to changes in functioning. Roth and Fonagy (1996) reviewed the research regarding therapeutic alliance and found that the expertise of the therapist, their skills and personal qualities in building a therapeutic alliance appeared to be more important than the experience of the therapist. Client factors also played a role in developing this alliance. The literature indicates that whilst knowledge of specific techniques is a good foundation, the therapist's expertise lies in being flexible when the clinical situation demands it. The aims of psychodynamic psychotherapy with people with ID are no different to those with non-intellectually disabled people.

The psychological impact of having intellectual disabilities

There may be direct psychological consequences associated with the experience of having ID (Sinason, 2004): emotional attachments may be fragile, and there may be a slower development of a sense of self and a realization of a lifelong dependency on others. It has been said that people with ID are thought to be more vulnerable to abuse (Sobsey, 1994; Brown and Turk, 1994) and therefore to psychological sequelae of abuse (Sequeira *et al.*, 2003). Separation and individuation from care givers may be significantly affected.

Department of Health guidelines

Valuing People (Department of Health, 2001) states the UK Government's aims of ensuring rights, independence, choice and inclusion for people with ID. The low current levels of service provision of psychodynamic treatments available to people with ID fall short of these aspirations. In reality they may have little or no treatment choice.

A recent council report from the Royal College of Psychiatrists on *Psychotherapy and Learning Disability* (2004) reports on a survey of services in UK and Ireland that included psychodynamic psychotherapy. There was a high perceived demand for psychotherapy. Barriers to accessing services were cited as negative attitudes of others and lack of training and supervision of staff, and what little is provided is often eclectic. The report recommended developing specialist expertise for effective psychotherapy for people with ID and suggested that the expertise required with any person was to be able to develop an effective language that worked with them in the therapeutic context. Additionally, the report provided models of how therapy could be expanded by training disability professionals in psychotherapy or offering 'top-up' training to mainstream psychotherapists. An unpublished study was described in which top-up training in working therapeutically was given to experienced bereavement counsellors. Using objective outcome measures, there were significant improvements in behaviour and mental health when bereaved clients attended between 8 and 30 counselling sessions.

New guidance in a report on *Organising and Delivering Psychological Therapies* (Department of Health, 2004) recommends changes in the delivery of psychological services for all client groups. It states that counselling and psychological therapy services are popular amongst service users and their families, and stresses the importance of mainstreaming psychological therapies and strengthening choice. It identifies patchy provision and says it is necessary to ensure that 'service delivery is not restricted by extraneous factors such as ethnicity, age, gender or diagnosis and [should] pay special attention to marginalized groups including people with learning disability'. The report acknowledges that accepting its recommendations might require a change in attitude in some localities. However, in policy terms there should no longer be any doubt that psychological therapies have a place in the range of effective treatments. The Department of Health report (2004) suggests that video conferencing provides a possible way to share expertise and give supervision. It also outlines the possibility of therapy being too long or too short; of the wrong type for the diagnosis; of the therapist lacking training and not being properly supported – all of which can lead to unsafe practices. The College working party found that some professionals appear to undertake psychological treatments for which they have not had adequate training, and it states standards should be at least as high as for general psychotherapy training, if not more exacting.

The report also notes that some services lack any type of psychological service for people with ID. Different professions may feel they must compete for resources, and fear that management will allocate psychological therapy services a low priority, more out of misinformation than ill will. This is more likely with psychodynamic psychotherapy provision, as the working party survey discussed above showed behavioural therapies were more widespread.

Some evidence (cited in the Department of Health, 2004, guidelines) suggests that these psychotherapies can be self-financing by reducing prescriptions, requiring less time to be spent in hospitals and more people entering employment.

Who can benefit?

A recent retrospective case-note review of an outpatient psychotherapy service for people with ID, which includes a small art therapy service, in South West London over a period from January 2000 to September 2003, looked at 100 consecutive referrals to the service (Parkes *et al.*, 2004). In a third of referrals, trauma and abuse were the reasons for referral, with high numbers also referred for loss and bereavement issues, challenging behaviour (unspecified, but usually involving problems with anger) and depression. A smaller number were referred for sexually inappropriate or offending behaviours or the consequences of institutional care and relationship difficulties. Referrers clearly saw psychodynamic psychotherapy as a treatment for these types of problems. After an initial assessment, high numbers were considered to be suitable for therapy.

Many studies have shown that people with ID are vulnerable to abuse, particularly sexual abuse, which can often remain hidden until therapy has been taking place over some time. Personality disorders can be diagnosed in people with ID, although this is much more difficult in people with more severe cognitive impairments.

Types of psychodynamic psychotherapy used with people with intellectual disabilities

Psychoanalytical therapy can be used with individuals, with groups or families, or to understand carer and staff group dynamics.

Systemic family therapy is available in some mental health teams for families where a member has a disability, looking at how presenting symptoms may be a way of maintaining a family system and helping families to think of alternatives. Two central issues often addressed are altered life-cycle patterns and continuing grief and mourning for all members of the family (Goldberg *et al.*, 1995). It is also suitable for people who live in groups that are not necessarily their family of origin, such as group homes, or where someone is dependent on staff support.

There is a long history of the use of art, music and drama therapies, often thought of as being particularly suitable for people with more severe ID. They can all involve a psychodynamic approach, using the developing relationship between client and therapist as a therapeutic tool.

All these therapies can be brief, medium or long term.

Indirect work such as staff consultation and work discussion groups can be a beneficial way of working psychodynamically with people with ID. Staff consultation can be used as an adjunct to the client's own therapy or as a stand-alone treatment. Key members of staff meet with a therapist on a regular basis and discuss problems and difficulties; and psychodynamic ideas and approaches can help staff to become more aware of the meaning of the person's interactions. Through this, staff can develop a greater understanding of the person's emotional life and modify the way in which they view the patient or react to them, thus modifying the person's own responses (Arthur, 2003). This kind of help can also mean staff feel more empowered to seek help and discuss problems or look for alternative strategies.

Work discussion groups, that meet weekly under the supervision of a qualified therapist, can be useful for staff working in community ID teams to think in depth about what is going on with their clients and to avoid common difficulties such as acting on counter-transference feelings, or feeling overwhelmed with the complexity of problems some people with ID present.

Particular differences in psychoanalytic technique

When people with ID are referred to psychotherapy they may not know that they have been referred or what psychotherapy is. A longer assessment period may be needed to explore issues of consent, and the idea of consent as a process must constantly be borne in mind by the therapist during treatment. Dropping out of therapy is sometimes seen as part of the consent process, once someone has had an experience of therapy and is aware of what it involves.

Transport and escorts need to be provided in most cases to enable therapy to occur, with these dependency needs increasing with the level of disability and functioning. One of the main reasons for someone with ID failing to engage in therapy is the failure of transport or of escorts to support the person to attend therapy sessions regularly and on time. All this needs to be considered at the assessment stage.

Approach to psychotherapy assessment

- Collect client from the waiting area on time, with or without their care provider.
- Ask if they would like to be seen.
- Therapists – introduce yourself using your first name.

Therapist	**Patient**
Do you know why you have come here today?	Usually says no.
Your carer/nurse/GP said you have got some worries. She thinks you need some help to think about your worries. Is that right?	Usually silent. Sometimes a nod.
You are brave coming to see us today (said with warmth). What are you worried about?	Often tearful – my Mum died or someone hurt me, or a non-verbal movement which suggests pain or avoidance.
That's upsetting – do you want to tell me more about this?	

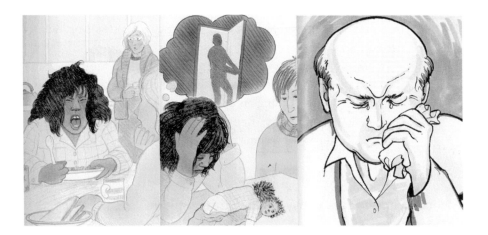

Note: this may be a good point to offer some pictures related to the presenting problem. The pictures may need a verbal prompt by the therapist, e.g. 'have you ever felt like that?', 'what do you think is happening in the picture?'.

Within 10–15 minutes:	Usually able to decide quite quickly.
Would you like to talk to someone about this? In a group or on your own with one other person?	
We will find a therapist for you. It may take some time to find the right person.	

With the permission of Hollins, S. and Sinason, V., Approach to Psychotherapy Assessment (unpublished). 2005.

The pictures above are taken from Books Beyond Words (Hollins *et al.*, 1998, and Hollins & Sireling, 2004), a counselling series of 30 books for people who find pictures easier to understand than words. See www.rcpsych.ac.uk/publications/bbw.

There are some differences or adaptations typically made to psychoanalytic technique when working with people with ID. More warmth and friendliness is needed to form a therapeutic alliance, as a lack of affect may be experienced as persecutory. Non-verbal communication is a powerful tool and has a greater role with this client group. Boundaries can be slightly looser, e.g. more time may be given at the end of a session if necessary, telephone calls to the wider network may be made in front of the client during session time to make explicit which information is shared and which is confidential as, often, people with ID have decisions made about them when they are not there and information is not fed back to them.

Attention is paid to all aspects of non-verbal communication including interpreting counter-transference. Confusion, helplessness and inadequacy can all be part of the counter-transference feelings of the therapists, mirroring the experience of the client. Therapy is more likely to take place face to face, which again aids the non-verbal aspects of communication. There is often more communication with the wider care network, which can be done during session time, as described above.

Three stages of therapy

There are three stages of therapy (Sinason, 1992). The first stage is a reduction in secondary handicap, described as the psychological defence of exaggerating one's impairments, e.g. wearing inappropriate clothing such as trousers that are too short, clothing and hairstyles more appropriate to a child.

The second stage is one of depression when the person is extremely vulnerable, having come face to face with having a disability.

The final stage is one of improvement in external and internal functioning.

People with ID can be passive and find it difficult to express any negative feelings towards people they depend on.

The handicapped smile is a smile at an inappropriate time, which masks any real feelings and is a defence against being different and a fear of the therapist or carer hating them.

Taboo subjects that are often not talked about outside of therapy are the disability itself, death, sexuality, dependency and fear of annihilation (Hollins and Sinason, 2000), also described by Sinason as the five mutative factors (Sinason, 2004).

Practice-based evidence

The evidence base for psychodynamic therapies in this population remains small. Many papers from the 1960s onwards in reviewing the literature have called for robust outcome research. Individual case reports, often very moving accounts, show the process of psychodynamic therapy in people with ID and that, anecdotally, people appear to benefit.

A recent evaluation of effectiveness of psychotherapy (Prout and Nowak-Drabik, 2003) reviewed 92 studies and concluded there was moderate effectiveness across theoretical approach. Nine of these studies were suitable for inclusion in a meta-analysis, all were behavioural, and other studies were not included, as they did not have an untreated control arm and data for calculation of effect size.

Beail and Warden (1996) reported significant reductions in symptoms of distress, increases in self-esteem and improved functioning for 20 adults following psychodynamic therapy. Beail (1998) studied 25 men referred over a three-year period with problem behaviours and mild ID. Treatment lasted between three to forty-three months with half receiving six months or less (this was open ended, dependent on client and therapist agreement). Aggression and offending behaviours disappeared altogether in 19 who completed treatment and in a further case the frequency of problem behaviour (repetitive questioning) was vastly reduced.

There is some evidence of psychodynamic psychotherapy being effective in preventing re-offending in men with ID (Beail, 2001). In a treatment group of thirteen men, none re-offended after six months of follow up and 11 had not re-offended at follow up four years later. Treatment length ranged from 4 months to 43 months. five men refused treatment and all re-offended within two years; three were given custodial sentences. Again these are small numbers.

In other case-series research, Frankish (1989) found a reduction in problem behaviours in a series of six people receiving psychodynamic psychotherapy. Bichard et al. (1996) used the Draw a Person Test (a projective test which works on the principle that we project aspects of our personality into ambiguous stimuli, which can be scored) to look at change before and after psychodynamic psychotherapy. If asked to draw a person we draw consistent figures; thus any change in a drawing is thought to reflect an inner change. The drawings of seven out of eight adults in psychotherapy became more detailed and sophisticated. In the waiting list controls only one client demonstrated an improvement in their scores. This corresponded with the views of carers as to whether clients' symptoms had worsened, stayed the same, improved or disappeared. All these studies represent practice-based evidence rather than an evidence base to inform practise. Large trials with random allocation to a control group are still absent from the literature.

Macdonald *et al.* (2003) looked at the satisfaction of persons with ID with group psychoanalytic therapy. Major themes were that people felt included and valued in the group. There were some negative themes such as finding talking upsetting. Overall it suggested that people with ID can engage meaningfully in group treatment and valued their experiences there.

Some researchers have argued that therapy centres should use the same evaluation and therapy outcome measures and pool results at a later stage, suggesting this is the only constructive way forward.

There is a lack of reliable and valid measures to evaluate change. It appears to be better to use a range of measures to be able to detect any change.

Future

More research is needed; whilst practice-based evidence is valuable, an evidence base needs to be built up to inform our practice. Funding can be a major problem, with funding bodies not seeing the value in these types of studies. People often cite ethical considerations as a reason for not funding projects. However as people with ID receive treatments, then it is unethical not to evaluate these treatments.

Conclusions

There is some evidence that psychodynamic treatment is an effective and useful tool for people with ID. At the moment there are only a few services in the UK which offer this treatment. Psychodynamic therapies need to be more widely available to people with ID. More research is needed using objective outcome measures, in particular using control groups. Whether in the future psychological therapies will come together and provide services for all populations or whether psychodynamic therapies will be provided within ID teams is still unknown. Probably each service will decide for itself rather than there being any nationwide consensus.

Summary points

- There may be direct psychological effects of having ID.
- Counselling and psychological therapies are popular with service users and their families.
- There are important differences in the techniques to be used with the ID and non-ID population: more warmth; greater non-verbal communication; slightly looser boundaries are indicated with the ID population.

- There are three stages in therapy: reduction of secondary handicap; depression; improvement in functioning.
- Practice-based evidence shows improvements in functioning and self-esteem and reductions of symptoms such as distress and aggressive and problem behaviours.
- Service provision is often patchy.
- There is a lack of reliable and valid measures to evaluate change.
- The evidence base needs to be built up.

REFERENCES

Arthur, A. (2003). The emotional lives of people with learning disability. *British Journal of Learning Disabilities*, **31**, 25–30.

Beail, N. (1998). Psychoanalytical psychotherapy with men with intellectual disabilities: a preliminary outcome study. *British Journal of Medical Psychology*, **71**, 1–11.

Beail, N. (2001). Recidivism following psychodynamic psychotherapy amongst offenders with intellectual disabilities. *The British Journal of Forensic Practice*, **3**(1), 33–7.

Beail, N. & Warden, S. (1996). Evaluation of a psychodynamic psychotherapy service for adults with intellectual disabilities: rationale, design and preliminary outcome data. *Journal of Applied Research in Intellectual Disabilities*, **9**(3), 223–8.

Bichard, S. H. Sinason, V. & Usiskin, J. (1996). Measuring change in mentally retarded clients in long-term psychoanalytic psychotherapy. *The National Association for Dual Diagnosis* **13**, 6–11.

Brown, H. & Turk, V. (1994). Sexual abuse in adulthood: Ongoing risks for people with learning disabilities. *Child Abuse Review*, **3**(1), 26–35.

Department of Health (1996). *A Review of Strategic Policy on NHS Psychotherapy Services in England*. London: NHS Executive.

Department of Health (2001). *Valuing People: A New Strategy for Learning Disability for the 21st Century*. London: Department of Health.

Department of Health (2004). *Organising and Delivering Psychological Therapies*. London: Department of Health.

Frankish, P. (1989). Meeting the emotional needs of handicapped people: a psycho-dynamic approach, *Journal of Mental Deficiency Research*, **33**, 407–14.

Goldberg, D., Magrill, L., Hale, J. *et al*. (1995). Protection and loss: working with learning-disabled adults and their families. *Journal of Family Therapy*, **17** (3) 263–79.

Hollins, S., Horrocks, C. & Sinason, V. (1998). *I Can Get Through It. Books Beyond Words*. London: Gaskell Press and St. George's Hospital Medical School.

Hollins, S. & Sinason, V. (2000). Psychotherapy, learning disabilities and trauma: new perspectives. *British Journal of Psychiatry*, **176**, 22–36.

Hollins, S. & Sireling, L. (2004). *When Mum Died*, 3rd edn. London: Co-published by Books Beyond Words, St. George's Hospital Medical School and Gaskell Press.

Macdonald, J., Sinason, V. & Hollins S. (2003). An interview study of people with learning disabilities experience of and satisfaction with group analytic therapy. *Psychology and Psychotherapy: Theory, Research and Practice*, **76**, 433–53.

Parkes, G., Mukherjee, R. A. S., Karagianni, E. *et al.* (2004). Characteristics and outcomes of referrals to a psychotherapy service for people with intellectual disabilities. *Journal of Intellectual Disability Research*, **48**, 291.

Prout, H. T. & Nowak-Drabik, K. M. (2003). Psychotherapy with persons who have mental retardation: an evaluation of effectiveness. *American Journal of Mental Retardation*, **108**(2), 82–93.

Royal College of Psychiatrists (2004). Psychotherapy and learning disability (Council Report CR116). London: Royal College of Psychiatrists.

Roth, A. & Fonagy, P. (1996). *What Works for Whom? A Critical Review of Psychotherapy Research*. New York: The Guildford Press.

Sequeira, H., Howlin, P., and Hollins, S. (2003). Psychological disturbance associated with sexual abuse in people with learning disabilities. *British Journal of Psychiatry*, **183**, 451–6.

Sobsey, D. (1994). *Violence and Abuse in the Lives of People with Disabilities: The End of Silent Acceptance?* Baltimore, MD: Paul H. Brooks.

Sinason, V. (1992). *Mental Handicap and the Human Condition: New Approaches from the Tavistock*. London: Free Association Books.

Sinason, V. (2004). Learning Disability as Trauma and the Impact of Trauma on Learning Disability. Unpublished Ph.D. thesis, Senate House, London.

Part IV

Policy and service systems

22

Mental health and intellectual disabilities: the development of services

Stuart Cumella

Introduction

There are limited data available to provide a comprehensive account on the development of services internationally for people with intellectual disabilities (ID). The historical study of intellectual disability is still in its infancy in many countries (particularly in the Third World), and generalization is made difficult by the substantial variations in the development of services between different countries (Holt *et al.*, 2000; European Intellectual Disability Research Network, 2003). Nevertheless, some general trends have been observed in many societies: the introduction of humane forms of treatment in the nineteenth century, the move towards incarceration in total institutions towards the end of the century, and the reaction to institutional care in the later years of the twentieth century.

The development of humane forms of care

There are still debates about whether pre-modern societies had a concept similar to that of 'intellectual disability' (Goodey, 2003), and Jacobson (1999) noted that most writers date the Western history of intellectual disability from about 1790 (Meyers & Blacher, 1987). However, Jacobson noted that some specialist services did exist before that date. These included the founding of an asylum by St Vincent de Paul in Austria (Barr, 1904/1973); the establishment of a hospital in Cairo in the middle ages; a form of group care in thirteenth-century Gheel, Belgium; and residential programmes in the early seventeenth century in Thuringen, Bavaria, and Austria (Kane & Rojahn, 1981; Meyers & Blacher, 1987).

The development of humane forms of care for people with ID in the early nineteenth century was inspired by two examples of heroic innovation:

Psychiatric and Behavioural Disorders in Intellectual and Developmental Disabilities, ed. Nick Bouras and Geraldine Holt. Published by Cambridge University Press. © Cambridge University Press 2007.

1. By Phillipe Pinel, who from 1793 reformed asylum care in Paris, to provide a safe environment, characterized by humane vigilance, planned treatment, recreation and vocational preparation, and the elimination of abuse, chains and indignities (Scheerenberger, 1983).

2. By the publication of *The Wild Boy of Aveyron* by Jean-Marc Itard in 1801 (Itard, 1962), which described how the author had worked with a 'feral' boy found running about on all fours in the woods. Itard described techniques which succeeded in engaging the attention of his subject and enabling him to learn some basic skills (Murray, 1988). Edouard Seguin, a protégé of Itard, generalized and expanded upon Itard's work (Meyers & Blacher, 1987), and developed a more extensive instructional methodology based on stimulation and training of the senses (Balthazar & Stevens, 1975). After founding the first educational programme for people with ID in France, Seguin also founded services in the USA.

   In the following decades, 'an almost religious movement, spread by evangelistic apostles' (Meyers & Blacher, 1987) promoted the establishment of educational facilities for people with ID, with the anticipation that many would re-enter society as productive citizens. Guggenbuhl set up the first residential centre in Switzerland (using a colony model); sheltered and church-sponsored homes were set up in Germany (Kane & Rojahn, 1981); while in the USA, Wilbur founded the first private school and Howe the first public programme (Meyers & Blacher, 1987). Programmes were set up by Saegert in Germany, by Guggenmoos in Salzburg, and by Reed in England. Between 1850 and 1900, community schools were founded in Germany and Sweden, and compulsory education statutes including some, but not all, children with ID were enacted in Norway and Saxony (Barr, 1904/1973; Kane & Rojahn, 1981). In the 40 years following Howe's first school for children with ID in Boston in 1848, 15 such state institutions were established in the USA.

The rise of the total institution

Despite this expansion, by 1850 only a small proportion of people with ID in Europe and North America attended special schools and similar establishments. A much greater number lived in almshouses, asylums, poorhouses, or with their families (Murray, 1988). Industrialization, the unprecedented growth in population in the century, coupled with the movement of millions of people between continents and from rural to urban areas, undermined informal care provisions (Meyers & Blacher, 1987). This led to a major increase in the size of many specialist facilities, which inevitably changed their character. Many of the places that eventually became total institutions had begun as small, community-related services. For instance, one German facility served 100 patients in 1871 and 920 in

1902 (Barr, 1904/1973). Many countries also began building large publicly funded institutions to house the growing number of people with ID accumulating in poor-law facilities.

By the beginning of the twentieth century, the incarceration of people with ID in large institutions had ceased to be just a regrettable necessity and had instead become an evangelical cause. The intellectual basis for this cause was the development of the theory of eugenics by Sir Francis Galton. This was based on an extension of Charles Darwin's theories to societies as a whole, which were conceptualized as 'races' in competition for survival. The theory proposed that a major threat to the survival of the 'race' was the disproportionate growth of 'moral imbeciles', a category that included people with ID who were seen to be particularly predisposed to engage in crime and sexual promiscuity. Eugenic theories were apparently supported by the research of the day. In England, the rejection of substantial numbers of recruits for service in the Boer War created a kind of moral panic, which supported the restrictive provisions of the 1913 Mental Deficiency Act (O'Connor, 1981).

Eugenics gave a peculiarly hostile and stigmatizing flavour to discussions of public policy, at worst viewing people with ID as sub-human. For instance, Henry Goddard, a prominent US expert in eugenics (who later recanted these views), proposed: 'The idiot is not our greatest problem. He is indeed loathsome . . . Nevertheless, he lives his life and is done. He does not continue the race with a line of children like himself . . . It is the moron type that makes for us our greatest problem'. (Goddard, 1912.)

The solutions to this problem were seen as being the lifetime incarceration of people with ID in sexually segregated and self-supporting 'colonies', isolated from the temptations of the city. For those people with ID who remained at large, compulsory sterilization was implemented in several countries. By the beginning of the twentieth century, 21 states in the USA had at least one institution, while serving 10 000 people nationally (Barr, 1904/1973); while by 1926, 23 US states had laws imposing sterilization (Meyers & Blacher, 1987). The logical extension of viewing people with ID as both sub-human and a threat to society was that they be denied the right to life, and systematic murder by the state was introduced by the Nazi regime in Germany.

Elsewhere, eugenics had a profound impact not just on the location, but also on the quality of care. Because people with ID were seen as a threat or at best a social nuisance, there was limited interest in research into their needs, or the development of improved techniques for education, treatment, or care (Greenland, 1963; Donaldson & Menolascino, 1977). The diverse physical and mental health needs of people with ID were not assessed, and little specialist medical treatment was provided even where large institutions were part of the healthcare system. As a result, many large residential institutions had very high mortality rates. Children with ID were assumed to be incapable of learning, a view seemingly supported by the application of intelligence testing (Gould, 1981).

The reaction to institutional care

Jacobson (1999) noted that the eugenics movement had met some public resistance from early in the twentieth century (Stainton, 2000), and that research in the 1920s had undermined claims of an association between ID and crime, alcoholism, prostitution, and pauperism. However, eugenic ideas only became discredited politically after 1945 because of the enthusiasm with which the Nazis had implemented them. The new political consensus emphasized instead the universality of human rights (as seen in the UN Universal Declaration of Human Rights and the European Convention of Human Rights), explicitly extended to disabled people in the later Declaration of Rights of Disabled People and the Declaration of Rights of Mentally Retarded Persons. Within democratic societies, politics became increasingly dominated by the demands for full social inclusion for racial and ethnic minorities, women, and people with disabilities.

In the case of people with ID, this took the form of hostility to large institutions, and was led by the new organizations set up by parents of people with ID (Jacobson 1999). These organizations increasingly managed their own alternative community-based services (Walmsley, 2000). Their campaigns were supported by a series of enquiries into severe neglect and brutality in large institutions, and by research showing the disabling effect of life in a total institution (particularly Goffman's influential work in 1960). Some of the first clinical effectiveness research in this field found that community-based units had better outcomes in terms of behaviour and self-care skills (Raynes & King, 1967). Renewed therapeutic optimism led to the increasing recruitment into services for people with ID of clinical psychologists, educationalists, occupational therapists and communication therapists, who had less personal investment in maintaining total institutions than medical and nursing staff.

The move from institutional care was promoted by the third great evangelical movement in the history of ID, based on the various competing theories of 'normalization'. The Scandinavian version of normalization emphasized the need for each disabled person to develop a sense of self-worth and adulthood by experiencing and passing over the various thresholds of challenge and growth common to all people (Nirje, 1972). The key role for public services was therefore to facilitate opportunities for disabled people to experience the same kinds of living environment as the general population, with similar opportunities for self-determination, for personal and sexual relationships, and for earning a living. Facilitation essentially involved compensating for a person's disabilities, such as providing staff to support a disabled person in carrying out domestic tasks, or specialized transport to help them get to town.

Wolfensburger's influential writings on normalization differed from this approach by emphasizing the need to overcome the social psychology of discrimination. He noted that disabled people suffer disadvantages not only in the form of overt discrimination, but also an unconscious process of denigration, and he observed how specialist services used derogatory labels or associated disabled people with other groups with low status in society. This confirmed to disabled people their inferior and dependent position in society, which they in turn expressed through their behaviour, thereby confirming the initial assumptions of their lower status. He proposed that a key objective of services should therefore be to enable disabled people to behave in ways that were socially valued rather than inferior, in order to assert their equal status and achieve acceptance by others in society. This could be attained by making staff aware of the way in which they and their workplaces can unconsciously devalue disabled people, by making every effort to place disabled people in positive social roles and to help them behave and appear in ways that are socially valued, by helping them develop their personal competencies, and by ensuring they take part in the valued social life of the rest of society. This involves living in 'normative housing within the valued community with valued people', attending the same schools, and being involved in a valued manner in work, shopping and leisure activities (Wolfensberger, 1969, 1972).

Normalization was implemented in various model services, of which the most influential was that of the Eastern Nebraska Community Office of Retardation (ENCOR). This pioneered the adaptation of ordinary houses to provide staffed residences for small groups of people with ID, together with a small staff team. In the UK, this model inspired the report *An Ordinary Life* (King's Fund, 1981), which came at the moment when changes in social security regulations inadvertently provided a massive expansion of public funds for resettling people from long-stay hospital care (Cumella 1998). Between 1971 and 2000, the number of people with ID in hospitals in England fell from over 50 000 to less than 2000 (Department of Health, 2001). Similar changes occurred elsewhere. The resident population in US institutions peaked in 1967, at 193 183 (Bachrach, 1981), falling to 63 258 in 1995 (Lakin *et al.*, 1996). Rates of annual decrease in the number of people with ID in large institutions between 1981 and 1991 were as high as 25% in the European Union and the USA, although a decline in institutional populations had yet to occur in Eastern Europe (Hatton *et al.*, 1995) (see also Chapter 23 by Davidson & O'Hara).

Mental illness and intellectual disabilities

Resettlement programmes usually found it easier and cheaper to resettle those residents in large institutions who were more able and had less complex needs. This group were also unlikely to require subsequent re-admission. As a result, the decline in the population of large institutions also changed their character, from being enclosed communities for the full range of people with ID, to smaller specialist services for people with ID and complex additional needs. This was a heterogeneous group, including those with profound disabilities, physical illness, and sensory impairments. However, the largest group that proved difficult to resettle were those with severe behavioural problems and/or a mental illness (Jacobson, 1982, 1988). This group with a 'dual diagnosis' had a high risk of re-admission to institutions even where local services were committed to community-based care (Kearney & Smull, 1992). This problem generated a new interest in research into the causes and treatment of 'challenging behaviour' and mental illness among people with ID.

Jacobson (1999) noted that instances of co-existing mental illness and ID had been described by Seguin as early as 1866, with more formal classification in the early twentieth century. But until the second half of the twentieth century there was little agreement in the professional literature about whether people with ID were susceptible to mental disorders and whether or how treatment should be offered. Research in this field was probably impeded by the eugenic view that mental illness and anti-social behaviour were an inherent characteristic of people with ID. However, a series of studies in different institutional populations began to estimate prevalence rates for psychiatric disorders (Craft, 1959), and there was recognition that behavioural problems and impoverished institutional environments and lack of support can aggravate mental disorders among people with ID living in the community (Menolascino, 1965; 1966).

There was a substantial delay before this greater awareness was converted into public policy. Although mental health clinics for people with ID were established from 1958 in the USA (Menolascino, 1965; Philips & Williams, 1975), policy-makers were reluctant to accept that people with ID needed more than just a uniform and undifferentiated set of services. For instance in the UK, it was not until 1979 that a government report concluded that people with ID had diverse needs, each requiring an array of specialist services (Department of Health and Social Security, 1979). A series of policy reports in the next two decades (Department of Health and Social Security, 1984; Department of Health, 1989, 1993; Lindsey, 1998) proposed various options for how services could be provided for what were eventually identified as three overlapping groups of people with ID: those with a mental illness; those with severe anti-social behaviours; and those who have committed offences against the law.

This eventually led in the UK to an uneven pattern of specialist services throughout the country, including specialist acute mental illness services (including some small inpatient admission units and community teams), a small number of inpatient forensic units, and a diverse range of 'challenging behaviour' services (Bouras *et al.*, 2003). The latter included specialist admission units, short-term behavioural intervention teams, domiciliary support for carers of people with a challenging behaviour, and an increasing use of supported living, in which individuals with severe behavioural problems live in what are essentially residential care homes with a single resident (Bailey & Cooper, 1997). The UK was a particularly favourable environment for developing services of this kind because services for people with ID had since 1948 been managed by the National Health Service. As the large hospitals reduced in size, sufficient funding could be transferred to maintain both specialist health and new community-based services.

Few if any other countries have even attempted to develop a comprehensive mental health service for people with ID. The most common pattern is for a limited number of specialist centres in larger population centres, with the expectation that people with ID and a mental illness will be admitted to generic psychiatric services (Holt *et al.*, 2000). However, access to generic services is often impeded by a lack of specialist skills among general psychiatrists in the diagnosis and treatment of mental disorders among people with ID, and by separate funding streams for ID and psychiatric services (Chaplin, 2004; Jacobson, 1999; Jacobson & Ackerman, 1988; Windle *et al.*, 1988). In some countries, the historical experience of adverse medically dominated institutions has led to a reluctance among policy-makers to consider any specialist health services for people with ID (Holt *et al.*, 2000) (see also Chapter 23 by Davidson & O'Hara).

Conclusion

Despite the uneven provision of mental health services for people with ID, something of an international consensus is developing (Bouras & Jacobson, 2002): that there is a high prevalence among people with ID of undiagnosed and untreated mental disorders, that mental illness among people with ID often presents in atypical ways, may co-exist with various developmental disorders, and that many people with ID have impaired communication and hence are unable to describe subjective symptoms (Lindsey, 2002, Chaplin & Flynn, 2000). Effective treatment therefore requires specialist clinical skills in communication, diagnosis and treatment, and these skills are at present rarely available in generic mental health services (Bouras *et al.*, 2003) (see also Chapter 25 by Costello *et al.*).

The key unresolved issue is the extent to which the solution lies in enhancing the skills of staff in generic mental health services in responding to the needs of people with ID, or developing a new specialist service. This may be a false opposite. Generic mental health services are most unlikely to sustain any skills in treating the relatively small number of people with ID, unless they have ready access to the advice of clinical teams that specialize in treating this group of patients (Gravestock & Bouras, 1997). There is in any case little sign that generic mental health services are pressing to treat more people with ID. Instead, as noted above, it often proves difficult to secure inpatient admission for people with ID and an acute mental illness. In the absence of specialist 'dual diagnosis' services, this group of patients may even be refused admission to both mental health and ID services. Specialist mental health services therefore also need to train staff in community-based ID services, to strengthen their ability to manage behavioural disorders and mental illness among their clients (Department of Health, 1993). There has been progress in developing accessible training packages to further this task (Holt *et al.*, 2005).

Summary points

- There is a growing interest in developing services for people with ID and mental illness in recent years.
- There is a tendency to use generic and mainstream mental health services for people with ID as far as possible. However, specialist services will remain a necessity. The challenge will be to identify the most appropriate model for specialist service and the extent of integration with generic mental health services.
- Whichever strategy is undertaken it should be based on high professional standards, involve the use of least-restrictive environments and appropriate treatments with established clinical effectiveness, and employ staff with an expertise and a personal commitment to the care of people with ID and a mental illness.
- Service user groups and carers will increasingly be involved with the design and planning of services.

Acknowledgments

This chapter is an update of the chapter by John Jacobson, in the first edition of this book.

REFERENCES

Bachrach, L. L. (1981). A conceptual approach to deinstitutionalization of the mentally retarded: a perspective from the experience of the mentally ill. In *Deinstitutionalization and Community Adjustment of Mentally Retarded People*, ed. R. H. Bruininks, C. E. Meyers, B. B. Sigford, & K. C. Lakin. Washington, DC: American Association on Mental Deficiency, pp. 51–67.

Bailey, N. M. & Cooper, S. A. (1997). The current provision of specialist health services to people with learning disabilities in England and Wales. *Journal of Intellectual Disability Research*, **41**, 52–9.

Balthazar, E. E. & Stevens, H. A. (1975). *The Emotionally Disturbed Mentally Retarded: a Historical and Contemporary Perspective*. Englewood Cliffs, NJ: Prentice-Hall.

Barr, M. W. (1904/1973). *Mental Defectives, their History, Treatment, and Training*. New York: Arno Press.

Bouras N., Cowley, A., Holt, G., Newton, J. T. & Sturmey, P. (2003). Referral trends of people with intellectual disabilities and psychiatric disorders. *Journal of Intellectual Disability Research*, **47**, 439–46.

Bouras, N. & Jacobson, J. (2002). Mental health care for people with mental retardation: a global perspective. *World Psychiatry*, **1**, 162–5.

Chaplin, R. (2004). General psychiatric services for adults with intellectual disability and mental illness. *Journal of Intellectual Disability Research*, **48**, 1–10.

Chaplin, R. & Flynn, A. (2000). Adults with learning disability admitted to psychiatric wards. *Advances in Psychiatric Treatment*, **6**, 128–34.

Craft, M. (1959). Mental disorder in the defective: a psychiatric survey among in-patients. *American Journal of Mental Deficiency*, **63**, 829–34.

Cumella, S. (1998). Community care. In Spurgeon, P. (ed.), *The New Face of the NHS*. Harlow: Longmans, pp. 253–69.

Department of Health (1989). *Needs and Responses. Services for Adults with Mental Handicap who are Mentally Ill, who have Behavioural Problems or who Offend. Report of a Department of Health Study Team*. London: Department of Health.

Department of Health (1993). *Services for People with Learning Disabilities and Challenging Behaviours or Mental Health Needs*. London: HMSO.

Department of Health (2001). *Valuing People: a New Strategy for Learning Disability for the 21st Century*. Cmd 5086. London: Department of Health.

Department of Health and Social Security (1979). *Report of the Committee of Enquiry into Mental Handicap Nursing and Care*. London: HMSO.

Department of Health and Social Security (1984). *Helping Mentally Handicapped Persons with Special Needs. Report of a DHSS Study Team. A Review of Current Approaches to Meeting the Needs of Mentally Handicapped People with Special Problems*. London: Department of Health and Social Security.

Donaldson, J. Y. & Menolascino, F. J. (1977). Past, current, and future roles of child psychiatry in mental retardation. *Journal of the American Academy of Child Psychiatry*, **16**, 38–52.

European Intellectual Disability Research Network (2003). *Intellectual Disability in Europe. Working Papers.* Canterbury: Tizard Centre.

Goddard, H. (1912). *The Kallikak Family: A Study in the Heredity of Feeble-Mindedness.* New York: MacMillan.

Goffman, E. (1960). *Asylums – Essays on the Social Situation of Mental Patients and Other Inmates.* Harmondsworth: Penguin.

Goodey, C. F. (2003). On certainty, reflexivity and the ethics of genetic research into intellectual disability. *Journal of Intellectual Disability Research,* **47**, 548–54.

Gould, S. J. (1981). *The Mismeasure of Man.* Harmondsworth: Penguin.

Gravestock, S. & Bouras, N. (1997). Survey of services for adults with learning disabilities. *Psychiatric Bulletin,* **21**, 197–9.

Greenland, C. (1963). The treatment of the mentally retarded in Ontario: an historical note. *Canadian Psychiatric Journal,* **8**(5), 328–36.

Hatton, C., Emerson, E. & Kiernan, C. (1995). People in institutions in Europe. *Mental Retardation,* **33**, 132.

Holt, G., Costello, H., Bouras, N. *et al.* (2000). BIOMED-MEROPE project: service provision for adults with intellectual disability: a European comparison. *Journal of Intellectual Disability Research,* **44**, 685–96.

Holt, G., Hardy, S. & Bouras, N. (2005). *Mental Health in Learning Disabilities: A Training Resource.* Brighton: Pavilion Publishing.

Itard, J.-M. (1962). *The Wild Boy of Aveyron.* New York: Appleton-Century-Crofts.

Jacobson, J. W. (1982). Problem behavior and psychiatric impairment in a developmentally disabled population. I: Behavior frequency. *Applied Research in Mental Retardation,* **3**, 121–39.

Jacobson, J. W. (1988). Problem behavior and psychiatric impairment in a developmentally disabled population. III: Psychotropic medication. *Research in Developmental Disabilities,* **9**, 23–38.

Jacobson, J. W. (1999). Dual diagnosis services: history, progress and perspectives. In *Psychiatric and Behavioural Disorders in Developmental Disabilities,* ed. N. Bouras. Cambridge: Cambridge University Press, pp. 329–58.

Jacobson, J. W. & Ackerman, L. J. (1988). An appraisal of services for mental retardation and psychiatric impairments. *Mental Retardation,* **26**, 377–80.

Kane, J. F. & Rojahn, J. (1981). Development of services for mentally retarded people in the Federal Republic of Germany: a survey of history, empirical research, and current trends. *Applied Research in Mental Retardation,* **2**, 195–210.

Kearney, F. J. & Smull, M. W. (1992). People with mental retardation leaving mental health institutions: Evaluating outcomes after five years in the community. In *Community Living for People with Developmental and Psychiatric Disabilities,* ed. J. W. Jacobson, S. N. Burchard & P. J. Carling. Baltimore, MD: The Johns Hopkins University Press, pp. 183–96.

King's Fund (1981). *An Ordinary Life. Comprehensive Locally-Based Residential Services for Mentally Handicapped People.* London: King's Fund Centre.

Lakin, K. C., Prouty, B., Smith, G. & Braddock, D. (1996). Nixon goal surpassed – twofold. *Mental Retardation,* **34**, 67.

Lindsey, M. (1998). *Signposts for Success in Commissioning and Providing Health Services for People with Learning Disabilities.* London: NHS Executive.

Lindsey, M. (2002). Comprehensive health care services for people with learning disabilities. *Advances in Psychiatric Treatment*, **8**, 138–48.

Menolascino, F. J. (1965). Emotional disturbance and mental retardation. *American Journal of Mental Deficiency*, **70**, 248–56.

Menolascino, F. J. (1966). The facade of mental retardation. *American Journal of Psychiatry*, **122**, 1227–35.

Meyers, C. E. & Blacher, J. (1987). Historical determinants of residential care. In *Living Environments and Mental Retardation*, ed. S. Landesman, P. M. Vietze & M. J. Begab. Washington, DC: American Association on Mental Retardation, pp. 3–16.

Murray, P. (1988). The study of the history of disability services: examining the past to improve the present and future. *Australia and New Zealand Journal of Developmental Disabilities*, **14**, 93–102.

Nirje, B. (1972). The right to self-determination. In W. Wolfensburger (ed.), *The Principle of Normalization in Human Services.* Toronto: National Institute on Mental Retardation.

O'Connor, N. (1981). British applied psychology of mental subnormality. *Applied Research in Mental Retardation*, **2**, 97–113.

Philips, I. & Williams, N. (1975). Psychopathology and mental retardation: a study of 100 mentally retarded children. *American Journal of Psychiatry*, **132**, 139–45.

Raynes, N. & King, R. (1967). Residential care for the mentally retarded. *First International Congress for the Scientific Study of Mental Deficiency.* Surrey: Montpellier. Reprinted in Boswell, D. and Wingrove, J. (1974). *The Handicapped Person in the Community. A Reader and Sourcebook.* London: Tavistock Publications in association with the Open University.

Scheerenberger, R. C. (1983). *A History of Mental Retardation.* Baltimore, MD: Paul H. Brookes.

Stainton, T. (2000). Equal citizens? The discourse of liberty and rights in the history of learning disabilities. In *Crossing Boundaries. Change and Continuity in the History of Learning Disability*, ed. Walmsley, J. Kidderminster: BILD Publications, pp. 87–102.

Walmsley, J. (2000). Straddling boundaries: the changing roles of voluntary organizations, 1913–1959. In *Crossing Boundaries. Change and Continuity in the History of Learning Disability*, ed. Walmsley, J. Kidderminster: BILD Publications, pp. 103–22.

Windle, C., Poppen, P. J., Thompson, J. W. & Marvelle, K. (1988). Types of patients served by various providers of outpatient care in CMHCs. *American Journal of Psychiatry*, **145**, 457–63.

Wolfensberger, W. (1969). The origin and nature of our institutional models. In *Changing Patterns in Residential Services for the Mentally Retarded*, ed. R. Kugel & W. Wolfensberger. Washington, DC: President's Committee on Mental Retardation, pp. 59–177.

Wolfensberger, W. (1972). *The Principle of Normalization in Human Services.* Toronto: National Institute on Mental Retardation.

23

Clinical services for people with intellectual disabilities and psychiatric or severe behaviour disorders

Philip W. Davidson and Jean O'Hara

Introduction

Kerker *et al.* (2004) reviewed 200 peer-reviewed articles, selected 52 based on stringent criteria, and concluded that between 5% and 12% of children and between 17% and 36% of adults with intellectual disabilities (ID) also had mental health disorders. Janicki, Davidson and colleagues (Janicki, *et al.*, 2002; Davidson, *et al.*, 2003) reported that prevalence rates of psychiatric diagnoses among adults with ID did not change with increasing age. A larger number may not actually have a formal psychiatric diagnosis but may be treated with psychotherapy, psychoactive medication or both by a mental health professional (Davidson *et al.*, 2003; Holland, 2003; Jacobson, 2003; Reiss, 1990). Reiss (1994) suggested that mental health disorders may be under-reported owing to the phenomenon of diagnostic overshadowing, i.e. the tendency to incorrectly attribute symptoms of frank mental illness to behavioural abnormalities associated with ID.

Behavioural or psychiatric disorders that may have been accepted by institutional staff are often not tolerated in community placements. Hence, the presence of additional mental health problems is a principal threat to social integration (Borthwick, 1988; Bruininks *et al.*, 1988; Bruininks *et al.*, 1987; Crawford *et al.*, 1979; Hill & Bruininks, 1984; Pagel & Whitling, 1978). As a consequence, the presence of mental health problems impairs the quality of life of persons with ID (Shalock & Keith, 1993), or cause regression of adaptive or developmental functioning (Russell & Tanguay, 1981). It may also create unnecessary escalation of family stressors and impair family functioning (Reiss, 1990).

The design of services for individuals with ID and mental health problems did not emerge as a major issue until the start of the deinstitutionalization movement in the latter third of the twentieth century. Until that point, persons with ID who developed severe behavioural problems lived in institutional settings and their

Psychiatric and Behavioural Disorders in Intellectual and Developmental Disabilities, ed. Nick Bouras and Geraldine Holt. Published by Cambridge University Press. © Cambridge University Press 2007.

disorders were easily managed by physical or pharmacological restraints. Those with recognized psychiatric illnesses were often removed from the ID system and maintained by the same treatments in psychiatric hospitals.

As more and more institutional beds were closed, persons with ID and mental health problems found themselves moving to less restrictive environments, or remaining longer with their families. In such community settings, it became clear that services from both the ID network and the mental health system were required. Unfortunately, inadequacies in service provision remained unrecognized for a long time. Notable contributory factors included a prevailing view in the 1970s that mental health need was over-exaggerated, and that most problems would be dealt with by generic services (Moss *et al.*, 1997). Even now, few localities have community-based programmes that provide comprehensive, integrated mental health and ID services that are fully accessible to persons with these disabilities. Within geographical areas there is a wide variation of services available. Sometimes, appropriate mental health services may not exist at all. More often, individuals with ID may be excluded from existing generic mental health services. This may be due to organizational issues, such as restrictions on providing services to persons with low IQs, or lack of expertise in addressing the needs of persons with ID and mental health problems. Exclusion may also stem from the belief by mental health professionals that persons with ID may not benefit from mental health interventions, owing either to an impaired ability to process information or to a lack of competence to participate in a therapeutic process.

In the last 15 years, mental health among people with ID has become a growing international concern (Moss *et al.* 2000). There has been an expansion of specialized community-based services as well as some recent developments in specialist inpatient facilities. The purpose of this chapter is to posit some benchmarks for such services, and review the few service models that have been field-tested and published, and assess them against the benchmarks.

Characteristics of comprehensive mental health services for people with ID

Conceptualizing service system models

Ever since people with ID have begun to depend upon community resources for diagnosing and treating mental health disorders, communities have been implementing services. Our review of the literature indicates a wide degree of variation in locations, service mix, financing options, and staffing patterns among those service models that have been reported. Moss *et al.* (2000) have provided a framework to conceptualize the factors that influence service development in this field. They propose a variant of the matrix model first described for non-disabled people with mental health problems by Thornicroft and Tansella (1999). The model is comprised of two dimensions, one determined by the level within the service system (e.g. national, local, or individual), and the other by the point in the temporal sequence of service provision (e.g. inputs to the service, the process of providing the service, and the resulting outcome). Using this model to characterize various approaches to service, Moss and colleagues observe that national priorities often vary from country to country and from culture to culture. These differences guide and influence inputs to the service system and ultimately affect the way a consumer is served, and the service products and outcomes. They also emphasize that inputs to every system at all levels are affected by the need for trained personnel to staff and administer the service. As we will see later in this chapter, there are significant shortages of skilled personnel at all levels in all service systems we reviewed, making training a very high priority for assuring the delivery of services that reduce or prevent mental health problems.

Barriers to comprehensive community services

In most of the service models described in the literature, there were both conceptual and operational gulfs between mental health and ID service systems. As a result, interagency communication was not well established and access to services across systems was limited. Reiss (1994) identified seven barriers to services for people with challenging behaviours. His list begins with a lack of community commitment to establishing special services, attributed to limited consumer advocacy, and a dearth of momentum-generating support from professional organizations. This lack of commitment and organizational resistance to change may be at the top of a cascade effect that limits access to existing systems of services and supports, and fiscal resources. It may confine mental health problems in people with ID to a low status among priorities to be addressed by governments and private voluntary groups.

Although social inclusion and the rights of people with ID to access mainstream as well as local specialist mental health services have been emphasized in the UK Government's strategy (Department of Health, 2001; NIMHE 2004) it still remains to be seen whether or not such ideals can be delivered.

Overcoming the barriers: characteristics of an idealized model

Established by consensus

Despite the presence of barriers to comprehensive care and supports, most of the models we describe successfully implemented community-based programmes. These programmes have overcome the barriers by different measures. Taken together, however, one can summarize these measures in terms of an idealized model programme. A number of models emphasized the need for consensus among providers, individuals, and funders in establishing a comprehensive service network for individuals with ID and mental health problems. Unless all sectors of the community agree on the need for such services and supports, what ensues may not achieve credibility, or it may not gain access to all components of the service system with which interfaces are required. Facilitating a consensus can be achieved by bringing all stakeholders together to sanction the need for, and the characteristics of, the service programme before it is established (Davidson et al., 1989; Hassiotis et al., 2000; Bouras & Holt, 2004).

The bringing together of stakeholders into Intellectual Disability Partnership Boards at every district level in the UK, has provided the opportunity to look at a range of social and primary health care issues affecting the lives of persons with ID (Department of Health (DoH), 2001) but there is still little evidence that their mental health needs are being adequately addressed (Department of Health, 1999a).

Establishing cross-system access

Persons with ID and mental health problems and their families may be primarily served by one service system (e.g. the ID system) and may not be known to other systems (the mental health or the social services system). For example, the initial presentation in the mental health system for such a person may be when they appear at a psychiatric emergency room. If an acute psychiatric disorder requiring inpatient treatment cannot be diagnosed, the emergency room staff may only be able to provide temporary stabilization of the behavioural component of the individual's problem (Beasley et al., 1992). Yet discharge to the original community setting may be complicated by an unwillingness of the ID agency staff to accept the person's ongoing behaviour problems, thus complicating the disposition (Marcos et al., 1986). Effective discharge planning may require a blending of resources and expertise through cross-system access and communication. This characteristic of co-ordinated comprehensive community-based mental health care for persons with ID is documented in the South East London Project reviewed below (Bouras & Drummond, 1989, 1990; Bouras et al., 1993; Bouras et al., 2003).

Cross-system access may be enhanced by staff trusted by both mental health and ID system personnel, who may act as an ombudsman. Such models are only recently reaching the policy agenda in the UK (Department of Health, 2001; NIMHE, 2004).

Comprehensive inter-disciplinary services

Challenging behaviours and mental disorders in persons with ID require an interdisciplinary approach by a team of professionals who can address both biomedical and environmental interventions, case management, and supports to families and consumers (Tufnell et al., 1985; Roy, 2000). The team should include members capable of consulting with generic service elements, including a psychiatric emergency department, an in patient unit, a community mental health centre, a psychiatric day treatment programme, an ID community residence or day treatment programme, or a sheltered workshop programme with equal facility.

Community-based services with tertiary links

Long-term resolution of behavioural or psychiatric disorders in persons with ID requires community-based activities, since most or all of the resources for habilitative and therapeutic services are community based. However, resolution of an acute crisis may require tertiary psychiatric or behavioural resources, often available only on a supra-district or regional basis. Tertiary centres such as university hospitals may offer such resources, including inpatient acute psychiatric evaluation and treatment service, specialized ambulatory psychiatric service, emergency respite service, or emergency behaviour stabilization services.

Credibility

Credibility with providers in both ID and mental health systems must be maintained in order to ensure cross-system access. The staff must be well trained and experienced in both ID and mental health systems, and the programme must be structured to permit them to easily access and provide effective service in both systems. The administrative structure should promote the staff's role as credible brokers, and should not impose any regulatory or bureaucratic constraints that upset the balance between mental health and ID systems. The service location will depend upon a consensus among the constituent stakeholders based on the ability to maintain and develop such a specialist service.

Direct funding

Beasley has made the point that some elements of the idealized service must depend upon direct funding, as third parties may not cover such services (Beasley *et al.*, 1992). Components such as crisis intervention, respite, or public education, may be too costly to remain viable in a fee-for-service or capitated system of reimbursement. In the UK there is an argument for the funding of such relatively small but highly specialist services to be funded more centrally from Strategic Health Authorities instead of at a locality or district level.

Training

The delivery of effective services to people with ID and mental health problems depends on the availability of personnel who can implement the services. This principle may seem simplistic, but as Geller and Pomeroy (2003) pointed out, specialized services require specialized personnel and very few resources exist in any country to prepare such personnel and to assure that positions they fill stay filled. Geller and Pomeroy (2003) have proposed a framework for providing comprehensive inter-disciplinary personnel preparation in the field. This model has been implemented in very few places because it requires long-duration training for clinical personnel, for whom there is very limited financing (see also Chapter 25 by Costello *et al.*)

Training pays off in returns at the service delivery level only if there are incentives to retain personnel once they complete their training. Such is rarely the case.

Examples of community-based and integrated inpatient service models

Attention to the growing need for services for persons with ID and mental health problems has lead to the development of community models for this population. The specifics of these models and the services offered vary from community to community. The following discussion describes community models for which established peer-reviewed material was available (see also Chapter 22 by Cumella).

European models

UK models

Allen (1998) examined services in Wales in the UK, over a 20-year period, as large institutions closed down in favour of community-based social and healthcare provision. He concluded that although the infrastructure of community services appeared to reduce the dependency on hospital provision, it did not completely eradicate the need for new long-stay admissions. However, the development of outpatient clinics helped to ensure that psychiatric advice and intervention continued to be provided, but within a framework of community support.

Bouras and his colleagues (Bouras & Holt, 2001; Bouras *et al.*, 2003) have described and evaluated a model for community mental health services for adults with ID that has been operating in southeast London for nearly 20 years. The service is comprised of outpatient clinics and a specialized inpatient unit based at a tertiary medical centre, coupled with outreach consultation and training in community agencies. The clinical team includes psychiatrists, community psychiatric nurses and administrative staff. Interfaces with other clinical disciplines including behavioural psychologists, social workers and occupational therapists are in place. The project also provides extensive university-based and outreach training from the Estia Centre (a local training, research and development resource now recognized internationally), to support the development of a competent work force at every level, from direct care staff to managers and organizations.

Adults with ID in this region of London are served through community-based teams. If an inpatient stay is warranted for an acute psychiatric crisis, admission is into the generic mental health facilities with consultative advice and support from MHiLD. Patients can also access a six-bed specialist unit at a tertiary level. The function of this unit is to provide comprehensive assessment of the mental health problems when these cannot be achieved in a community setting or within generic mental health services, to make recommendations and implement therapeutic interventions and to ensure the appropriate care plans are transferred to the community setting on discharge. Care is delivered and co-ordinated via a person-centred, Care Programme Approach (CPA) (Department of Health (DoH), 1999a; DoH 1999b) to help ensure effective links with the full range of psychiatric health and social care services. The CPA consists of single assessment and treatment processes, risk assessments, care planning and reviews, crises and contingency plans. The current debate is the threshold of mental health need before patients benefit from CPA, particularly where one presents with behavioural problems with no identified underlying psychiatric illness (Roy, 2000). In the MHiLD Service, those patients that are admitted to the specialist unit, in contrast to those admitted to a generic inpatient unit, showed a significant decrease in psychiatric symptoms, an increase in overall level of functioning, a reduction in severity of their mental health problems, and an improvement in behavioural function on discharge, at six and 12 months following discharge (Xenitidis *et al.*, 2004). Longer-term follow up data are awaited.

Alexander *et al.* (2001) describe two models of community and inpatient services in two London districts, both with well-developed community ID teams and consultant psychiatrists in ID who had been in their post for more than ten years. One district used designated beds in a general psychiatric unit for the assessment and treatment of patients with borderline, mild and moderate ID, and referred those with more severe disabilities to a supra-district tertiary care facility. The other had a purpose-built unit, which catered for persons with all levels of disability, although access to a supra-district facility was also available. During the three-year study period, residential status at the time of the admission was the only predictor of length of admission, with those from residential homes tending to stay longer. The authors found that a purpose-built facility allowed for admission of persons with severe and profound disabilities, as well as those with autistic spectrum disorder when compared to the use of beds in a general psychiatric unit.

Southeast London's Mental Impairment Evaluation and Treatment Service (MIETS) is a 13-bedded inpatient unit at the Bethlem Royal Hospital in Kent. As a tertiary service, it takes referrals from outside its immediate locality. It offers a multidisciplinary assessment and treatment service for people with mild to moderate ID and severe challenging behaviours (Xenitidis *et al.*, 1999; Murphy *et al.*, 1991; Murphy & Clare, 1991), with its main outcome measure being a return to a community placement. However, this outcome appeared to be a reflection of the willingness of local communities and local services to accept people with severe challenging behaviours back into their communities. The MIETS found the only characteristic that differed significantly between good and poor outcome groups was fire-setting behaviour. At the time of writing, there was no data available regarding the length of time people remained in their community placement after discharge.

Chaplin (2004) found no conclusive evidence to favour the use of general or specialist inpatient units. Whilst acknowledging the limitations of the review, he nevertheless points to a number of clear clinical implications and calls for studies in community general psychiatry to report the outcomes of persons with ID in separate analyses from those without ID.

Assertive community treatment (ACT) is a service model developed in the USA in an attempt to avoid fragmentation in service delivery for persons with severe and persistent mental illness and little community support. Although its efficacy in the UK remains debatable, its existence is now an integral part of mainstream mental health services. However, in a chance finding, Hassiotis and colleagues (2001) found that a subset (20%) of those included in the UK 700 Study, with borderline intellectual functioning, appeared to benefit significantly from intensive case management. Martin and colleagues (2005) have attempted to compare the effectiveness of ACT in ID (ACT-ID) with standard community treatments, but failed to find any significant difference. However, this preliminary finding may have more to do with similarities between ACT and the well-developed community services recruited into the study rather than being a comment on the model itself. A randomized controlled trial by Oliver and colleagues (2005) has also encountered similar difficulties.

Other European models

Few models outside of the progressive efforts in the UK have been reported. Holt and colleagues (2000) reported the results of the BIOMED-MEROPE project, designed to review, describe and evaluate service models in five European countries, including Greece, Ireland, England, Spain and Austria. As would be predicted by the matrix model described earlier, each country's unique historical perspective and national philosophies about care for people with ID drive different service models. In general, community-based services began to appear as deinstitutionalization proceeded, with an increased reliance on family, voluntary and private organizations to provide for long-term care. Where emphasis has been on treatment in the community, there is a growing recognition of the need for additional specialist services as well as help to access services (Costello *et al.*, 2001). The review concluded that legislation and policy in the five countries tended to separate ID and mental health, resulting in unmet needs remaining largely invisible, to the detriment of people with ID and mental health problems, their families and carers. Similarly, Weinbach (2004) published a condensed overview of service profiles across Europe (including Belgium, England, Germany, Greece, Spain, Sweden and the Netherlands) in an attempt to describe the systems of care and support available for people with ID. These two examples of cross-national comparisons is a fundamental step towards identifying common service dimensions and developing common methods and models for comparing and evaluating health programmes.

Raitasuo and colleagues (1999) describe a 5-bedded specialist psychiatric inpatient facility in southwest Finland, covering a catchment area of 435 000 with 1878 persons with ID. Admission was seen as 'the last resort'. Therapy meetings (sessions between the patient, primary carers and the multiprofessional team from the specialist unit) were an essential component of their treatment approach. This helped improve understanding of the person's situation, the assessment process and follow-up treatment. It enabled a psycho-educative approach for primary carers, particularly where there were persistent and long-term psychiatric symptoms. The service was found to fill the gap that existed in the Finnish psychiatric care system, but the authors imply there is little consideration given to what services are necessary for persons with ID and mental health problems.

In contrast, van Minnen and colleagues (1997) found that outreach treatment represented an effective and efficient alternative to hospital treatment in the Netherlands, and on the basis of their small controlled study, the Dutch Government is reported to be supporting a policy of non-hospitalization and financing outreach treatment for persons with mild or borderline ID and severe psychiatric problems.

Models from outside the European community

Australia

The *Queensland Model* began with conducting a survey on the nature and distribution of disruptive behaviour among the registered clients of the Developmental Disability Services, which is the state agency for people with ID in Queensland (Attwood & Joachin, 1994). The survey identified a range of factors that included overcrowding, lack of privacy, frustration stemming from poor communication skills, lack of stimulation, lack of attention and affection, poor interpersonal skills, institutionalization effects, and behaviours related to specific conditions.

A small working party was formed to provide recommendations on the prevention and management of seriously disruptive incidents. The recommendations were training programmes for all staff; including protective actions to minimize injuries to staff, administrative review after each seriously disruptive incident, and strategies to reduce the risk of a similar incident occurring again. Owing to the fact that staff and services span over 200 km, a train-the-trainer approach was adopted.

The Victorian Dual Disability Service (VDDS)

The VDDS is a publicly funded state initiative, managed through the department of psychiatry at St Vincent's Hospital in Melbourne (Bennett, 2000). Like the southeast London model, the service offered is secondary consultation around specific patients, and the development of training and education programmes. However, there are no inpatient facilities and limited capacity for direct clinical management of patients. The service consists of four senior clinicians (from psychology and psychiatric nursing) as well as a full-time consultant psychiatrist, a psychiatric trainee, a clinician/manager and an administrative officer. Each of the four senior clinicians took on the main liaison worker role for five to six Area Mental Health Services (AMHS), of the 21 AMHS in Victoria. Unfortunately, each AMHS was unable to reciprocate in kind.

In its first year, VDDS received 217 referrals – 66% from AMHS, 16% from disability services and the remaining 20% for a variety of other sources. Many referrals were dealt with by phone: immediate advice and guidance, redirection to other agencies or inappropriateness of referral were recorded as outcomes of these telephone-based secondary consultations. All were reviewed in a multidisciplinary team meeting the next day, providing peer review, supervision and ensuring consistency of service delivery. In total, 94 were seen for assessment, often in conjunction with an AMHS. As the VDDS was unable to undertake primary treatment, this joint approach allowed for a transfer of skills and a dialogue about differences of opinion. Assessments were carried out over up to three visits, and recommendations made. These were followed up in the form of a case conference or video link, but VDDS found that differences in opinion and lack of resources or skills meant that many recommendations were not acted upon. Major disagreement about service roles among the different agencies involved also meant that these could not be addressed through video conferencing, as was initially planned. This model is not a simple programme of intervention provided directly to a patient but a set of refinements to an already complex service system. Often the referral is complex too, involving clarification of diagnosis, working with severe communication deficits, complex medical issues and self-harming or aggressive behaviours outside the range of those found in an average AMHS caseload. As in other countries, there is debate about who should manage patients with autistic features, particularly when their IQ scores mean they are ineligible for acceptance by disability services.

The provision of training (skills provision) and education (raising knowledge and awareness) are core functions of the service and and are linked into AMHS, the Disability Services Branch and university courses. The VDDS also has a statewide role and is well placed to guide policy development and service initiatives to address the issues that impede the needs of this population being met.

North American models

The Greater Boston START model

The START model was rooted in the philosophy that no one specific diagnosis or treatment modality will work with all clients (Beasley *et al.*, 1992). The acronym START stands for *Systemic, Therapeutic, Assessment, Respite and Treatment*. It was developed as a crisis intervention and prevention service funded by the Massachusetts Department of Mental Retardation in the northern region of Greater Boston. The programme provided emergency assessments and respite care for people with ID who evidenced acute behavioural and emotional experiences. Staffing for the clinical team included a part-time psychiatrist, three full-time masters-degree clinicians, and six full-time bachelor-degree clinicians. Doctoral-degree psychology consultants and licensed social workers were available to provide consultation regarding their field such as behavioural psychology, neuropsychology, and family advocacy.

Each referral received a comprehensive clinical assessment, achieved via the crisis team members collecting the historical information from and then working with community caregivers to collect the necessary behavioural data. Ideally the crisis team served as a facilitator for the diagnostic process by co-ordinating data collection and networking with clinicians involved in the case. The team was also available to co-ordinate outpatient services. Respite was available to referrals and served several functions, including diffusing crises that stemmed from environmental stressors; stabilizing a client who was too disturbed to remain at home; and help in the transition from inpatient settings to the community. Inpatient mental health services, including discharge planning, were facilitated by the crisis team members. Additional services provided by the crisis team included educating community care providers and clinicians regarding mental health needs of persons with ID. Workshops and trainings on various topics such as psychiatric diagnosis, positive behaviour programming, and psychotropic drug therapy were provided.

The Massachusetts experience (Mikkelsen, 2001) involved discrete programmes of care, which, though not specifically linked to one another, provide an overall continuum of psychiatric services, which could be accessed by clinicians, families and individuals. These consisted of:

- Specialized outpatient services – and the establishment of a higher reimbursement rate for 'complex' psychiatric outpatient visits, which allowed for the complex nature of presentation, the time spent and the need to communicate with multiple service providers including residential staff, day programme staff, case managers and family members.
- Partial hospitalization (Shedlack, 2001) – an inpatient setting which allowed for skilled observation and gradual evaluations of psychopharmacological

interventions and behaviour therapies over a more extensive time frame, coupled with nights and weekends at the patient's own community residence.

- Inpatient psychiatric hospitalization (Charlot *et al.*, 2001) – consisting of three separate units, each with a specific subspecialty capability, one located within a major university teaching hospital thus making it possible to carry out sophisticated assessment of comorbid and /or contributory medical problems.

The Toronto MATCH project

The Metro Agencies Representatures' Council (MARC) in Toronto implemented the Continuum of Service for persons with dual diagnosis, also known as the MATCH programme (Puddephatt & Sussman, 1994). The acronym MATCH stands for the Metro Agencies Treatment Continuum for Health, and MARC is an association of over 40 agencies in the Metro Toronto area with commitments to providing services for persons with ID. This model for providing services for persons with ID and mental health problems began as a pilot project. The project was funded jointly through the Ministry of Community and Social Services and the Ministry of Health. It was designed specifically to serve the needs of this dually diagnosed population. Assessment and treatment planning is a main focus for this programme. Services are provided across a continuum, covering: prevention/early intervention in the form of education and training; assessment and treatment planning provided in inpatient, outpatient and crisis response settings; crisis intervention to secure containment and for stabilization; treatment in community-based outpatient settings, day treatment programmes, specialized residential treatment and inpatient psychiatric care; long-term care and support via high levels of support to residential community-living settings, appropriate day treatment and vocational programmes, family support networks, and respite services for parents.

The Rochester crisis intervention model

The model developed in Rochester, New York emerged through a series of planning stages, including a formal needs assessment, a survey of existing resources and a community-based consensus planning conference (Davidson *et al.*, 1995). The model was implemented based on the recommendations developed at the consensus planning conference. Services offered through the Rochester model included: an inter-disciplinary crisis intervention team, acute inpatient psychiatric services, outpatient services provided through a specialized Mental Retardation/Developmental Disabilities Psychiatric clinic, specialized residential services, family support services including residential respite, prevention services providing staff education and training, and family-centred case management.

Funding for the crisis intervention component of this programme came from annual grants from the New York State Office of Mental Retardation and Developmental Disabilities (OMRDD). The programme was a joint effort between the University of Rochester Medical Center and OMRDD's local district office. The treatment team consisted of a programme director, two behaviour modification specialists, a part-time licensed psychologist and a part-time consulting psychiatrist. Persons eligible for services were individuals with ID living with families or living in community-based supervised or independent living situations in the Monroe County Area of New York. There was no fee for service. Services were also accessed by agencies providing services for these individuals such as schools, sheltered workshops, day treatment programmes, supported work programmes and supported living programmes.

Crisis intervention services were available on a 24-hour per day basis for acute behavioural crises. Specific services available from the crisis team covered a continuum of services including: service co-ordination; participation in inpatient treatment and discharge planning; follow-up consultation to ID service agencies and families; identification of at-risk consumers; in-home counselling to families of at risk individuals; consultation to community agencies serving at-risk individuals; and staff training for all involved parties.

The Young Adult Institute HMO model

The Young Adult Institute is a private voluntary agency providing residential and day programmes to people with ID in the New York metropolitan area. It is one of the largest non-governmental community agencies in the United States. Its community-based health maintenance organization (HMO) is one of the few examples of a community-wide specialized HMO in the nation. Levy (2001) summarized the HMO's comprehensive mental health service programme, which resembles a community mental health centre. However, its funding derives from third-party payers under ID insurance mechanisms. Unlike the southeast London project, it does not have its own inpatient unit. Its success in serving individuals with ID and mental health problems probably accrues to its accessibility, large customer base, and availability and access to other well-established generic community mental health services unique to large cities like New York City. Although Levy and Levy did not report a programme evaluation, we mention this project because of its sheer size and applicability to other large metropolitan areas.

The Minnesota model crisis intervention program

Rudolph and colleagues (1998) described a community behavioural support and crisis response demonstration project based in a suburb of Minneapolis and which serves five counties in western Minneapolis. This programme provides outreach services in the individual's normal environment. The second part of the programme is to provide short-term crisis placement in a specialized unit. These services are provided through a multidisciplinary approach to the assessment and intervention strategies. Rudolph and colleagues reported that, much like the southeast London and the Rochester projects, the Minnesota project reduced loss of placements and psychiatric hospitalizations, and saved resources, making it cost effective.

The Ulster County comprehensive mental health model

Community agencies working with individuals with ID in Ulster County, New York, worked in conjunction with Ulster County Mental Health Services to develop a multi-year, comprehensive plan to address the needs of the dually diagnosed population, which began with a comprehensive needs assessment (Landsberg *et al.*, 1987). The model for services included a continuum of residential facilities from supervised living programmes to independent living situations, comprehensive mental health outpatient services from diagnosis to day treatment, occupational and vocational treatment and experience (sheltered employment, placement, vocational testing), access to short- and long-term inpatient psychiatric care, training and education for staff of mental health and ID agencies, and a mechanism to co-ordinate and guide programme development.

For a continuum of residential facilities to be available in Ulster County, there was a need to create more specialized residential beds. In order to reach this goal, ten beds were set aside in existing community residences for those with ID and mental health problems and a 14-bed specialized facility was developed. To increase mental health clinical services, the county mental health outpatient programme was asked to seek additional staffing to increase outpatient services and to provide services at work sites. In addition to these other steps, the establishment of a specialized day treatment programme was needed. Specifically, a 40-client day treatment facility with the county mental health centre providing specialized care and consultation was suggested.

The Interface model

Interface, the name for the collaborative undertaking of the Hamilton County Community Mental Health Board and the University Affiliated Cincinnati Center for Developmental Disorders, set forth to develop multi-system services for individuals with ID and mental health problems (Woodward, 1993). This joint effort was funded by the Hamilton County Community Mental Health Board and administered by the University Affiliated Cincinnati Center for Developmental Disorders. This arrangement removed the focus of responsibility away from both the mental health board and the mental retardation/intellectual disabilities office. Community service committees were convened to develop and implement individual

service plans, obtain needed mental health and ID services, maintain networking and team characteristics, and gather data. Mental health and ID professionals
worked together on the committees.

Three outcomes resulted: there was an increase in community mental health
services; a mental health intermediate care facility/ID community residential setting
was built and run collaboratively by county mental health and ID boards; a multi-
system community and inpatient crisis intervention system was developed. The
crisis intervention system consisted of three behaviour management specialists
with expertise in ID and with services available seven days a week. This community
mobile crisis team had links to outpatient psychiatric emergency services, inpatient
psychiatric wards, and hospitalization discharge follow-up.

The Eastern Virginia Mental Retardation and Emotional Disturbance Project

Eastern State Hospital, the southeastern Virginia Training Center, the Community Services Division of the Virginia Department of Mental Health and Mental
Retardation, and nine community services boards in eastern Virginia began discussions around the Mental Retardation and Emotional Disturbance (MR/ED) Project
(Parkhurst, 1984). They identified the following objectives: develop a survey to the
MR/ED population in the area who have sought, but not received services; conduct
a region-wide needs assessment; survey existing service components that could
be expanded; survey programmes for the dually diagnosed nationwide and assess
applicability; develop a service system to co-ordinate services at the community and
institutional levels, accessible for both rural and urban populations; estimate costs,
personnel requirements, location, and potential funding sources; develop legislative
and policy recommendations for delivery of services to MR/ED population; and
gather data and service information to develop the public education and prevention
component.

Outcomes consisted of recommendations for crisis centres accessible throughout
eastern Virginia for persons with ID and mental health problems, special staff training for the treatment of mental health in ID, and to address the lack of community
living arrangements by developing community-based residences.

The Rock Creek model

This comprehensive community support system was developed over a decade ago
by the Rock Creek Foundation (RCF) in the Metropolitan Washington, DC area
(Smull *et al.*, 1994). They endorsed the developmental model and view mental health
problems as conditions separate and distinct from ID. They valued the recognition
of basic human worth and dignity and endorsed normalization.

Services involve many different components. Psychotherapeutic services
include medication evaluation, individual, group, family, and behaviour therapy;

psychiatric and psychological evaluations; and expressive arts therapies. Day treatment programmes had both psychiatric and behavioural programming. Outpatient psychotherapeutic services and 24-hour crisis services were available. Social survival services included life skills training in money, time, communication and public transportation training. Vocational services included both prevocational and vocational development. Psychosocial rehabilitation programmes existed for those who still needed structure but do not need intensive day treatment. Residential services had the capacity to programme for maladaptive behaviour within the residential setting.

Programming began in a treatment habilitation and planning process where the consumer was viewed within the context of the environment and service system. Programmes were adapted to individual consumer needs. The surrounding community worked with the treatment team to develop strategies for integration. The consumer gave meaningful input into their plan to the degree feasible. Variable and creative funding sources were obtained in order to enable the programme to develop in response to the individual consumer needs.

The Eastern Region Diversion and Support Program

The Eastern Region Diversion and Support Program was a collaborative effort among the State of North Carolina Department of Human Resources, 13 area mental health programmes, and the Department of Psychiatric Medicine at East Carolina University (Antonacci *et al.*, 1996). This programme embraced a person-centred approach to treatment. Services strived to be flexible, accessible, mobile and integrated. It served a predominately rural area where interagency collaboration is essential.

Services included inter-disciplinary team intervention. The team consisted of a full-time psychiatrist, a clinical social worker, a psychologist and a behaviour specialist. They provided support to existing community systems via comprehensive integrated assessments and recommendations. Crisis stabilization was provided and co-ordinated. The crisis was defined through functional assessment. The individual was advocated for and support was provided to the systems involved. The team was not administratively tied to any one system in the region.

Inpatient psychiatric services were accessed in the community where the individual lived. The team was available for consultation and training for any hospital in North Carolina that provided treatment for persons with ID and mental illness. A specialized psychiatric inpatient unit was established via a collaborative effort between the Department of Psychiatric Medicine at the Eastern Carolina University and the University Medical Center of Eastern Carolina Pitt County. The inpatient unit was staffed by a separate team from the consultation team.

Ongoing training and education was provided to persons who provide services for individuals with ID and mental health problems. Training and education was approached through providing general education around specific cases or by providing broader-based educational inservice training and workshops.

The ENCOR programme

The Eastern Nebraska Community Office of Retardation in Omaha, Nebraska demonstrated that it is both possible and cost-beneficial to serve individuals with ID and mental illness in their home communities (Menolascino, 1994). The programme developed over two decades and included community involvement and citizen advocacy in designing it. They were prepared to serve all individuals regardless of level of ID. The specialized clinical staff also provided direct teaching to care givers. The programme made use of existing community services, including family support services, and integrated job placements, which had been encouraged through liaison with local industries.

A Developmental Maximation Home for individuals with more severe and multiple disabilities existed at one end of the continuum of services (Menolascino, 1989). Other services included integrated pre school services, in-home teachers, crisis assistance programmes, specialized group homes, alternative living units, and work stations in industry.

ENCOR's consumers were grouped into three different levels of involvement. Level I included persons who present daily behavioural management problems; individuals classified as Level II displayed occasional behavioural problems; and those at Level III had only infrequent behavioural problems. This classification by levels as opposed to specific diagnoses allowed for accurate assessment of the type of personnel, supports and back-up services required to provide appropriate services for the individual.

ENCOR was governed at the community level by five elected county commissioners providing a direct link to parents, neighbours, employers, and the public at large. There was also a well organized and active parent advisory committee. The managerial system had public accountability; this facilitated constant improvements in service models, quality of care and opportunities for integration.

The Fairbanks, Alaska programme

A pilot project was begun within the Fairbanks community utilizing the existing primary mental health agency (Rambow & Arnold, 1996). A partnership between mental health and ID service providers was the goal of this project. By utilizing the existing agency in the community the pilot project was provided with cost effective administrative support and clinical supervision. A collaboration with integrated psychiatric care to prescribe and monitor any needed psychotropic medications was provided as well. A commitment was made to serve all persons with ID and mental health needs. Services were systematically designed to meet the individual needs of the client. Having a single/central comprehensive service plan outlining all of the services needed for a given individual was emphasized, and safeguarded against duplication of service. The model supported prevention and early intervention strategies.

Funding sources were combined from both the mental health and the ID budgets. Consumer needs were met via an inter-disciplinary team, which was selected by the consumer. The individual was directly involved in designing their services. In this model, the role of the clinician was expanded to include advocacy, service co-ordination, staff training, community relations, and consultation. The clinician had the ability to offer long-term individual therapy rather than being limited to brief therapy or group models. Therapy was provided in community settings such as the consumers' homes, the local mental health centre, or in other providers' agencies. The continuum of services and supports that an individual received was often co-ordinated by a case manager working in another agency.

Conclusion

We have reviewed a number of innovative model programmes that have been developed to meet the needs of people with ID and mental health problems. These have included a range of community and inpatient services, using both generic and local specialist facilities, and a variety of cross-agency partnerships. It is clear that the reported prevalence of mental health problems in persons with ID would suggest that as institutional closures progress, such programmes will be necessary in all communities where people with ID will reside. The alternative may be numerous failures of community integration caused by lack of appropriate treatment and supports.

The models we reviewed all fall short of achieving the idealized hypothetical mental health programme. Problems and solutions are often contextual and dependent on local resources as well as service histories and policies. At the same time, there has never been a test of a hypothetical model community-based service addressing the complex needs presented by persons with ID and mental health problems. Of those models we reported, very few data were available measuring their impact on service users, families, carers and service systems. The field would profit from more research evaluating the different service models in operation; their aims, structures, processes, interfaces, interventions and outcomes.

We are aware of numerous local efforts to establish and operate community-based programmes for people with ID and mental health problems for which no literature exists. There is a need to disseminate such experiences and efforts, as many of the obstacles to service/programme design and delivery are shared across countries.

Finally, the field will advance if and only if we undertake comparative studies that evaluate, side by side, the effectiveness of inter-disciplinary, integrated community models and traditional mental health alternatives. It is on the basis of such comparisons that the rationale for change will be identified.

Summary points

- The mental health needs of people with ID are inadequately met by mainstream mental health services.
- A range of community and inpatient services has developed in response to these perceived inadequacies.
- The level of development of specialist mental health services for people with ID varies considerably within and between countries.
- All the models reviewed in this chapter fall short of the idealized model.
- Research in this field is urgently needed to provide the evidence base to develop and maintain effective mental health services for people with ID.
- Such research will need to address comparisons with the proliferation of mainstream community mental health services for the general population.
- In line with ordinary life principles and the normalization philosophy, services exist to complement and support mainstream services, whilst at the same time having the capacity to offer a full range of specialist services to those with the most complex needs.
- The interfaces and refinements that are required on top of an already complex health and social care system means it is not a simple case of delivering a package of care directly to an individual.
- Training and educational packages need to be developed and delivered in such a way as to address the prevailing cultures, attitudes and practices which impede the development and delivery of effective services.
- Specialist services have a vital role in providing the evidence which shapes and develops the policy agenda, both locally and at a higher level.

Acknowledgments

P. W. Davidson's *preparation of this paper was supported by a University Center for Excellence in Developmental Disabilities (UCEDD) Core grant to the University of Rochester from the US Administration on Developmental Disabilities.*

REFERENCES

Alexander, R. T., Piachaud, J. & Singh, I. (2001). Two districts, two models: inpatient care in the psychiatry of learning disability. *British Journal of Developmental Disability*, **47**:1, No. 93. 105–10.

Allen, D. (1998). Changes in admissions to a hospital for people with intellectual disability following development of alternative community services: a brief report. *Journal of Applied Research in Intellectual Disabilities*. **11**: No. 2. 155–65.

Antonacci, D. J., Hurley, G., Johnson, G., Rota, J. & White, S. (1996). Crisis prevention and community support for individuals who are dually diagnosed: a model program for open systems consultation. In R. Friedlander & D. Sobsey (eds.), *Conference Proceedings of the National Association for the Dually Diagnosed – Through the Lifespan*, November 13–16, Kingston, NY: The National Association for the Dually Diagnosed.

Attwood, T. & Joachin, R. (1994). The prevention and management of seriously disruptive behavior in Australia. In N. Bouras (ed.), *Mental Health in Mental Retardation: Recent Advances and Practices*, Cambridge: Cambridge University Press.

Beasley, J., Kroll, J. & Sovner, R. (1992). Community-based crisis mental health services for persons with developmental disabilities: The S. T. A. R.T model. *The Habilitative Mental Healthcare Newsletter*, **11**(9), 55–7.

Bennett, C. (2000). The Victorian Dual Disability Service. *Australasian Psychiatry*. **8**(3), 238–43.

Borthwick, S. (1988). Maladaptive behavior among the mentally retarded: The need for reliable data. In J. Stark, F. Menolascino, M. Albarelli & V. Gray (eds.), *Mental Retardation and Mental Health: Classification, Diagnosis, Treatment Services*. New York: Springer-Verlag, pp. 30–40.

Bouras, N. & Drummond, C. (1989). Community psychiatric service in mental handicap. *Health Trend*, **21**, 72.

Bouras, N. & Drummond, C. (1990). Diagnostic and treatment issues for adults in community care. In A. Dosen, A. Van Gennep & G. Zwanikken (eds.), *Treatment of Mental Illness and Behavior Disorder in the Mentally Retarded*. Proceedings of the International Congress, May 3–4. Amsterdam: Logon Publications.

Bouras, N., Cowley, A, Holt, G., Newton, T. J. & Sturmey, P. (2003). Referral trends of people with intellectual disabilities and psychiatric disorders. *Journal of Intellectual Disability Research*, **47**, 439–46.

Bouras, H. and Holt, G. (2001). Psychiatric treatment in community care. In *Treating Mental Illness and Behaviour Disorders in Children and Adults with Mental Retardation*, Dosen, A. and Day, K. (eds), pp. 493–502. Washington, DC: American Psychiatric Press.

Bouras, N. and Holt, G. (2004). Mental health services for adults with learning disabilities *(editorial) British Journal of Psychiatry* **184**:291–92.

Bouras, N., Kon, Y. & Drummond, C. (1993). Medical and psychiatric needs of adults with a mental handicap. *Journal of Intellectual Disability Research*, **37**, 177–82.

Bruininks, R. Hill, B. & Morreau, L. (1988). Prevalence and implications of maladaptive behaviors and dual diagnosis in residential and other service programmes. In J. Stark, F. Menolascino,

M. Albarelli & V. Gray (eds.), *Mental Retardation and Mental Health: Classification, Diagnosis, Treatment Services*. New York: Springer-Verlag, pp. 3–29.

Bruininks, R., Rotegard, L., Lakin, K. & Hill, B. (1987). Epidemiology of mental retardation and trends in residential services in the United States. In S. Landesman & P. Veitze (eds.), *Living Environments and Mental Retardation*. Washington, DC: American Association on Mental Retardation, pp. 17–42.

Chaplin, R. (2004). General psychiatric services for adults with intellectual disability and mental illness: a review. *Journal of Intellectual Disability Research*, **48**(1), 1–10.

Charlot, L., Silka, V. R. and Bonney-Kuropatkin, B. (2001). A short-stay inpatient psychiatric unit for adults with developmental disabilities: one year's experience. In *Proceedings of the National Association for the Dually Diagnosed International Congress IV*, pp. 68–74. Kingston, NT: National Association for the Dually Diagnosed Press.

Costello, H., Bouras, N. and Holt, G. (2001). Dual diagnosis services in five European countries. *Tizard Learning Disability Review*, European Issue. 11–16.

Crawford, J., Aiello, J. & Thompson, D. (1979). Deinstitutionalization and community placement: Clinical and environmental factors. *Mental Retardation*, **17**, 59–63.

Davidson, P. W., Cain, N. N., Sloane-Reeves, J. E. *et al.* (1995). Crisis intervention for community-based individuals with developmental disabilities and behavioral and psychiatric disorders. *Mental Retardation*, **33**(1), 21–30.

Davidson, P., Peloquin, L. J., Salzman, L. *et al.* (1989). Planning and implementing comprehensive crisis intervention for people with developmental disabilities. In J. Levy, P. Levy & B. Nivis (eds.), *Strengthening Families: New Directions in Providing Services to People with Developmental Disabilities and Their Families*. New York: YAI Press, pp. 203–10.

Davidson, P. W., Prasher, V. and Janicki, M. P. (2003). Introduction. In P. W. Davidson, V. Prasher & M. P. Janicki (eds.), *Mental Health, Intellectual Disabilities, and the Aging Process*. Oxford: Blackwell Science, pp. 1–6.

Department of Health (1999a). National Service Framework for Mental Health: Modern Standards and Srvice Models for Mental Health. London: HSC 1999/223 HMSO.

Department of Health (1999b). Effective Care Co-ordination in Mental Health Services: modernizing the CPA. London: DoH.

Department of Health (1999c). Facing the facts – services for people with learning disabilities. A policy impact study of social case and health services. London: HMSO.

Department of Health (2001). Valuing People: A New Strategy for Learning Disabilities in the 21st Century. London: HMSO.

Geller, L. L. & Pomeroy, J. C. (2003). Community education and prevention strategies. In P. W. Davidson, V. Prasher & M. P. Janicki (eds.), *Mental Health, Intellectual Disabilities, and the Aging Process*. Oxford: Blackwell Science, pp. 214–22.

Hassiotis, A., Barron, P. and O'Hara, J. (2000). Mental health services for people with learning disabilities (editorial). *British Journal of Medicine*, **321**, 583–4.

Hassiotis, A., Ukoumunne, O. C., Byford, S. *et al.* (2001). Intellectual functioning and outcome of patients with severe psychotic illness randomized to intensive case management: report from the UK 700 case management trial. *British Journal of Psychiatry*, **178**, 166–71.

Hill, B. & Bruininks, R. (1984). Maladaptive behavior of mentally retarded people in residential facilities. *American Journal of Mental Deficiency*, **88**, 380–7.

Holland, A. J. (2003). Assessment of behavioral and psychiatric disorders. In P. W. Davidson, V. Prasher & M. P. Janicki (eds.), *Mental Health, Intellectual Disabilities, and the Aging Process.* Oxford: Blackwell Science, pp. 38–50.

Holt, G., Costello, H., Bouras, N. *et al.* (2000). BIOMED-MEROPE project: service provision for adults with intellectual disability: a European comparison. *Journal of Intellectual Disability Research,* **44**(6), 685–96.

Jacobson, J. (2003). Prevalence of mental and behavioral disorders. In P. W. Davidson, V. Prasher and M. P. Janicki (eds.), *Mental Health, Intellectual Disabilities, and the Aging Process.* Oxford: Blackwell Science, pp. 9–21.

Janicki, M. P., Davidson, P. W., Henderson, C. M. *et al.* (2002). Health characteristics and health services utilization in older adults with intellectual disabilities living in community residences. *Journal of Intellectual Disability Research,* **46**, 287–98.

Kerker, B. D., Owens, P. L., Zigler, E. & Horwitz, S. M. (2004). Mental health disorders among individuals with mental retardation: challenges to accurate prevalence estimates. *Public Health Reports,* **119**, 409–17.

Landsberg, G., Fletcher, F. & Maxwell, T. (1987). Developing a comprehensive community care system for the mentally ill/mentally retarded. *Community Mental Health Journal,* **23**(2) 137–42.

Levy, P. (2001). Meeting the Mental Health Needs of People with Mental Retardation and Developmental Disabilities. Paper presented at the Annual Meetings of the American Psychological Association, San Francisco, California, August 23–27.

Marcos, L., Gil, R. & Vasquez, K. (1986). Who will treat psychiatrically disturbed developmentally disabled patients? A health care nightmare. *Hospital and Community Psychiatry,* **37**(2), 171–4.

Martin, G., Costello, H., Leese, M. *et al.* (2005). An exploratory study of assertive community treatment for people with intellectual disability and psychiatric disorders: conceptual, clinical and service issues. *Journal of Intellectual Disability Research,* **49**, 516–24.

Menolascino, F. (1989). Model services for treatment/management of the mentally retarded-mentally ill. *Community Mental Health Journal,* **25**(2), 145–55.

Menolascino, F. J. (1994). Services for people with dual diagnosis in the USA. In N. Bouras (ed.), *Mental Health in Mental Retardation Recent Advances and Practices,* Cambridge: Cambridge University Press.

Mikkelsen, E. J. (2001). Creating a continuum of intensive psychiatric services for individuals with dual diagnosis: a perspective on the Massachusetts experience. *The National Association for the Dually Diagnosed Bulletin,* Jan/Feb 4: **1**, 3–4.

Moss, S., Bouras, N. & Holt, G. (2000). Mental health services for people with intellectual disability: a conceptual framework. *Journal of Intellectual Disability Research* **44**, 97–107.

Moss, S., Emerson, E., Bouras, N. & Holland, A. (1997). Mental disorders and problematic behaviours in people with intellectual disability: future directions for research. *Journal of Intellectual Disability Research,* **41**(6), 440–7.

Murphy, G. and Clare, I. (1991). 1. MIETS: a service option for people with mild mental handicaps and challenging behaviour or psychiatric problems. 2. Assessment, treatment, and outcome for service users and service effectiveness. *Mental Handicap Research,* **4**: 180–206.

Murphy, G., Holland, A., Fowler, P. & Reep, U. (1991). MIETS: a service option for people with mild mental handicaps and challenging behaviour or psychiatric problems.1: Philosophy, service and service users. *Mental Handicap Research*, **4**, 41–66.

NIMHE (2004). Green Light: How Good are your Mental Health Services for People with Learning Disabilities? A Service Improvement Toolkit. National Institute for Mental Health (NIMHE) (England), UK.

Oliver, P. C., Piachaud, J., Tyrer, P. *et al.* (2005). Randomised controlled trial of assertive community treatment in intellectual disability: the TACTILD study. *Journal of Intellectual Disability Research*, **49**(7), 507–15.

Pagel, S. E. & Whitling, C. A. (1978). Readmissions to a state hospital for mentally retarded persons: Reasons for community placement failure. *Mental Retardation*, **16**, 164–6.

Parkhurst, R. (1984). Need assessment and service planning for mentally retarded-mentally ill persons. In F. J. Menolascino & J. A. Stark (eds.), *Handbook of Mental Illness in the Mentally Retarded*, New York: Plenum Press.

Puddephatt, A. & Sussman, S. (1994). Developing services in Canada: Ontario vignettes. In N. Bouras (ed.), *Mental Health in Mental Retardation: Recent Advances and Practices*. Cambridge: Cambridge University Press.

Raitasuo *et al.* (1999). Inpatient care and its outcome in a specialist psychiatric unit for people with intellectual disability: a prospective study. *Journal of Intellectual Disability Research*, **43**(2) 119–27.

Rambow, T. R. & Arnold, M. (1996). Individualized/homogenized/cost effective service model: 'It's time for a professional awakening'. National Association for the Dually Diagnosed Newsletter, **13**(6), 1–4.

Reiss, S. (1990). Prevalence of dual diagnosis in community-based day programs in the Chicago metropolitan area. *American Journal of Mental Retardation*, **94**(6), 578–85.

Reiss, S. (1994). *Handbook of Challenging Behaviors: Mental Health Aspects of Mental Retardation.* Worthington, OH: IDS Publishing Corporation.

Roy, A (2000). The Care Programme Approach in Learning Disability Psychiatry. *Advanced Psychiatric Treatment*, **6**, 380–7.

Rudolph, C., Lakin, K. C., Oslund, J. M. & Larson, W. (1998). Evaluation of outcomes and cost-effectiveness of a community behavioral support and crisis response demonstration project. *Mental Retardation*, **36**(6), 187–97.

Russell, A. T. & Tanguay, P. E. (1981). Mental illness and mental retardation: Cause or coincidence. *American Journal of Mental Deficiency*, **85**, 570–4.

Shalock, R. L. & Keith, K. D. (1993). *Quality of Life Questionnaire Manual.* Worthington, OH: IDS Publishing Corporation.

Shedlack, K. (2001). Creating a continuum of intensive psychiatric services for individuals with dual diagnosis: a perspective on the Massachusetts experience. II. Partial hospitalization. *The National Association for the Dually Diagnosed Bulletin*, Jan/Feb. **4**(1) 5–6.

Smull, M. W., Fabian, E. S. & Charteau, F. B. (1994). Value-based programming for the dually diagnosed: the Rock Creek model. In F. J. Menolascino & J. A. Stark (eds.), *Handbook of Mental Illness in the Mentally Retarded*, New York: Plenum Press.

Thornicroft, G. & Tansella, M. (1999). *The Mental Health Matrix: A Manual to Improve Services.* Cambridge: Cambridge University Press.

Tufnell, G., Bouras, N., Watson, J. & Brough, D. (1985). Home assessment and treatment in a community psychiatric service. *Acta Psychiatrica Scandianvia*, **72**, 20–8.

Van Minnen, A., Hoogduin, C. A. L. & Broekman, T. G. (1997). Hospital vs outreach treatment of patients with mental retardation and psychiatric disorders: a controlled study. *Acta Psychiatrica Scandinavica* **95**, 515–22.

Weinbach, H. (2004). Comparing Structure, Design and Organisation of Support of People with Learning Disabilities in Europe: The Work of the Intellectual Disability Research Network (IDRESNET). *Tizard Learning Disability Review*, **9**(1) 2–6.

Woodward, H. L. (1993). One community's response to the multi-system service needs of individuals with mental illness and developmental disabilities. *Community Mental Health Journal*, **29**(4), 347–59.

Xenitidis, K., Gratsa, A., Bouras, N. *et al.* (2004). Psychiatric inpatient care for adults with intellectual disabilities: generic or specialist units? *Journal of Intellectual Disability Research*, **48**, 11–18.

Xenitidis, K., Henry, J., Russell, A. J., Ward, A. & Murphy, D. G. M. (1999). An inpatient treatment model for adults with mild intellectual disability and challenging behaviour. *Journal of Intellectual Disability Research*, **43**(2), 128–34.

24

Staff supporting people with intellectual disabilities and mental health problems

Chris Hatton and Fiona Lobban

Introduction

Staff supporting people with intellectual disabilities (ID) constitute a significant workforce. Although precise statistics are unavailable, there were an estimated 83 000 staff in England working with people with ID in 1999 (Ward, 1999); estimates for the USA in 2000 were well over 600 000 support staff (Hewitt & Lakin, 2001). Given the relatively high proportion of people with ID who also experience mental health problems and the general lack of mental health services for people with ID in the UK and elsewhere (Bailey & Cooper, 1997; Bouras and Holt 2004), a significant proportion of staff will be supporting at least one person with ID and a mental health problem (Quigley *et al.*, 2001).

In many countries around the world, services supporting people with ID have shifted from predominantly state-run institutional services to community-based services provided by diverse agencies (Braddock *et al.*, 2001). This shift has led to a workforce characterized by:

- Large proportions of unqualified staff (75% estimated in England; Ward, 1999; 73% in the USA; Larson *et al.*, 1998).
- Support staff being predominantly young, inexperienced at supporting people with ID, female, and without dependants (Hatton *et al.*, 1999b; Larson *et al.*, 1998).
- High staff turnover and vacancy rates. In UK residential services, staff annual turnover rates have been estimated between 18% and 25%, with services reporting vacancy rates of 6%–10% (Ward, 1999). In the USA, staff annual turnover rates are much higher, particularly in independent sector services (e.g. 50%–75% independent sector versus 20%–25% state-run; Larson *et al.*, 2002), with correspondingly high vacancy rates (e.g. 12%; Larson *et al.*, 1998).

Psychiatric and Behavioural Disorders in Intellectual and Developmental Disabilities, ed. Nick Bouras and Geraldine Holt. Published by Cambridge University Press. © Cambridge University Press 2007.

- Low pay, particularly amongst unqualified staff working in independent sector services. For example, in the USA, staff in non-state service earned an average of $7.33 per hour compared with $9.49 per hour in state operated services (Polister *et al.*, 2003). There are no comparable figures available for the UK, although staff commonly report inadequate income (Hatton *et al.*, 1999b) (see also Chapters 22 by Cumella and 23 by Davidson & O'Hara).

Staff well-being

UK studies have consistently found high levels of distress amongst support staff working with people with ID: 30% or more of staff report clinically significant levels of general psychological distress (Hatton *et al.*, 1999a) compared with 18% of UK employed adults and 27% of UK health service staff (Borrill *et al.*, 1996). However, levels of staff distress vary considerably across services, suggesting that staff distress is not an inevitable feature of the support role (Hatton *et al.*, 1999a).

The research literature on specific work-related distress, conceptualized as burnout, is more encouraging. Burnout is typically defined as a state of physical, emotional and mental exhaustion that occurs when workers feel overburdened by the demands of long-term involvement in emotionally demanding situations. Burnout comprises three distinct elements: feelings of being exhausted emotionally; loss of feelings of accomplishment on the job; and negative, cynical and depersonalizing attitudes towards service users (Innstrand *et al.*, 2002; Maslach & Jackson, 1981).

A systematic review of 18 studies concluded that staff supporting people with ID reported lower levels of depersonalization, and similar levels of emotional exhaustion and personal accomplishment, than normative studies of staff in human services (Skirrow & Hatton, in press). Furthermore, more recent studies report lower levels of emotional exhaustion and depersonalization than older studies. Studies of staff in community mental health services report higher levels of staff distress and burnout compared with services for people with ID (Oliver & Kuipers, 1996; Prosser *et al.*, 1999; Wykes *et al.*, 1997), although levels of staff burnout in hospital-based services may be relatively low (Carson *et al.*, 1999).

What influences staff well-being and staff turnover?

Staff well-being can vary greatly across different services supporting people with ID and people with mental health problems. Although much of the relevant research literature is fragmented and uses very different theoretical assumptions and methods (Hatton *et al.*, 2004), a coherent picture is beginning to emerge of the different constellations of factors that influence staff distress/burnout, staff job satisfaction, and staff turnover/intended turnover.

Many studies have investigated factors potentially associated with staff distress/burnout, although few have used research designs that allow for causal inference or included a comprehensive range of variables to allow the exploration of mediator and moderator effects (Hastings, 2002; Hatton *et al.*, 2004; Skirrow & Hatton, in press). Factors commonly associated with staff distress/burnout are predominantly organizational (similar findings exist in mental health services, Oliver & Kuipers, 1996)), and include:

- Staff lacking qualifications and feeling that they require more training.
- Poor working conditions associated with a low-status job, such as long working hours, low pay, poor career prospects, and staff feeling unrewarded.
- Staff having a negative perception of the job and a lack of commitment to the organization.
- Poor support from colleagues, supervisors and managers.
- Staff feeling unclear about their role, and being subject to conflicting demands.
- Maladaptive staff coping strategies in response to people with ID, such as wishful thinking or disengagement.

Although job satisfaction has been less researched than staff distress, there is evidence that a consistent set of factors are associated with job satisfaction, particularly when the personal accomplishment dimension of burnout is considered as a job satisfaction measure (Hatton *et al.*, 1999a; Skirrow & Hatton, in press). It is worth noting that these factors involve spending more time with service users, within an organizational context that supports staff to engage in positive activities:

- Being in a role with more direct contact with service users, particularly when staff members report positive relationships with service users.
- Staff having positive perceptions of and commitment to their job.
- More positive and engaged staff coping strategies.
- Staff having more control over their job, being clear about what their job is and being subject to fewer conflicting demands.
- More support from colleagues, supervisors and managers.

Staff turnover/intended turnover in services for people with ID has been robustly associated with the following factors across several studies (Hall & Hall, 2002; Hatton *et al.*, 2001; Larson *et al.*, 1998), and reflects the broader literature concerning staff turnover in human services (Barak *et al.*, 2001). These factors focus on the characteristics of staff that make them more employable elsewhere and organizational factors that make alternative employment more attractive:

- Staff factors, notably younger age, better education and shorter tenure in the service.
- Working conditions, notably low income and increased alternative employment opportunities locally.

- Greater dissatisfaction with the job and the organization, a lack of commitment to the job and the organization, and greater job stress.
- A mismatch between the expectations and values of staff and those of the organization.
- Poor support from colleagues and poor management practices, including supervisory practices.

In summary, various characteristics of the staff member and their working conditions within the organization seem to be important determinants of staff well-being and turnover.

Staff working with people with ID and mental health problems will be subject to all these potential risk factors for poor staff well-being and high staff turnover, and may be at higher risk of experiencing some of the determinants of high staff distress and burnout. For example, staff supporting people with ID are unlikely to have received training in mental health issues as part of their training and report a need for further training in this area (Costello, 2004; Quigley *et al.*, 2001). Consequently, staff are likely to have poor knowledge and awareness of mental health issues in people with ID (Costello, 2004; Moss *et al.*, 1996), particularly in terms of the under-recognition of internalizing mental health problems (e.g. depression) compared to more visible and disruptive mental health problems such as psychotic behaviour (Edelstein & Glenwick, 1997, 2001). Such an under-recognition is likely to lead to the behaviour of people with ID and mental health problems being viewed negatively, or as unpredictable and possibly frightening to staff members, resulting in maladaptive staff coping strategies such as wishful thinking and disengagement and consequent staff distress and burnout.

When staff do have an awareness of mental health problems, it is likely that working with people with ID and mental health problems will create uncertainties, ambiguities and conflicting demands for staff, all associated with poorer staff well-being. Staff commonly report considerable uncertainty about appropriate ways of working with people with ID and mental health problems (Costello, 2004; Kon & Bouras, 1997), and can report negative attitudes towards the application of mental health interventions for people with ID (Christian *et al.*, 1999).

Effect of staff well-being on people with ID and mental health problems

Whilst staff well-being is an important issue in its own right, staffing issues have often been investigated with the assumption that aspects of staff well-being have direct and indirect effects on the lives of the people with ID using the service. However, very few studies have empirically demonstrated associations between staff well-being and staff behaviour in services for people with ID. These studies have consistently reported associations between poor staff morale (high distress, anxiety, depression or emotional exhaustion) and lower levels of positive interactions between staff and service users (Lawson & O'Brien, 1994; Rose *et al.*, 1994, 1998a). A lack of positive interactions is itself associated with negative aspects of service user lifestyle such as lower levels of positive engagement in constructive activities (Felce & Emerson, 2004).

Much more research attention has been paid to hypothesized mediators between staff well-being and staff behaviour. Within the ID field, these studies have largely used self-reported responses to vignettes rather than investigating actual staff behaviour. They have also focused on staff responses to active challenging behaviours rather than staff responses to mental health problems amongst people with ID, particularly internalizing mental health problems that may be less noticeable to staff (Hatton *et al.*, 2004).

Particular research attention has been devoted to staff attributions, or beliefs about the causes for a service user's behaviour. These use typical attributional dimensions such as whether the behaviour is caused by factors internal or external to the person, whether the behaviour occurs across a range of settings or only in particular settings (global vs. specific), whether the behaviour reliably occurs over time or not (stable vs. unstable), and whether the behaviour is seen as controllable by the person or not (controllable vs. uncontrollable) (Hatton *et al.*, 2004).

Extending an attributional approach, in theories such as Weiner's model of helping behaviour (Weiner, 1980), attributions determine emotional responses, which in turn determine the extent to which staff will offer help. In particular, if the service user is assumed to be in control of their challenging behaviour and the behaviour is stable over time, then staff will experience greater anger and less sympathy, resulting in rejection, avoidance or a punitive response. This model has generated a large literature concerning staff working with people with ID (Mossman *et al.*, 2002), which has often added additional hypothesized mediators such as optimism (e.g. Dagnan *et al.*, 1998; Stanley & Standen, 2000). Although studies have consistently reported associations between various components of Weiner's theory, support for the theory as a whole is weak. Furthermore, a recent study investigating associations between staff attributions, emotional responses and observed interactions with people with ID, reported associations in the opposite directions to those reported in vignette research (Bailey *et al.*, 2006).

Research within the mental health field has also focused on attributions as determinants of staff responses. This work has developed as a result of associations between attributional styles and high levels of Expressed Emotion (EE) in family carers. EE is a measure of the emotional response of the relative towards the individual experiencing mental health problems and is a reliable predictor of outcome in psychosis (Butzlaff & Hooley 1998). High EE can be characterized by high levels of hostility, criticism, or emotional over-involvement. Relatives with marked criticism and/or hostility make more attributions to factors personal to and controllable by the person with psychosis than other relatives (Brewin *et al.*, 1991) and make causal attributions that are more internal to and controllable by the person (Barrowclough *et al.*, 1994). Research with a range of paid staff in mental health services has generally reported low levels of staff EE, and an absence of emotional over-involvement (Barrowclough *et al.*, 2001a). However, high levels of critical comments have been associated with poorer outcomes for mental health service users in residential services (Ball *et al.*, 1992; Barrowclough *et al.*, 2001a; Snyder *et al.*, 1994) and amongst care managers (Tattan & Tarrier, 2000). Furthermore, staff criticism is associated with service users' perceptions of poor relationships with staff (Barrowclough *et al.*, 2001a; Van Humbeeck *et al.*, 2001), and also with staff attributions of service users' problems being internal, stable and under the service users' voluntary control (Barrowclough *et al.*, 2001a).

More comprehensive theories of interactions between cognitive appraisals, emotional responses and behaviour may be worth investigating when considering staff working with people with ID and mental health problems. For example, the self-regulation model has been applied to carers of people with mental health problems (Barrowclough *et al.*, 2001b; Lobban *et al.*, 2003). This model focuses on appraisals of a mental health problem, along the dimensions of *identity* (label and signs/symptoms), perceived *consequences* (physical, social and behavioural), likely *causes* of the problem, the potential for *control/cure* (personal and treatment) and a *timeline* (sense of how long the problem will last for). The model also contains an emotional representation arm in parallel with (rather than mediating) cognitive appraisals.

Such an integrative theoretical model may have considerable potential in understanding staff responses to people with ID and mental health problems. For example, staff are likely to have a poor illness identity for some mental health problems, leading to under-recognition or the misapprehension that behaviours are signs of functional challenging behaviours rather than a mental health problem. Appraisals of the cause of the mental health problem might lead staff to hold unhelpful beliefs about the potential for intervention. Appraisals of consequences and timeline might lead to staff avoidance and withdrawal, and appraisals of control might lead to critical and hostile staff behaviour and a consequent poor relationship with the service user. Emotional reactions would be linked to these cognitive appraisals, but other factors such as staff burnout and organizational factors could also have impact on staff emotions.

Finally, for service users with ID and mental health problems, staff identification and beliefs about appropriate referral strategies are important determinants of staff behaviour (Costello, 2004). Whilst direct care staff often report positive attitudes towards people with ID and mental health problems (Costello, 2004), staff are more likely to identify externalizing behaviours as indicators of mental health problems than less disruptive behaviours and to consequently recommend referral to mental health professionals (Costello, 2004; Edelstein & Glenwick, 1997, 2001). However, it is worth noting that the only study to longitudinally investigate associations between staff awareness/attitudes and later receipt of mental health services by people with ID found no association (Costello, 2004), indicating the importance of more complex organizational factors (see also Chapter 25 by Costello *et al.*).

Interventions to improve staff well-being

Despite the well-recognized importance of staff stress, burnout and turnover in organizational psychology (DeFrank & Cooper, 1987), research concerning the effectiveness of interventions to improve staff well-being and reduce staff turnover in services for people with ID or mental health problems is remarkably sparse (Edwards & Burnard, 2003; Fothergill *et al.*, 2004; Rose *et al.*, 1998b).

One popular set of stress management interventions is at the level of individual staff, such as relaxation training and stress management workshops for staff. Although these can have a positive effect on staff morale in human services (Edwards & Burnard, 2003), more thorough analysis of staff roles and management of organizational change seems to be required to effect lasting changes in staff well-being, turnover and behaviour towards service users (Innstrand *et al.*, 2004; Reid *et al.*, 1989; Rose *et al.*, 1998b; Strouse *et al.*, 2003)

Training, for example in behavioural and therapeutic techniques, has been reported to reduce stress in mental health nurses (Edwards & Burnard, 2003), but mental health training for staff supporting people with ID has been reported to have no effect on staff stress (Costello, 2004).

The evidence reviewed above suggests that future interventions need to focus on change at a number of different levels including: organizational factors to address staff working conditions and pay, staff support, and staff control over their jobs; general training in awareness and understanding of mental health problems; and individualized staff interventions to modify attributions about individual behaviour associated with hostility and criticism.

Conclusion

This chapter has hopefully demonstrated that poor staff morale and high staff turnover can be a major problem in services for people with ID, although they are not an inevitable consequence of working with people with ID and mental health problems. Often, poor working conditions are combined with unsupportive organizations to produce a distressed and burned out workforce. The research literature consistently suggests that organizations have a major impact on staff well-being, although reports of interventions to improve staff well-being are urgently needed.

Staff working with people with ID and mental health problems may face particular challenges, including the identification of a mental health problem (particularly an internalizing mental health problem), being able to appropriately and effectively refer the service user to the right service, and the management of positive on-going relationships with the service user. For support staff to effectively meet these challenges will require effective training, clear referral pathways that result in effective mental health interventions for the service user, and on-going effective management and support to help support workers maintain positive relationships with the service user. This is a demanding agenda for organizations, but one which cannot be ignored if people with ID and mental health problems are to receive effective and valued services.

Summary points

- The direct support staff workforce in community services for people with ID is largely inexperienced, poorly paid and without professional or vocational qualifications.
- Support staff in community services are highly likely to be working with a person with ID and mental health problems.
- Staff in services for people with ID report relatively high levels of distress but average levels of burnout compared to staff in other human services.
- Staff distress and burnout are largely influenced by organizational factors such as a lack of training, poor working conditions, a lack of support from others and a lack of clarity about the role.
- Greater staff job satisfaction is associated with spending more time with service users and working within a supportive service environment.
- Staff turnover is largely influenced by the characteristics of staff that make them more employable elsewhere and organizational factors that make alternative employment more attractive.
- High staff stress and burnout are associated with less positive interactions between staff and service users.
- Staff beliefs and emotional responses to people with ID and mental health problems are likely to have an impact on identification, referral and on-going relationships between support staff and service users.
- Evidence concerning the effectiveness of interventions designed to improve the well-being of support staff is urgently needed.

REFERENCES

Bailey, N. M. & Cooper, S.-A. (1997). The current provision of specialist health services to people with learning disabilities in England and Wales. *Journal of Intellectual Disability Research*, **41**, 52–9.

Bailey, B. A., Hare, D. J., Hatton, C. & Limb, K. (2006). Care staff attributions, emotions and responses to challenging behaviour. *Journal of Applied Research in Intellectual Disabilities*, **50**, 199–211.

Ball, R. A., Moore, E. & Kuipers, L. (1992). EE in community care facilities: A comparison of patient outcome in a nine-month follow-up of two residential hostels. *Social Psychiatry and Psychiatric Epidemiology*, **27**, 35–9.

Barak, M. E. M., Nissly, J. A. & Levin, A. (2001). Antecedents to retention and turnover among child welfare, social work, and other human service employees: What can we learn from past research? A review and meta-analysis. *Social Service Review*, **75**, 625–61.

Barrowclough, C., Haddock, G., Lowens, I. *et al.* (2001a). Staff expressed emotion and causal attributions for client problems on a low security unit: an exploratory study. *Schizophrenia Bulletin*, **27**, 517–26.

Barrowclough, C., Johnston, M. & Tarrier, N. (1994). Attributions, expressed emotion, and patient relapse: an attributional model of relatives' responses to schizophrenic illness. *Behaviour Therapy*, **25**, 67–88.

Barrowclough, C., Lobban, F., Hatton, C. & Quinn, J. (2001b). Investigation of models of illness in carers of schizophrenia patients using the Illness Perception Questionnaire. *British Journal of Clinical Psychology*, **40**, 371–85.

Borrill, C., Wall, T. D., West, M. A. *et al.* (1996). *Mental Health of the Workforce in NHS Trusts: Phase 1 Final Report*. Sheffield: Institute of Work Psychology.

Bouras, N. and Holt, G. (2004). Mental Health Services for Adults with Learning Disabilities. *British Journal of Psychiatry*, **184**, 291–2.

Braddock, D., Emerson, E., Felce, D. & Stancliffe, R. (2001). The living circumstances of children and adults with MR/DD in the United States, Canada, England and Wales, and Australia. *Mental Retardation and Developmental Disabilities Research Reviews*, **7**, 115–21.

Brewin, C. R., MacCarthy, B., Duda, K. & Vaughn, C. E. (1991). Attribution and expressed emotion in the relatives of patients with schizophrenia. *Journal of Abnormal Psychology*, **100**, 546–54.

Butzlaff, R. L. & Hooley, J. M. (1998). Expressed emotion and psychiatric relapse. *Archives of General Psychiatry*, **55**, 547–52.

Carson, J., Maal, S. *et al.* (1999). Burnout in mental health nurses: Much ado about nothing? *Stress Medicine*, **15**, 127–34.

Christian, L., Synycerski, S. M. & Singh, N. N. (1999). Direct service staff and their perceptions of psychotropic medication in non-institutional settings for people with intellectual disability. *Journal of Intellectual Disability Research*, **43**, 88–93.

Costello, H. (2004). *Does Training Carers Improve Outcome for Adults with Learning Disabilities and Mental Health Problems?* Unpublished Ph.D. Thesis, King's College, University of London.

Dagnan, D., Trower, P. & Smith, R. (1998). Care staff responses to people with learning disabilities and challenging behaviour: A cognitive-emotional analysis. *British Journal of Clinical Psychology*, **37**, 59–68.

DeFrank, R. S. & Cooper, C. L. (1987). Worksite stress management interventions: their effectiveness and conceptualisation. *Journal of Managerial Psychology*, **2**, 4–10.

Edelstein, T. M. & Glenwick, D. S. (1997). Referral reasons for psychological services for adults with mental retardation. *Research in Developmental Disabilities*, **18**, 45–59.

Edelstein, T. M. & Glenwick, D. S. (2001). Direct-care workers' attributions of psychopathology in adults with mental retardation. *Mental Retardation*, **39**, 368–78.

Edwards, D. & Burnard, P. (2003). A systematic review of stress and stress management interventions for mental health nurses. *Journal of Advanced Nursing*, **42**, 169–200.

Felce, D. & Emerson, E. (2004). Research on engagement in activity. In E. Emerson, C. Hatton, T. Thompson & T. R. Parmenter (eds.), *The International Handbook of Applied Research in Intellectual Disabilities* (pp. 353–68). Chichester: Wiley.

Fothergill, A., Edwards, D. & Burnard, P. (2004). Stress, burnout, coping and stress management in psychiatrists: Findings from a systematic review. *International Journal of Social Psychiatry*, **50**, 54–65.

Hall, P. S. & Hall, N. D. (2002). Hiring and retaining direct-care staff: After 50 years of research, what do we know? *Mental Retardation*, **40**, 201–11.

Hastings, R. P. (2002). Do challenging behaviors affect staff psychological well-being? Issues of causality and mechanism. *American Journal on Mental Retardation*, **107**, 455–67.

Hatton, C., Emerson, E., Rivers, M. *et al.* (1999a). Factors associated with staff stress and work satisfaction in services for people with intellectual disabilities. *Journal of Intellectual Disability Research*, **43**, 253–67.

Hatton, C., Emerson, E., Rivers, M. *et al.* (2001). Factors associated with intended staff turnover and job search behaviour in services for people with intellectual disability. *Journal of Intellectual Disability Research*, **45**, 258–70.

Hatton, C., Rivers, M., Emerson, E. *et al.* (1999b). Staff characteristics, working conditions and outcomes in services for people with intellectual disabilities: results of a staff survey. *Journal of Applied Research in Intellectual Disabilities*, **12**, 340–47.

Hatton, C., Rose, J. & Rose, D. (2004). Researching staff. In E. Emerson, C. Hatton, T. Thompson & T. R. Parmenter (eds.), *The International Handbook of Applied Research in Intellectual Disabilities* (pp. 581–605). Chichester: Wiley.

Hewitt, A. & Lakin, K. C. (2001). *Issues in the Direct Support Workforce and their Connections to the Growth, Sustainability and Quality of Community Supports*. Minneapolis, MN: Research and Training Center on Community Living, University of Minnesota.

Innstrand, S. T., Espnes, G. A. & Mykleun, R. (2002). Burnout among people working with intellectually disabled persons: A theory update and an example. *Scandinavian Journal of Caring Sciences*, **16**, 272–9.

Innstrand, S. T., Espnes, G. A. & Mykletun, R. (2004). Job stress, burnout and job satisfaction: An intervention study for staff working with people with intellectual disabilities. *Journal of Applied Research in Intellectual Disabilities*, **17**, 119–26.

Kon, Y. & Bouras, N. (1997). Psychiatric follow-up and health services utilisation for people with learning disabilities. *British Journal of Learning Disabilities*, **18**, 20–6.

Larson, S. A., Lakin, K. C. & Bruininks, R. H. (1998). *Staff Recruitment and Retention: Study Results and Intervention Strategies*. Washington, DC: American Association on Mental Retardation.

Larson, S. A., Lakin, K. C. & Hewitt, A. (2002). Direct support professionals. In R. L. Schalock, P. Baker & M. D. Crosser (eds.), *Embarking On A New Century: Mental Retardation at the End of the 20th Century* (pp. 203–20). Washington, DC: American Association on Mental Retardation.

Lawson, D. A. & O'Brien, R. M. (1994). Behavioral and self-report measures of burnout in developmental disabilities. *Journal of Organizational Behavior Management*, **14**, 37–54.

Lobban, F., Barrowclough, C. & Jones, S. (2003). A review of the role of illness models in severe mental illness. *Clinical Psychology Review*, **23**, 171–96.

Maslach, C. & Jackson. S. E. (1981). The measurement and experience of burnout. *Journal of Occupational Behaviour*, **2**, 99–113.

Moss, S., Prosser, H., Ibbotson, B. & Goldberg, D. (1996). Respondent and informant accounts of psychiatric symptoms in a sample of patients with learning disability. *Journal of Intellectual Disability Research*, **40**, 457–65.

Mossman, D. A., Hastings, R. P. & Brown, T. (2002). Mediators' emotional responses to self-injurious behavior: an experimental study. *American Journal on Mental Retardation*, **107**, 252–60.

Oliver, N. & Kuipers, E. (1996). Stress and its relationship to expressed emotion in community mental health workers. *International Journal of Social Psychiatry*, **42**, 150–59.

Polister, B., Lakin, K. C. & Prouty, R. (2003). *Wages of Direct Support Professionals Serving Persons with Intellectual and Developmental Disabilities: A Survey of State Agencies and Private Residential Trade Associations*. Policy Research Brief 14 (2). Minneapolis, MN: Research and Training Center on Community Living, University of Minnesota.

Prosser, D., Johnson, S., Kuipers, E. *et al.* (1999). Mental health, 'burnout' and job satisfaction in a longitudinal study of mental health staff. *Social Psychiatry and Psychiatric Epidemiology*, **34**, 295–300.

Quigley, A., Murray, G. C., McKenzie, K. & Elliot, G. (2001). Staff knowledge about symptoms of mental health in people with learning disabilities. *Journal of Learning Disabilities*, **5**, 235–44.

Reid, D. H., Parsons, M. B. & Green, C. W. (1989). *Staff Management in Human Services*. Springfield, IL: Charles C. Thomas.

Rose, J., Jones, F. & Fletcher, B. (1998a). Investigating the relationship between stress and worker behaviour. *Journal of Intellectual Disability Research*, **42**, 163–72.

Rose, J., Jones, F. & Fletcher, B. (1998b). The impact of a stress management programme on staff well-being and performance at work. *Work and Stress*, **12**, 112–24.

Rose, J., Mullan, E. & Fletcher, B. (1994). An examination of the relationship between staff behaviour and stress levels in residential care. *Mental Handicap Research*, **7**, 312–28.

Skirrow, P. M. & Hatton, C. (in press). The prevalence and correlates of burnout amongst direct care workers: A systematic review. *Journal of Applied Research in Intellectual Disabilities*.

Snyder, K. S., Wallace, C. J., Moe, K. & Liberman, R. P. (1994). EE by residential care operators' and residents' symptoms and quality of life. *Hospital and Community Psychiatry*, **45**, 1141–3.

Stanley, B. & Standen, P. J. (2000). Carers' attributions for challenging behaviour. *British Journal of Clinical Psychology*, **39**, 157–68.

Strouse, M. C., Carroll-Hernandez, T. A., Sherman, J. A. & Sheldon, J. B. (2003). Turning over turnover: The evaluation of a staff scheduling system in a community-based program for adults with developmental disabilities. *Journal of Organizational Behavior Management*, **23**, 45–63.

Tattan, T. & Tarrier, N. (2000). The expressed emotion of case managers of the seriously mentally ill: The influence of expressed emotion on clinical outcomes. *Psychological Medicine*, **30**, 195–204.

Van Humbeeck, G., Van Audenhove, C., Pieters, G. *et al.* (2001). Expressed emotion in staff-patient relationships: the professionals' and residents' perspectives. *Social Psychiatry and Psychiatric Epidemiology*, **36**, 486–92.

Ward, F. (1999). *Modernising the Social Care Workforce – the first national training strategy for England: Supplementary report on learning disability*. Leeds: Training Organisation for the Personal Social Services (TOPPS).

Weiner, B. (1980). A cognitive (attribution) – emotion – action model of helping behavior: An analysis of judgments of help giving. *Journal of Personality and Social Psychology*, **39**, 1142–62.

Wykes, T., Stevens, W. & Everitt, B. (1997). Stress in community care teams: will it affect the sustainability of community care? *Social Psychiatry and Psychiatric Epidemiology*, **32**, 398–407.

25

Professional training for those working with people with intellectual disabilities and mental health problems

Helen Costello, Geraldine Holt, Nancy Cain, Elspeth Bradley, Jennifer Torr, Robert Davis, Niki Edwards, Nick Lennox and Germain Weber

Introduction

Life in the community for individuals with intellectual disabilities (ID) implies new roles and responsibilities for professionals providing mental health care to this population. A diverse range of mental health service models have emerged both nationally and internationally to meet these needs. In some cases, emphasis is on the provision of generic mainstream services to individuals with ID, while in others specialist services have been developed, either working independently of or in tandem with generic teams. This variability implies that a variety of professional groups require specialist knowledge for assessing, treating and managing mental health problems in individuals with ID. Very little is written about the education of professionals providing mental health care for this group and there is a lack of recognition of the need for formalized training in mental health and ID from a national and international perspective. Many training programmes appear ad hoc, with the availability and content of most educational initiatives being largely determined by the specific interests of those individuals providing and undergoing training. This chapter reviews the training programmes of three groups of health care professionals (psychiatrists, psychologists and primary care physicians) available in five countries (UK, USA, Canada, Australia and Austria) in relation to mental health problems in individuals with ID. The role of specific institutions and key individuals in increasing the profile of mental health problems in this population is highlighted, factors hindering the development of professional training are identified and recent innovations in curricula are described. Finally, some recommendations are made for the future development of training initiatives.

Psychiatric and Behavioural Disorders in Intellectual and Developmental Disabilities, ed. Nick Bouras and Geraldine Holt. Published by Cambridge University Press. © Cambridge University Press 2007.

Psychiatrists

In the UK, specialist psychiatric training is six to seven years in duration and consists of basic professional training and higher training in a chosen psychiatric specialty or specialties. All training schemes must be approved by the Royal College of Psychiatrists. Basic training lasts for three years and leads to the MRCPsych examination. This exam includes questions and cases in the psychiatry of ID, and recent innovations include the participation of people with ID in the curriculum as trainers. Completion of a six-month attachment in either the psychiatry of ID or child and adolescent psychiatry (or a combination of the two) to provide a developmental perspective is necessary to move on to higher training.

Higher training leads to the Certificate of Completion of Specialist Training (CCST) – a mandatory qualification for all consultants in the NHS since 1997. Aimed at developing and deepening diagnostic, therapeutic and management skills, trainees attend weekly academic meetings, gain teaching experience, plan and execute an original research project and obtain management experience by serving on committees and participating in clinical audit, as well as working clinically. It takes three years to gain a CCST in the psychiatry of ID, of which one year can be spent in general psychiatry or another appropriate psychiatric specialty and the remaining time being in the specialty of psychiatry of ID. Dual training programmes, lasting from four to five years, are also possible where a trainee gains a CCST in the psychiatry of ID and another speciality such as general adult psychiatry. Postgraduate training of all doctors in the UK, including those training in psychiatry, is currently under review (Bhugra and Holsgrove, 2005). This will have implications for both those wishing to specialize in the field of psychiatry of ID and those requiring a working knowledge of this area (Bhugra, 2005).

Most psychiatric training programmes in the USA still do not include any education about assessing and treating people with ID and mental health problems although there are recommendations for including it in the curriculum. In 1995, a syllabus for teaching trainee psychiatrists about people with ID and mental health problems was written and disseminated via the American Psychiatric Association (King *et al.*, 1995). Even so, very few programmes offer any extended or supervised experience with people with ID and mental health problems (Reinblatt *et al.*, 2004). Exceptions include the psychiatry departments at the University of Rochester and Zucker Hillside Hospital in New York City. Although highly valued within their institutions, reductions in funding threaten the development and maintenance of these programmes. The curriculum in child psychiatry often includes more information about ID, as well as an understanding of child development.

Ultimately, most of the psychiatrists working with people with ID and mental health problems in the USA have been self-taught, often through a part-time job at an agency providing services for individuals with ID. Reading any available literature, going to workshops and seminars, and essentially trying what worked in general psychiatry, often enhance such experiences. There have been exceptions to this as occasionally a psychiatrist interested in the field has had an opportunity to develop training at his or her university. Two such individuals, Ludwig Szymanski, M.D. at Harvard and Frank Menolascino, M.D. at the University of Nebraska, became mentors for many of the psychiatrists practising today.

In Canada, specialty training (Royal College of Physicians and Surgeons of Canada) in psychiatry requires five years of approved training after undergraduate medical studies. In the goals and objectives of this training, only fleeting mention is made of ID and research has highlighted inadequacies in many programmes, particularly with regard to adolescents and adults with ID (Lunsky & Bradley, 2001). Although some didactic opportunities are usually available, supervised clinical opportunities are rare and mostly optional. Training programmes describing mandatory clinical and didactic components generally have at least one psychiatrist specializing in ID who has an academic affiliation with the local university Department of Psychiatry. Such programmes also tend to exist in provinces where a clear need for services for persons with ID had been declared at a provincial level.

There have been two chairs in ID in Canada, both in Ontario (at the University of Western Ontario and Queen's University) and each, until recently, remained vacant (following retirement) for several years, in the absence of candidates to fill these positions. The sustained efforts of the previous incumbents of these chairs (Professors Goldberg and McCreary) has facilitated, in recent years, a network across Canada of clinicians, researchers and consumers, concerned about the health care of persons with ID (Peppin *et al.*, 2001). This network is providing a national forum for discussion, national meetings/conferences and opportunities for collaborative education and research activities (see www.heidiresearch.ca; www.autismtraining.ca; http://meds.queensu.ca/ ciddda). Concern by clinicians and consumers in Ontario have resulted in two teaching texts (Brown and Percy, 2003; Griffiths *et al.*, 2002).

Few Australian psychiatrists possess adequate knowledge about ID, with most acknowledging inadequate training and a poor standard of care for this population (Lennox & Chaplin, 1996). Some Australian psychiatrists have received training in ID psychiatry in the United Kingdom. The Royal Australian and New Zealand College of Psychiatrists encourages trainees to develop skills and expertise in the psychiatry of ID (Royal Australian and New Zealand College of Psychiatrists, 2003).

However, without specialist services and a critical mass of expert psychiatrists, training cannot at this time be mandatory. Elective subjects in psychiatry of ID are offered in Victoria and New South Wales as part of the academic programmes for psychiatry trainees. There are few clinical posts in ID for psychiatry trainees in Australia. The Victorian Department of Human Services provided 12 months pilot funding for three half-time positions in 2003–2004, however this funding is not ongoing. The Queensland Centre for Intellectual and Developmental Disability and the Centre for Developmental Disability Health Victoria host a half-time psychiatry training position.

Over the last decade academic centres of excellence in developmental disability have been established within university settings in Queensland, Victoria, New South Wales and South Australia. These centres provide tertiary clinical services, in addition to education and research activities. There has been continuing progress in the inclusion of developmental disability at the undergraduate level within these states (Lennox & Diggens, 1999). At the postgraduate level, educational programmes in the mental health of people with ID have targeted primary care physicians, psychiatry trainees and allied health professionals. Clinical services provided by the centres, although limited, create crucial training opportunities for health professionals. The centres continue to advocate for training programmes within the medical colleges.

Training for psychiatrists in Austria is regulated by the decree 'physician's training curriculum' of 1994, updated in 1998 (ÄAO, 1998) and the number of training positions is limited for each accredited training institution (e.g. university hospitals, larger regional psychiatric hospitals). Training takes a minimum of six years, generally comprising major and minor subjects. Accordingly, a psychiatrist trains for four years in psychiatry (major) and for two years in compulsory minor subjects (here defined as 12 months training in the special field of internal medicine and another 12 months training in neurology – appendix 36 of ÄAO). The training is run as a supervised 'on-the-job-training' with additional accompanying theoretical instructions. The curriculum for postgraduate training in psychiatry does not refer to ID and, with the exception of childhood and youth, training in psychiatry is not formally structured according to specific target groups. In addition, psychiatric hospitals lack departments for people with ID (Holt *et al.*, 2000).

On completion of postgraduate training in psychiatry, additional training in areas like genetics, clinical pharmacology and neuropsychiatry of childhood and youth can be taken. At the Medical University of Vienna the chair for neuropsychiatry of childhood and adolescence includes issues of pervasive developmental disorders and disability. Training in neuropsychiatry of childhood and youth, which takes an additional three years, covers biological developmental issues with additional focus on psychological and sociological aspects. This includes knowledge of early intervention and care for disabled children or children at risk of disability and basic understanding of special education methods.

Psychologists

In the UK, psychologists undertake a postgraduate three-year university course leading to a doctoral degree in clinical psychology, approved by the British Psychological Society (BPS, 1994). Under the direct supervision of approved senior professional staff, trainees follow an academic programme that includes lectures on ID encompassing development; causes and characteristics; aspects of care (assessment and monitoring, interventions, skills development); service issues (normalization, staff support, service provision) and organization and policy (Powell *et al.*, 1993). Students also learn research skills and must carry out a clinically relevant piece of original research. Academic teaching is integrated with periods of practical clinical experience in a variety of service specialities and across the full age spectrum. Trainees may opt to complete a six-month clinical placement in ID services.

In the USA, compared with other professions, psychologists have been much more involved in the care of individuals with ID and behaviour problems. While the Ph.D. curriculum does not usually include training about ID, many psychologists train in applied behaviour analysis and work for agencies caring for individuals with ID. There are also a number of pre- and postdoctoral fellowships and some of these include experience with individuals with ID and mental health problems. The American Psychological Association has a large section for psychologists specializing in ID, many of whom focus on research and training about ID, but this rarely includes ID and mental health problems.

Requirements for practice and registration of psychologists in Canada are set by the Colleges of Psychologists in each province and territory. Designation as a psychologist requires a doctoral degree, or in some cases a master's degree, from a programme of study with a primary focus in psychology, a period of supervised practice and successful completion of written and oral examinations. Across Canada there are 51 graduate programmes in psychology. Specific exposure or experience in ID is not required, although some graduate level courses in some psychology programmes provide opportunities in ID to the interested trainee. More recently, several provinces have been developing programmes for children with autism and these will likely raise more general awareness and interest in ID, particularly as some components of these programmes will require psychologists in supervisory roles. In common with psychiatrists and family physicians, psychologists are required by their colleges to participate in a programme of maintenance of certification, ongoing quality assurance and professional development activities. While these requirements represent further opportunities for ID teaching, such opportunities currently remain mostly dormant.

Psychologists working in the field of ID in Australia are generally involved in cognitive assessments and management of behaviour disorders. The Australian Psychological Society College of Clinical Psychology (Australian Psychological Society College of Clinical Psychologists, 2003) requires clinical psychologists to be trained in the principles and methods of behavioural, psychometric and clinical assessment of significant psychological problems, as well as the principles, procedures and techniques of psychological intervention and rehabilitation and primary prevention of psychological disturbance. This applies to people across their lifespan in diverse clinical settings and do not mention the needs of specific groups apart from Aboriginal and Torres Strait Islanders. The emphasis on intellectual and developmental disabilities varies from course to course.

In Austria, postgraduate training in clinical and health psychology, regulated by law since 1991 (Psychologengesetz, 1990), comprises theoretical and practical components. The theoretical part is offered by four training institutions (one of which is university based), all accredited by the Council of Psychologists located at the National Ministry of Health. It consists of a minimum of 120 hours of instruction and covers areas such as health prevention and health facilitation, clinical psychological assessment and intervention strategies, rehabilitation, psychiatry and psychopharmacology, ethical considerations and institutional and legal frameworks. Organized on a continuous education model, training modules are usually one and a half days in duration and offered during weekends, thus allowing trainees to follow practical training during the week. It has a minimum duration of 1480 hours and achieving professional competence is linked to psychological actions delivered in a supervized format in health and social care institutional settings. Registration of clinical and health psychologists is controlled by the Council of Psychologists. As in the case of postgraduate training in psychiatry, the curriculum for psychologists does not formally refer to ID, training programmes lack a track record of specializing in ID and few are involved in intellectual disability research activities at an academic level. In 2004, a chair for special education was set up at the University of Vienna, Faculty of Philosophy and Education, with research being centred on issues of integration of children with ID into the educational system.

Primary health physicians

Currently in the UK there is no formal training in ID for primary health physicians. Principal responsibility for medical student training rests with the departments of psychiatry, child health, family and community medicine. A senior academic presence in the field in each medical school is required to organize and co-ordinate the programme (Hollins, 1988). The Royal College of Psychiatrists recommends a minimum core training of 12–15 hours of undergraduate teaching in ID for medical students (Royal College of Psychiatrists, 1986).

At a postgraduate level, teaching in ID remains ad hoc and essentially dependent upon the interests and enthusiasms of individual primary health physicians, local service providers and postgraduate training departments. Ultimately, a more systematic approach on a national basis is needed and there is evidence that many primary health physicians would welcome this (Singh, 1997).

Training initiatives include local postgraduate courses, distance learning guides and conferences provided by bodies such as the Royal Society of Medicine's Forum on Learning Disability, the Royal College of General Practitioners Learning Disability Working Group and university departments. Launched at the Houses of Parliament in 2002, 'Learning About Intellectual Disabilities & Health' is a web-based learning resource for medical and health care students and practitioners that provides up-to-date information about the health needs of people with ID (www.intellectualdisability.info).

Most medical schools in the USA have no lectures, let alone formal courses about individuals with ID and mental health problems. Even education about individuals with ID is limited. Following graduation, physicians undergoing specialty training in internal medicine or gynaecology usually only learn about ID and mental health problems if they happen to have individuals with these disabilities in their practice. Specialty training for practitioners in family medicine may include some informal education, but only if there are faculty members with an interest in the psychiatry of ID. Paediatricians get the most education as there are more options for them.

Nationally funded programmes that provide research and training in ID and mental health problems have been in place in the USA since 1963 (The Developmental Disabilities Services and Facilities Construction Act, 1963; The Mental Retardation Facilities and Community Mental Health Centers Construction Act, 1963). About half of these University Affiliated Programs (UAPs) were developed in departments of paediatrics and generally focused on children. The others were associated with Departments of Education that had no connection with medical education. There is also a developmental paediatrics sub-specialty which focuses on the medical care for individuals with ID and mental health problems. These programmes include experience in the treatment of problem behaviours, but rarely in the assessment and treatment of psychiatric disorders. Another training opportunity available for any interested physician is the **L**eadership **E**ducation in **N**eurodevelopmental and Related **D**isabilities (LEND) programme. This programme provides long-term, graduate level, inter-disciplinary leadership training to health professionals. Such programmes operate within a university system and most have collaborative arrangements with local university hospitals, children's hospitals, and/or health care centres.

In Canada, medical students interested in family medicine enter a two-year community-based training programme after completing their medical degree. College of Family Physicians Certification (a programme of study followed by written and oral examinations) is then required to enter into practice as a family physician. In this certification there is no specific requirement for training in the area of ID, nor are there any specific standards about ID in the accreditation standards for family medicine training programmes. Formal teaching and clinical practice in the area of ID for the family medicine resident (as for medical students) is a rather 'hit and miss' affair depending on whether there is local interest (often a local 'champion') in pushing forward this agenda into existing curricula.

Primary care physicians in Australia report gaps in their training, particularly in the assessment and management of behavioural and mental health problems of people with ID (Phillips *et al.*, 2004). Aspects of mental health, including assessment and management of psychiatric and behaviour disorders, are covered in the Management Guidelines for People with Developmental Disabilities (Lennox *et al.*, 2005), and the Mental Health in Adult Developmental Disability guidelines (Edwards *et al.*, 2003). Nonetheless it has been a major challenge to engage primary care physicians in addressing the mental and physical health needs of this population. There have been few enrolments in distance education subjects and modules targeting general practitioners developed by the Centre for Developmental Disability Victoria. Educational presentations at general practice conferences have raised awareness and interest in further education.

In general, the knowledge and competences of general physicians in Austria in the area of ID is poor and in extreme cases quasi non-existent. Training for primary care physicians, defined within a life-span model, aims to develop skills in health promotion as well as in the detection and treatment of disorders of all kinds, independent of age, sex and type of health dysfunction. During this three years of on the job training, a minimum of six months are spent within primary medical sector services and a maximum of 12 months are spent in the secondary medical sector. The curriculum comprises eight compulsory areas, each with a specified minimum duration. Neither ID nor disability in general is formally addressed in the curriculum and its guidelines. However, within paediatrics the physician acquires skills in assessing the development and maturity of children, and within psychiatry the physician focuses on groups with special risks for mental health issues such as those with ID. Primary care physicians also receive training in primary and secondary prevention and rehabilitation, with rehabilitation being related in Austria closely to the topic of disability. The 1994 training decree, amended in 1998 (BGBl, 1998/169), refers to psychosocial competences and knowledge structures such as counselling, social integration measures and to structural institutional knowledge.

Conclusion

A review of education programmes for psychiatrists, psychologists and primary care physicians in five countries reveals that the majority of professional groups providing mental health care receive little formal training in the assessment and care of individuals with ID and psychiatric and behaviour disorders. Of the countries included in the review, only the UK includes ID training as a mandatory component in training programmes for psychiatrists. Elsewhere, ID training is not a requirement, although it is usually an option for interested trainee psychiatrists, with its availability restricted to certain areas and dependent on the presence of psychiatrists specializing in this area. Similarly, although sometimes incorporated in the academic programmes for psychologists in the countries reviewed, clinical exposure to individuals with ID is optional and more likely to be gained following qualification.

The skills of primary care physicians in detecting mental health problems and making appropriate referrals underpin the effective delivery of mental health services to individuals with ID living in the community. Despite this critical role, formal training in ID was not a compulsory component in the training of primary care physicians in any of the countries reviewed.

Overall, professional training in ID struggles at many different levels. Nevertheless, some progress in raising the profile of mental health problems in individuals with ID on the training agenda is evident within each country. Educational materials, such as academic textbooks and distance-learning tools, focusing on this topic and targeting specific groups, are now widely available. A broad range of related training events, and national and international conferences are routinely offered. For example, based on materials mainly developed in the UK (Bouras & Holt, 1997; Moss, 2002; Holt *et al.*, 2005) efforts have been made in Austria to develop training packages on mental health issues and ID for front-line carers as well as professionals, psychiatrists and psychologists (Weber & Fritsch, 2003). These training packages, though not integrated in the continuous education programme of the Austrian Physicians Academy or the Austrian Professional Association of Psychologists, are continually requested by health and social care institutions.

Examples of good training practice are also apparent. In the UK, the participation of individuals with ID as trainers in the education of psychiatrists is a promising development, which warrants replication in the training of other professional groups and in other countries. Careful consideration is needed to ensure that professional training is not an aversive experience. Trainee attitudes towards certain service-user groups influence both the choice of specialty pursued and the therapeutic relationship (Benham, 1988). A survey by Burge *et al.* (2002) of psychiatry trainees in Canada reported inadequacies in training in ID at the undergraduate and residency levels. Similarly, in the UK, Graham *et al.* (2004) report that many trainee psychiatrists in ID experience feelings of impotence, hopelessness, disempowerment and feel unskilled. In addition, they felt a sense of alienation, both from the individuals with ID and from other professionals working in the field. Promoting the participation of individuals with ID in training activities may be especially valuable in helping mould trainee attitudes, reducing negative emotions, providing a positive experience of working with this group and helping them to feel more skilled. Enriching the experiences of trainees during their placements in ID is therefore an important step in improving recruitment to and retention within the specialty.

Summary points

- Many, and in some countries most, health care professionals receive little training in the assessment, treatment and management of mental health problems in people with ID.
- In the UK, ID is a compulsory component of the training of psychiatrists. This is not the case in the USA, Canada, Australia and Austria.
- ID is included in some training programmes for psychologists, but clinical experience in the field is less available, is optional and usually post-qualification.
- Primary care physicians in all the countries reviewed receive little or no exposure to the health care needs of people with ID, including mental health, at both an undergraduate and postgraduate level.
- Positive developments in training were evident in all the countries reviewed. These often are linked to charismatic individuals who pioneer the initiatives.
- An infrastructure is necessary to support training, including national standards of care for people with ID and mental health problems, to drive accreditation and certification of courses, together with secure career paths.

Acknowledgments

Elspeth Bradley would like to acknowledge her dialogues with Drs Friedlander (British Columbia), Carpenter (Alberta), Hennen (Manitoba), Holden (Ontario), Summers (Ontario), Sullivan (Ontario) and Miss Gitta (Ontario) and Korossy (Ontario), in the preparation of the Canadian contribution to this chapter.

REFERENCES

ÄAO – Ärzte-Ausbildungsordnung (decree on the general physician's training) (1998). Decree by the National Ministry of Health and Social Affairs on the training of general practitioners and specialised physicians (physician's training curriculum). BGBl – Bundesgesetzblatt (National Act Register), 1994/152 in the updated form of 1998/169.

Australian Psychological Society College of Clinical Psychologists (2003). Course Approval Guidelines. APS College of Clinical Psychologists. http://www.psychology.org.au/study/studying/clinical_guidelines.pdf: Australian Psychological Society.

Benham, P. K. (1988). Attitudes of occupational therapy personnel towards persons with disabilities. *American Journal of Occupational Therapy*, **42**, 305–11.

BGBl (*Bundes-Gesetz-Bl*att) (National Register of Law) (1998/169). Ärzte-Ausbildungsordnung (decree on the general physician's training) BGBl. 1994/152 actualized in BGBl. 1998/169.

Bhugra, D. (2005). Training for consultants in 2020. Response to Drs Mukherjee and Nimmagadda. *Psychiatric Bulletin*, **29**, 46.

Bhugra, D. & Holsgrove, G. (2005). Patient-centred psychiatry. Training and assessment: the way forward. *Psychiatric Bulletin*, **29**, 49–52.

Bouras, N. & Holt, G. (1997). *Mental health in learning disabilities: A training pack for staff working with people who have a dual diagnosis of mental health needs and learning disabilities*. Brighton: Pavilion Publishers.

British Psychological Society (1994). *Everything you need to know about training in psychology*. Leicester: British Psychological Society.

Brown, I. and Percy, M. E. (2003). *Developmental disabilities in Ontario*. Toronto: Ontario Association on Developmental Disabilities.

Burge, P., Ouellette-Kuntz, H., McCreary, B., Bradley, E. & Leichner, P. (2002). Senior residents in psychiatry: views on training in developmental disabilities. *Canadian Journal of Psychiatry*, **47**, 568–71.

Edwards, N., Lennox, N., Holt, G. & Bouras, N. (2003). *Mental Health in Adult Developmental Disability: Education and Training Kit for Professionals and Service Providers*. Queensland Centre for Intellectual and Developmental Disabilities.

Graham, S., Herbert, R., Price, S. & Willaims, S. (2004). Attitudes and emotions of trainees in learning disability psychiatry. *Psychiatric Bulletin*, **28**, 254–6.

Griffiths, D. M., Stavrakaki, C. & Summers, J. (2002). *Dual Diagnosis: An Introduction to the Mental Health Needs of Persons with Developmental Disabilities*. Ontario: Habilitative Mental Health Resource Network.

Hollins, S. (1988). How mental handicap is taught in UK medical schools. *Medical Teacher*, **10**, 289–96.

Holt, G., Costello, H., Bouras, N. *et al.* (2000). BIOMED-MEROPE project: service provision for adults with intellectual disability: a European comparison. *Journal of Intellectual Disability Research*, **44**, 685–96.

Holt, G., Hardy, S. & Bouras, N. (2005). *Mental Health in Learning Disabilities: A Training Resource*. Brighton: Pavilion Publishers.

King, B. H., Szymanski, Ludwik, S. *et al.* (1995). *Psychiatry and Mental Retardation: A Curriculum Guide.* Washington, DC: American Psychiatric Association Committee on Psychiatric Services for Persons with Mental Retardation and Developmental Disabilities.

Lennox, N., Beange, H., Davis, R. *et al.* (2005). *Management Guidelines Developmental Disability Version 2.* Melbourne: Therapeutic Guidelines Ltd.

Lennox, N. & Chaplin, R. (1996). The psychiatric care of people with intellectual disabilities: The perceptions of consultant psychiatrists in Victoria. *Australia and New Zealand Journal of Psychiatry*, **30**, 774–80.

Lennox, N. & Diggens, J. (1999). Knowledge, skills and attitudes: Medical schools' coverage of an ideal curriculum on intellectual disability. *Journal of Intellectual and Developmental Disability*, **24**, 341–7.

Lunsky, Y. & Bradley, E. (2001). Developmental disability training in Canadian psychiatry residency programs. *Canadian Journal of Psychiatry*, **46**, 138–43.

Moss, S. (2002). *The Mini PAS-ADD Interview Pack.* Brighton: Pavilion Publishing.

Peppin, P., McCreary, B. D., Stanton, B. & Queen's University (Kingston, Ont.) (2001). *Catalysts for University Education in Developmental Disabilities.* Developmental Consulting Program, Ontario: Queen's University, Kingston.

Phillips, A., Morrison, J. & Davis, R. W. (2004). General practitioners' educational needs in intellectual disability health. *Journal of Intellectual Disability Research*, **48**, 142–9.

Powell, G. E., Young, R. & Frosh, S. (eds.) (1993). *Curriculum in Clinical Psychology.* Leicester: British Psychological Society Publications.

Psychologengesetz (Psychlogist's Act) (1990). Bundesgesetz: Psychologengesetz (National Act: Psychologist's Act. BGBl – Bundesgesetzblatt (National Act Register), 1990/151.

Reinblatt, *et al.* (2004). General Psychiatry Residents' Perceptions of Specialized Training in the Field of Mental Retardation. *Psychiatric Services*, **55**, 312–14.

Royal Australian and New Zealand College of Psychiatrists (RANZCP) (2003). RANZCP Training and Assessment Regulations, 2003.

Royal College of Psychiatrists (1986). Undergraduate Training in Mental Handicap. Section for the Psychiatry of Mental Handicap. *Bulletin of The Royal College of Psychiatrists*, **10**, 292.

Singh, P. (1997). Prescription for Change: *A Mencap Report on the Role of GPs and Carers in the Provision of Primary Care for People with Learning Disabilities.* London: Mencap.

The Developmental Disabilities Services and Facilities Construction Act of 1963 (1963). Pub. L. No. 91–517, UAPDD.

The Mental Retardation Facilities and Community Mental Health Centers Construction Act of 1963 (1963). Pub. L. No. 88–164.

Weber, G. & Fritsch, A. (2003). *Psychische Störungen und Verhaltensstörungen bei erwachsenen Menschen mit intellektueller Behinderung: Ein Trainingsmanual (Psychiatric Disorders and Behavioural Disorders in Adult People with Intellectual Disabilities: A Training Manual).* Wien (Vienna): Universität Wien, Autoren (University of Vienna, authors).

www.autismtraining.ca

www.heidiresearch.ca

www.intellectualdisability.info

http://meds.queensu.ca/ciddda

Index